Epidemics in Moder

MW00694803

Epidemics have played a critical role in shaping modern Asia. Encompassing two centuries of Asian history, Robert Peckham explores the profound impact that infectious disease has had on societies across the region: from India to China and the Russian Far East. The book tracks the links between biology, history, and geopolitics, highlighting the interdependencies of infectious disease with empire, modernization, revolution, nationalism, migration, and transnational patterns of trade. By examining the history of Asia through the lens of epidemics, Peckham vividly illustrates how society's material conditions are entangled with social and political processes, offering an entirely fresh perspective on Asia's transformation.

ROBERT PECKHAM is Associate Professor in the Department of History and co-Director of the Centre for the Humanities and Medicine at the University of Hong Kong.

New Approaches to Asian History

This dynamic new series publishes books on the milestones in Asian history; those that have come to define particular periods or to mark turning points in the political, cultural and social evolution of the region. The books in this series are intended as introductions for students to be used in the classroom. They are written by scholars whose credentials are well-established in their particular fields and who have, in many cases, taught the subject across a number of years.

Books in the series

1 Judith M. Brown, *Global South Asians: Introducing the Modern Diaspora*
2 Diana Lary, *China's Republic*
3 Peter A. Lorge, *The Asian Military Revolution: From Gunpowder to the Bomb*
4 Ian Talbot and Gurharpal Singh, *The Partition of India*
5 Stephen F. Dale, *The Muslim Empires of the Ottomans, Safavids, and Mughals*
6 Diana Lary, *The Chinese People at War: Human Suffering and Social Transformation, 1937–1945*
7 Sunil S. Amrith, *Migration and Diaspora in Modern Asia*
8 Thomas David DuBois, *Religion and the Making of Modern East Asia*
9 Susan L. Mann, *Gender and Sexuality in Modern Chinese History*
10 Tirthankar Roy, *India in the World Economy: From Antiquity to the Present*
11 Robin R. Wang, *Yinyang: The Way of Heaven and Earth in Chinese Thought and Culture*
12 Li Feng, *Early China: A Social and Cultural History*
13 Diana Lary, *China's Civil War: A Social History, 1945–1949*
14 Kiri Paramore, *Japanese Confucianism: A Cultural History*
15 Robert Peckham, *Epidemics in Modern Asia*

Epidemics in Modern Asia

Robert Peckham

University of Hong Kong

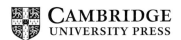
CAMBRIDGE
UNIVERSITY PRESS

CAMBRIDGE
UNIVERSITY PRESS

University Printing House, Cambridge CB2 8BS, United Kingdom

Cambridge University Press is part of the University of Cambridge.

It furthers the University's mission by disseminating knowledge in the pursuit of education, learning and research at the highest international levels of excellence.

www.cambridge.org
Information on this title: www.cambridge.org/9781107084681

© Robert Peckham 2016

First published 2016

Printed in the United Kingdom by TJ International Ltd, Padstow, Cornwall

A catalog record for this publication is available from the British Library

ISBN 978-1-107-08468-1 Hardback
ISBN 978-1-107-44676-2 Paperback

For Michael and Catherine

Contents

Figures

Maps

Preface

There is, perhaps, no better place to begin a history of the global than with the hyper-local: the view over Victoria Harbour towards Tai Mo Shan, Hong Kong's highest summit, from my office at the University of Hong Kong. Across the water to the north, Stonecutters Island juts out of the Kowloon peninsula. Acquired by the British from the Qing dynasty in 1860, along with Kowloon, Stonecutters Island has served over the years as a quarry, a military depot, the site of a prison, a smallpox hospital, and a quarantine station. As a result of land reclamation in the 1990s, it was joined to the mainland and today houses a large sewage treatment facility with a naval base operated by the People's Liberation Army (PLA).

Many Hongkongers are likely to be unaware of the history of Stonecutters Island, just as they may be unfamiliar with the history of Taipingshan, in Hong Kong's Central and Western District, where an epidemic of bubonic plague broke out in 1894, often taken to mark the onset of the third plague pandemic. From southern China and Hong Kong, plague diffused along shipping routes to India, Australia, South Africa, North America, and Europe. Perhaps as many as 15 million people died worldwide. Today, hard-surface ball courts and a small public garden mark the spot where, following the Taipingshan Resumption Ordinance in September 1894, the British demolished the crowded Chinese tenements at the epicenter of the outbreak.

The contemporary landscape of Hong Kong, like many other Asian cities, has been shaped by disease episodes of the past. Yet most accounts of the transformations that have taken place across the region over the last few centuries focus exclusively on political, social, economic, and cultural upheavals. For the most part, disease is mentioned only as a backdrop to more momentous events, relegated to a footnote, or overlooked altogether. The aim of this book is to write epidemics back into history, examining the transformative role that disease has played in making modern Asia, and suggesting how the threat of infection continues to influence societies across the region today.

Epidemics in Modern Asia proposes a new transnational approach to modern Asian history and global modernity; one that places emphasis on connections and continuities over space and across time – as well as on discontinuities – and, in so doing, resituates the experience of epidemics at the heart of Asian history. The book challenges previous histories that have tracked the diffusion of epidemics westwards from their origins in the East and emphasized the counter-migration of knowledge and technological know-how eastwards from the West. It argues that examining the causes and consequences of epidemics in history can transform our understanding of the past and the emergence of the modern world. In recent years, there has been a surge of interest in cross-cultural contacts and transmissions across Asia. With a few notable exceptions, disease has been largely and inexplicably absent from this literature. Although there is now a substantive scholarship on the history of medicine, health, and disease in Asia – particularly in South Asia, but increasingly in East Asia – the study of epidemics has not, on the whole, been sufficiently integrated into a broader, interregional framework. Research on the history of disease in India, for example, has remained typically disconnected from histories of Southeast Asia, just as artificial boundaries are apt to be drawn between Southeast Asia, China, and Japan. As a result, regions that for centuries have been characterized by cultural, political, and economic exchange, vanish from view. The purpose of this book is to offer a much-needed corrective to this sequestration, furnishing a fresh comparative vantage of analysis, while providing suggestions for future directions of research.

In her ethnographic exploration of the conflicts over the future of the rainforests in South Kalimantan, on Indonesian Borneo, the anthropologist Anna Tsing enquires: 'How does one do an ethnography of global connections?'[1] In this book, I recast the question to ask: How does one write a history of disease that explores continuities but simultaneously takes cultural differences seriously? The view across Victoria Harbour – one of the busiest ports in the world – onto a former quarantine station that now serves as a base for the PLA is a poignant reminder of the complex and sometimes violent interactions that have shaped this post-colonial port city. To borrow Tsing's phrase, Hong Kong is 'a zone of awkward engagement,' a global hub that is also a place of 'friction.' This is a book, then, about disease, cultural interactions, and global networks of power and trade. It investigates epidemics as unstable phenomena that

---

[1] Anna Lowenhaupt Tsing, *Friction: An Ethnography of Global Connection* (Princeton, NJ: Princeton University Press, 2005), p.xi.

are produced when global processes become entangled with highly local circumstances.

There are, of course, many challenges in writing a history of epidemic disease in Asia. First, and most obviously, are the impediments presented by the sheer geographical and chronological scale of such a project. In focusing on the macro-level there is a danger that the particularities of specific places at specific times may be overlooked, with the consequence that epidemic histories are inadvertently abstracted and de-territorialized. Second, is the linguistic challenge that the task poses, since a trans-Asian history requires proficiency in many languages – too numerous, certainly, for any individual scholar to acquire. Third, and relatedly, is the sheer quantity and variety of sources. And fourth, are the gaps in existing knowledge and the patchiness of the archives. Given the lack of systematic and reliable statistical data, estimating morbidity and mortality is often no more than guesswork. While the book draws on my own archival research, it is also necessarily a work of synthesis informed by the research of many other scholars. I am profoundly beholden to colleagues whose writing has stimulated me to think in fresh ways about modern Asia. Wherever possible, I have sought to acknowledge this debt clearly in the main text. At the end of the book, a brief guide to further reading identifies work that I have found particularly helpful. Although this is an English bibliography, the books and articles that are referenced contain abundant additional material in Asian languages.

Epidemics in Modern Asia is organized into five cross-cutting chapters that pivot on specific themes: mobility, cities, the environment, war, and globalization. These are not watertight categories, but rather provisional frames for interrogating specific epidemic events, with frequent crossovers and switchbacks. In this sense, the themes are approached as questions rather than fixed conceptual anchors. One aim of the book is to introduce readers to larger historiographical issues and in so doing to contribute, on a more theoretical level, to discussions about the methods and scope of history. Each chapter is structured around three or four case studies. A conclusion summarizes the main arguments and the critical questions that the chapters have raised. The book also includes a select timeline, maps, and a glossary, where essential terms are defined. Plates and maps provide a visual narrative that emphasizes the spatial and visual dimension of the epidemics under discussion. Throughout, text boxes introduce key concepts, topics, and illustrative readings from a range of primary and secondary sources.

I am grateful to the Research Grants Council of Hong Kong for generously supporting research for sections of this book with a grant from the

General Research Fund ('Infective Economies: Plague and the Crisis of Empire' HKU752011H). A work such as this, which reaches across terrains, is inevitably a collaborative process. The arguments developed in the book have been tested in a large cross-faculty undergraduate course at the University of Hong Kong entitled 'Contagions: Global Histories of Disease' (CCGL9003). *Epidemics in Modern Asia* was written first and foremost with my students in mind. While there is an expansive literature on the history of disease in the West, it is relatively recently that academic work has begun to appear in English on disease in East Asia. Much of this specialist literature is dispersed across journals and difficult to access. A practical aim in writing this book has been to make existing scholarship more accessible, bringing together area-specific research to highlight broader themes. I should like to thank my students for encouraging me to write this book, for helping me to draw connections between the past and the present, for challenging many of my assumptions about Hong Kong and modern Asia, and for reminding me how important history can be for understanding the contemporary world. I am grateful to Amy Tsui, Ian Holliday, Gwyn Edwards, Gray Kochhar-Lindgren, and the members of the Common Core Committee for espousing transdisciplinary, research-based teaching in the new curriculum, and to my colleague Carol Tsang who helped with the course materials and provided much useful feedback. A special thank you to Nancy Yang and to all the students involved in Beyond the Pivot (BTP), a student-led NGO that I am privileged to have mentored: their humanitarian work in rural China has shaped my own understanding of the health challenges facing the region, and their commitment and enthusiasm have given me hope. Thanks to my postgraduate students Mark Clifford, Angharad Fletcher, Maurits Meerwijk, and Georges Papavasiliou, who have kept me on my toes.

I am grateful to Lucy Rhymer at Cambridge University Press for her encouragement and support, to Rosalyn Scott and the production team, to Frances Peck for copyediting, and to the three anonymous readers for providing invaluable comments and suggestions; they have certainly helped to strengthen the arguments, although any remaining shortcomings are obviously my responsibility alone. The ideas in this book have been shaped by numerous discussions with friends and colleagues, and it is a pleasure to acknowledge them here: Thomas Abraham, Sunil Amrith, Warwick Anderson, David Arnold, Roberto Bruzzone, Christopher Bayly, James Beattie, Lisa Cartwright, L. C. Chan, Stephen Davies, Amy Fairchild, Didier Fassin, Richard Fielding, Staci Ford, Mark Ravinder Frost, Sander Gilman, Miriam Gross, Marta Hanson, Faith Ho, Frédéric Keck, Nick King, Gray Kochhar-Lindgren,

Shigehisa Kuriyama, Heidi Larson, Alan Lester, Shao-hua Liu, Christos Lynteris, Laurence Monnais, Projit Bihari Mukharji, Christopher Munn, Rosanna Peeling, Malik Peiris, Peter Piot, Anne Marie Rafferty, Charles Schencking, Mark Seltzer, Ria Sinha, Facil Tesfaye, Andrew Thompson, Chung To, Joe Tucker, and Zhou Xun. My thanks to Alison Bashford for encouraging me to rethink the spaces of quarantine; to the late Anthony Hyman, for his mentorship and an unforgettable trip through the Sindh; to Mark Jackson for commissioning me to write on cholera and empire in Southeast Asia and China; to Sayeed Khan for his hospitality in Pakistan; to Carlos Rojas for expeditiously dispatching 'homesickness'; to the late Aziz Siddiqui for pointing to the map and, in difficult times, offering me a ride to Jalalabad; and to Priscilla Wald for conversations over six years about contagion, globalization, and the need for an expanded vision of health.

At the University of Hong Kong, I thank all of my colleagues in the Department of History. I have benefitted greatly from conversations with Frank Dikötter, whose insights have informed my thinking, and from the encouragement of John Carroll and David Pomfret. Over the last few years, Helen Siu and Angela Ki Che Leung at the Hong Kong Institute for the Humanities and Social Sciences have been generous interlocutors and my warm thanks to them. I am grateful to Daniel Chua who was instrumental in establishing the Centre for the Humanities and Medicine, which I have been fortunate to co-direct since 2009. In the Li Ka Shing Faculty of Medicine, Gabriel Leung has been a champion of the 'big picture' view of disease and medicine and a passionate advocate for history. I owe a unique debt to Maria Sin for her encouragement, ingenuity, and indispensable support during the writing of this book. Her acumen and energy have also ensured the success of the Global Histories of Disease and Medicine project, which has provided a vibrant forum for exploring many of the ideas and issues examined in this book.

For help with sourcing the images, thanks to Anita Austin, Iris Chan, Jack Eckert, Stephen Greenberg, Akiko Kasiwara, Mattias Klum, Ako Matsuo, Michael Sappol, Joanna Skeels, Charlotte Todd, and Michael Wolf. My thanks to Dick Yeung for the maps. I gratefully acknowledge the permission granted to reproduce the copyright material in this book. Every effort has been made to trace copyright holders and to obtain their prior permission for the use of copyright material. I apologize in advance for any errors or omissions and if notified of any corrections will ensure that they are incorporated in future editions of this book.

Finally, *Epidemics in Modern Asia* could not have been written without the support of my wife, Rebecca, with whom I have shared many adventures in Asia, including six special months in Tokyo. Our children Lily

Mei and James – Hongkongers both – were wonderful antidotes to contagious preoccupations. Exchanges with Oriana were always a joy. This book is dedicated with appreciation and love to my parents, Michael and Catherine, truly doctors without borders.

ROBERT PECKHAM
Hong Kong, October 2015

Abbreviations

ARC	American Red Cross
ASEAN	Association of Southeast Asian Nations
CDC	US Centers for Disease Control and Prevention
CER	Chinese Eastern Railway
CIA	US Central Intelligence Agency
DDT	Dichlorodiphenyltrichloroethane
EIC	East India Company
EID	Emerging infectious disease
ENSO	El Niño Southern Oscillation
EVD	Ebola virus disease
FAO	UN Food and Agriculture Organization
FATA	Federally Administered Tribal Areas
FCR	Frontier Crimes Regulation
GHSI	Global Health Security Initiative
GPEI	Global Polio Eradication Initiative
GPHIN	Global Public Health Intelligence Network
HIV/AIDS	Human immunodeficiency virus/acquired immune deficiency syndrome
IMCS	Imperial Maritime Customs Service
INSEP	Intensified Smallpox Eradication Program
ISIL	Islamic State of Iraq and the Levant
JE	Japanese encephalitis
KP	Khyber Pakhtunkhwa
MERS	Middle East respiratory syndrome
NiV	Nipah virus
NTD	Neglected tropical disease
OIE	*Office International des Epizooties* (World Organisation for Animal Health)
PLA	People's Liberation Army
PRC	People's Republic of China
ProMED	Program for Monitoring Emerging Diseases
SARS	Severe acute respiratory syndrome

STI	Sexually transmitted infection
TCM	Traditional Chinese medicine
UAV	Unmanned aerial vehicle
UNICEF	United Nations Children's Fund
VOC	*Vereenigde Oostindische Compagnie* (United East India Company)
WCS	Wildlife Conservation Society
WHO	World Health Organization
WTO	World Trade Organization

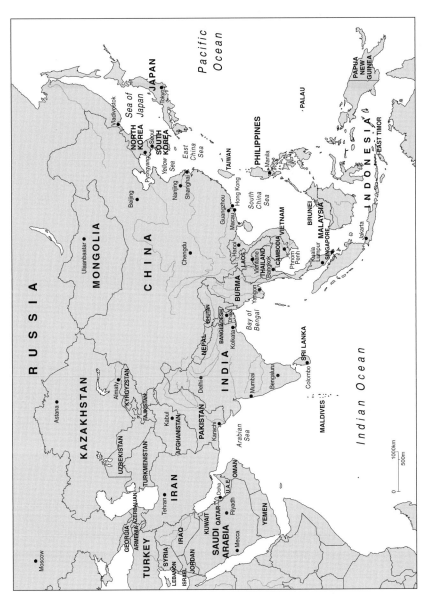

Map 0.1. Contemporary Asia

Introduction: Contagious histories

Throughout 2014, an epidemic of Ebola virus disease (EVD) in West Africa dominated the global media. While the World Health Organization (WHO) declared the epidemic a public health emergency, images of makeshift quarantines, field-laboratories, and bagged bodies fueled panic in many countries around the world. The high mortality rate of up to 90 percent, together with graphic details of the symptoms, which may include internal and external bleeding, added to public concerns. In Hong Kong, health authorities stepped up surveillance and rushed to implement Ebola contingency plans. Travelers from West Africa who showed symptoms of fever were quarantined and tested. Authorities in the People's Republic of China (PRC), conscious of the large numbers of Chinese workers in Africa, heightened border controls.

Two other viral infections also caused alarm across Asia. Middle East respiratory syndrome (MERS), a highly pathogenic viral illness, was first reported in 2012 in Saudi Arabia. The Saudi Arabian economy is dependent on some nine million non-national residents, many of them migrant workers from South and Southeast Asia. Every year millions of pilgrims from across Asia converge on Saudi Arabia for the *hajj*, the annual Islamic pilgrimage to Mecca. In May 2015, an outbreak of MERS in South Korea led to the imposition of quarantine measures, the closing of schools, and – amidst public panic – the establishment of specialist MERS clinics in major cities. By mid July 2015, there had been 186 confirmed cases of infection with 36 deaths (Figure 0.1).

Meanwhile, in March 2013, human cases of the novel avian influenza virus H7N9 were reported in China. A WHO announcement about the new virus, which was posted on Twitter, prompted up to 500 retweets per hour.[1] By December 2013, there had been 143 laboratory-confirmed

---

[1] Sara E. Davies, 'Internet Surveillance and Disease Outbreaks.' In: Simon Rushton and Jeremy Youde, eds., *Routledge Handbook of Global Health Security* (Abingdon and New York: Routledge, 2015), pp.226–238 (226).

1

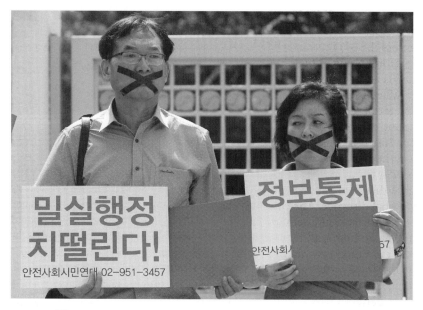

Figure 0.1. 'MERS in South Korea, June 4, 2015.' Photograph by Yang Ji-Woong. Courtesy: EPA.

MERS: Panic and protest in Korea

An outbreak of MERS in South Korea in 2015 brought to the fore many of the themes explored in this book: global interconnectedness, the particular social and cultural circumstances that shape responses to novel infections, as well as an epidemic's political and economic ramifications. MERS is a viral respiratory disease caused by a coronavirus (MERS-CoV) and leads to death in approximately 36 percent of those infected. While the disease appears to have been introduced to Korea from the Middle East, it was widely claimed in the media that overcrowded hospital facilities, as well as the practice of 'doctor shopping,' facilitated its spread. The epidemic in South Korea sparked panic across the country and criticism was leveled at the government for playing down the risks and failing to act decisively. In Figure 0.1, two protesters attending an anti-government rally in Seoul hold up red cards. A placard reads: 'Total incompetence of the government for sluggish response!' South Korea is Asia's fourth-largest economy and the epidemic impelled the country's central bank to cut interest rates amidst fears of the economic fallout from MERS.

human cases of H7N9 with 45 deaths. A 36-year-old Indonesian domestic helper, who had visited a live poultry market and slaughtered a chicken across the border in Shenzhen, became the first confirmed H7N9 patient in Hong Kong. This sparked a ban on poultry imports from Shenzhen farms and a heightened alert in hospitals.

What do these epidemics have in common, aside from the fact that they are zoonoses – that is, infections of animal origin? What can they tell us about contemporary Asia? In this book, I explore many of the themes contained in this brief overview of current epidemic threats: South and Southeast Asians in the Middle East; an Indonesian helper crossing the border from Hong Kong to mainland China to visit a 'wet market'; a Chinese diaspora in Africa; the plotting of scattered events as symptoms of a global disorder. The book considers this interconnected but splintered world through the lens of infectious disease, tracing the consequences of new and old interdependencies across Asia: historic networks of trade and culture, mass migrations, booming cities where expanding industry is drawing low-wage workers, as well as growing Asian interests outside Asia. We examine the role of the state in epidemic surveillance, the tensions between national interests and transnational flows, and investigate the asymmetries of a world where globalization is espoused at the same time as the foreign is stigmatized; where epidemics are often ascribed to cultural practices rather than to deeper social and biological causes.

Recent infectious disease outbreaks demonstrate how current threats are often viewed in relation to past events. Responses to Ebola, MERS, and H7N9 have been shaped by the experiences of other epidemics, including severe acute respiratory syndrome (SARS) in 2002 and 2003. Allusions to history pervade media coverage of these epidemics, most obviously in recurrent fears about the coming plague. What if Ebola should become airborne? Supposing the influenza virus mutated or different flu strains 'reassorted' to allow effective human-to-human transmission? Accounts of the present repeatedly evoke the future in terms of the past. Could Ebola, or MERS, or H7N9 become the next pandemic, like the 'Spanish flu' in 1918–1919, which killed perhaps 50 million people or more globally, the majority in Asia?

Since the 1980s, particularly with the identification of the human immunodeficiency virus and acquired immune deficiency syndrome (HIV/AIDS), there has been a renewed focus on the threats posed to human societies by infectious disease. Today, Asia is regarded by many commentators as a frontline in the global 'war' against novel pathogens, notably those of animal origin. Experiences of avian influenza from the late 1990s, as well as the outbreak of SARS in southern China, have drawn attention to the region's vulnerabilities. Over 30 percent of the world's population resides in East and Southeast Asia, with 1.36 billion in China alone. Even though there has been a significant shift from communicable to chronic degenerative diseases as causes of death in recent decades, Southeast Asia still accounts for over a quarter of the global burden of infectious and parasitic diseases, and remains 'an acknowledged hotspot for risk.'[2] According to the WHO, there are six million annual deaths attributable to infectious diseases across the region (Figure 0.2).[3]

The rapid growth of Asian economies has put increasing pressure on natural resources from industry and consumers. Urban expansion, the intensification of agriculture, demands for wood and water, as well as mineral extraction and infrastructural projects, including damming for hydroelectric power and road construction, have all impacted upon landscapes, altering habitats and influencing inter-species interactions.[4] Particularly over the last two decades, Southeast Asia has been viewed as a 'biodiversity hotspot where exceptional concentrations of endemic species are undergoing exceptional loss of habitat' under the pressure of development.[5] Disruptions to ecosystems are understood to have implications for the emergence and spread of infectious diseases. Deforestation and forest encroachment, for example, may drive species that serve as viral reservoirs into new proximity with humans. This was the case with the Nipah virus (NiV), first identified in Malaysia in 1999, which was transmitted to humans via pigs infected by fruit bats flushed out of their natural forest habitat (Chapter 3).

In part as a result of these transformations, Asia is habitually represented in the Western media as a region of teeming megacities, degraded environments, unscrupulous mass-farming practices, and particular cultural habits and behaviors that render it susceptible to lethal infection with upshots for the global order. Political instability, corruption, and uneven development are viewed as contributory factors driving epidemics. In this calamitous history, Asia's biophysical volatility (earthquakes, tsunamis, volcanoes, epidemics) provides the ground for other kinds of catastrophic violence: riots, revolution, and dictatorship. As the journalist Alan Sipress asserts in his book *The Fatal Strain*, Asia 'is

---

[2] Richard J. Coker, et al., 'Emerging Infectious Diseases in Southeast Asia: Regional Challenges to Control,' *Lancet*, vol.377, no.9765 (February 12, 2011): 599–609 (607).

[3] Jai P. Narain and R. Bhatia, 'The Challenge of Communicable Diseases in the WHO South-East Asia Region,' *Bulletin of the World Health Organization*, vol.88, no.3 (2010): 162.

[4] Peter W. Horby, et al., 'Drivers of Emerging Zoonotic Infectious Diseases.' In: Akio Yamada, et al., eds., *Confronting Emerging Zoonoses: The One Health Paradigm* (Dordrecht: Springer, 2014), pp.13–26 (17).

[5] Norman Myers, et al., 'Biodiversity Hotspots for Conservation Priorities,' *Nature*, vol.403, no.6772 (February 24, 2000): 853–858.

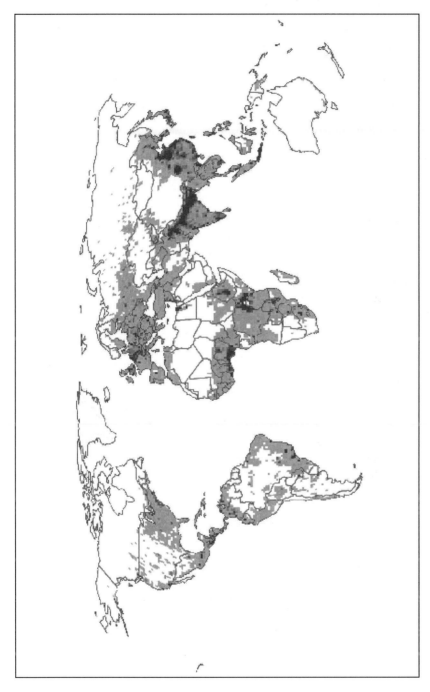

Figure 0.2. 'Global hotspots for emerging infectious diseases that originate in wildlife.'

Zoonoses: Global hotspots

Over 60 percent of new emerging infectious diseases (EIDs) are zoonotic, including HIV/AIDS, SARS, Ebola, and pandemic influenza. Many other diseases that affect humans, such as smallpox and measles, evolved from animal infections. Socio-economic, ecological, and behavioral factors are understood to be the principal drivers of EIDs and the vast majority of zoonotic diseases have been spillovers from wildlife. Equatorial regions, notably in sub-Saharan Africa and Southeast Asia, are commonly identified as 'hotspots' for zoonotic EIDs with a wildlife origin, on account of their 'human pathogen species richness.' Global distribution models suggest that regions in higher latitudes – including Western Europe – are also at risk, given their dense populations. Figure 0.2, adapted from a 2008 paper in *Nature*, shows the risk from EIDs caused by zoonotic pathogens from wildlife, with darker shades indicating higher risk. The map is based on the 'temporal emergence' of 335 EIDs between 1940 and 2004. Maps play a key role in biosurveillance, in assessing the risk of EID outbreaks, and in helping to quantify the burden of disease. Today, innovations in automated data collection, including Internet text mining and health reporting systems, such as ProMED (Program for Monitoring Emerging Diseases), are enabling new ways of visualizing data to provide a baseline for disease risk assessments. HealthMap acquires and processes data hourly from electronic media sources to provide a view of the global state of infectious disease online and via mobile devices.

Kate E. Jones, et al., 'Global Trends in Emerging Infectious Diseases,' *Nature*, vol.451, no.7181 (February 21, 2008): 990–993.

Simon I. Hay, et al., 'Global Mapping of Infectious Disease,' *Philosophical Transactions of the Royal Society B: Biological Sciences*, vol.368, no.1614 (2013): 20120250.

defined by poverty, superstition, unregulated development, and corrupt, parochial politics.' The WHO's headquarters in the leafy outskirts of Geneva – 'a citadel of efficiency, social order, and good government' – are a far cry from this Asian battleground. The cover of Sipress's book accentuates the message graphically by pinpointing Asia as the locus of influenza emergence. On a map that cuts off the Americas and most of

Western Europe, the islands of Southeast Asia and the eastern Eurasian landmass from Delhi to Vladivostok are covered with clusters of red push-pins, suggesting an 'unfriendly terrain,' or what Sipress calls the 'theater of conflict that is Asia.'[6]

Although diseases such as Nipah are labeled 'emerging' or 're-emerging' in the scientific literature – since they are 'rapidly increasing in incidence or geographic range' (WHO) – Asia has in fact long been viewed in the Western imaginary as a source of contagion: from the Black Death in the mid fourteenth century, attributed to the westward expansion of the Mongol Empire, to epidemics of 'Asiatic' cholera in the nineteenth century, the scourge of smallpox, and more recently, avian influenza. From the eighteenth century, images of smallpox patients, which had been produced in China to assist in the diagnosis and treatment of the disease, circulated in Europe, where they were taken as illustrative of China's unwholesome and backward character. In Western medical discourse, particularly during the nineteenth century, Chinese identity became linked to pestilence with the country imagined as the 'cradle of smallpox' and the homeland of plague. Prevalent Western perceptions of China as the 'sick man of Asia' were interpolated by late Qing commentators, who employed a similar language of pathology and dysfunction to describe China's enfeebled condition.[7] Likewise, from the 1840s – and particularly after the Indian Rebellion of 1857 – cholera was progressively 'Asianized' as Western observers sought to locate the infection's origin in the East, invariably tracing its 'home' to the Delta of the rivers Ganges and Brahmaputra.[8] As recent epidemic events have shown, dormant historical associations may be easily reactivated and inserted into contemporary contexts. During the SARS outbreak in 2003, Chinese-owned businesses in some North America cities were boycotted as sites of possible infection, even though there had been no cases of disease there.[9]

Western epidemic narratives frequently hinge on a geopolitical asymmetry, wherein the origins of infection are tracked to the global South and East, and the expertise to combat this incipient menace is deemed

---

[6] Alan Sipress, *The Fatal Strain: On the Trail of Avian Flu and the Coming Pandemic* (New York: Viking, 2009), p.7.

[7] Larissa N. Heinrich, *The Afterlife of Images: Translating the Pathological Body between China and the West* (Durham, NC: Duke University Press, 2008), pp.14–37.

[8] Christopher Hamlin, *Cholera: A Biography* (Oxford: Oxford University Press, 2009), pp.39–46.

[9] Huiling Ding, 'Transnational Quarantine Rhetorics: Public Mobilization in SARS and in H1N1 Flu,' *Journal of Medical Humanities*, vol.35, no.2 (2014): 191–210 (201–203); Laura Eichelberger, 'SARS and New York's Chinatown: The Politics of Risk and Blame During an Epidemic of Fear,' *Social Science & Medicine*, vol.65, no.6 (2007): 1284–1295.

to reside in the North and West.[10] This dynamic is reprised in contemporary pandemic thrillers, such as Steven Soderbergh's *Contagion* (2011), where a fictional pathogen wreaks havoc in the United States. The MEV-1 virus in the movie, like the real-life NiV, is the result of environmental despoliation that has pushed the virus's natural hosts – in this case fruit bats – into fatal contact with domesticated animals. While pandemic thrillers may serve to dramatize pandemics in ways that shock the public out of its complacency, they also shape public perspectives and expectations. In *Contagion*, a delirious young man staggers through the bustling streets of Hong Kong; a Japanese businessman keels over in a crowded commuter bus in Tokyo; an epidemiologist dispatched by the WHO to investigate the deadly disease outbreak in southern China is abducted by fearful locals. Asia is represented in the movie through an accumulation of such feverish scenes as the ground zero of infectious disease: it is a high-risk region of violence, capitalist speculation, and the unethical exploitation of the environment. Significantly, Beth Emhoff (played by Gwyneth Paltrow), the 'super spreader' in the movie who works for the global corporation AIMM Alderson, contracts MEV-1 on a business trip to a Macau casino. The association of the casino's gaming tables with infection intimates a prevailing view of Asia as 'the genetic roulette table' for influenza mutations.[11] From the early 1990s, when the term 'emerging infections' gained currency to describe novel pathogens, such as HIV/AIDS (Chapter 5), the pandemic thriller became a popular Hollywood genre. Asia has invariably been imagined in such films as a weak link in global health security. A BBC Horizon documentary on SARS in 2003 articulated a prevalent Western view of Asia, when over the image of a writhing snake in a Chinese wet market, the narrator intoned forebodingly that 'something deadly' was stirring in the East.

What have the consequences been of this geopolitical framing of disease? Conceptualizing Asia as a source of infection that threatens global security has obscured the profound role that disease episodes have played in shaping modern Asia itself. Global histories of disease often include no more than gestural references to Asia. Although the region is singled out as a pandemic epicenter, little attention is paid to the fallout there. Instead, the emphasis is on transmission pathways and on the social and economic shocks produced in the destination countries of the West. The extensive literature on the 1918–1919 influenza pandemic is a case in point. While much has been written about the impact of the

---

[10] Priscilla Wald, *Contagious: Cultures, Carriers, and the Outbreak Narrative* (Durham, NC: Duke University Press, 2008), p.34.

[11] Michael T. Osterholm, 'The Next Contagion: Closer Than You Think,' *New York Times* (May 9, 2013).

deadly influenza virus in the United States and Europe after the First World War, considerably less study has been made of the infection's eastward trajectory, even though the Asia-Pacific region was the hardest hit by the pandemic. In his comprehensive and popular history, *The Great Influenza*, John Barry devotes less than two pages to India, despite declaring: 'In the Indian subcontinent alone, it is likely that close to 20 million died, and quite possibly the death toll exceeded that number.'[12] Equivalently, although there is an extensive literature on the cholera epidemics that swept nineteenth-century Europe and North America, there are no commensurate studies focusing on the cholera's spread eastwards from 1817 to Indonesia, the Philippines, China, the Korean peninsula, and Japan. One aim of this book is thus to offer a postcolonial critique that decenters Western history and the assumptions about infection that have been built into it – 'provincializing' Europe, in the words of the historian Dipesh Chakrabarty – and thereby offering new perspectives on the inter-dynamics of people, environments, and diseases across Asia.[13]

Certainly, over the last 20 years a substantive body of work has been published on the history of medicine and health in South Asia, particularly in relation to epidemics. More recently, there has been a similar focus on East Asia – as attested by the bibliography included at the end of this book. It is not so much, then, that epidemics in Asia have been ignored but that they have not been well integrated into mainstream political history, into wider interregional and transnational histories of disease, or reframed in the context of concerns about the nature and meaning of globalization. Concurrently, political and social histories persist in their tendency to view epidemics as epiphenomena: part of the historical backdrop to more significant political, social, and economic conditions and events. Many history textbooks allude only cursorily – if at all – to infectious diseases. Jonathan Spence's magisterial 700-page overview of modern China from the collapse of the Ming dynasty in the seventeenth century to the present, for example, contains fleeting mention of epidemics, even though we are told that Chinese chroniclers noted of one destructive pestilence between 1642 and 1643 that it 'caused many communities to suffer losses of half or more of their inhabitants.' An observer in Henan province remarked of a devastated city that 'there were few signs of human life in the streets and all that was heard was the buzzing

[12] John M. Barry, *The Great Influenza: The Story of the Deadliest Pandemic in History* (New York: Penguin, [2004] 2009), p.365.
[13] Dipesh Chakrabarty, *Provincializing Europe: Postcolonial Thought and Historical Difference* (Princeton, NJ: Princeton University Press, 2000).

of flies.'[14] Why is disease so conspicuously left out of Asia's political and social history, despite the fact that epidemics have overwhelmed communities in this way? How should historians grapple with this often absent disease context? What would the past look like if we inverted the emphasis, rethinking the history of Asia through the prism of epidemics?

Histories of Asia have tended to focus on the evolution of political and economic systems, social transitions, and military conflict. Transnational approaches have stressed the mercantile and cultural connections across stretches of Asia, emphasizing flows of people, commodities, and ideas. My aim in this book is to write disease back into history. In other words, disease is not viewed as an extraneous phenomenon but is resituated within dynamic political, economic, social, and cultural milieus. At the same time, the book endeavors to integrate area-specific perspectives into a broader interregional framework. I argue that studying epidemic diseases contextually in this way can help us understand critical themes in Asian history: shifting relations between local and state authorities, the causes and after-effects of migration, the expansion of interregional trade networks, modernization, and the development of new forms of citizenship.

In accentuating disease in this way, there is, of course, a risk that predominant Western views of Asia as a singularly pathological space – a disease 'hotspot' in the parlance of contemporary epidemiology – are reinforced rather than critiqued. To suggest that Asian societies are facing unprecedented epidemic threats may imply that the pathogenic menace has in some way been produced by Asian societies themselves. In other words, epidemics may be taken to reflect a society's underlying condition, serving as an index of its health. This has certainly been a recurring theme in Western assessments, where epidemics have often been intuited as the damaging fallout of progress. Outbreaks are signs of a modernizing society out of kilter; of a world gone awry. 'In one sense, this ironic and persistent emphasis on the role of civilization in the causation of disease is no more than a cliché,' the historian Charles E. Rosenberg has observed, 'a variation of traditional primitivistic notions, endless evocations of lost worlds in which humankind had not been corrupted by wealth and artifice – all versions and reiterations of the Garden of Eden's Faustian bargain recast in epidemiological terms.' Epidemic histories may function, then, as a genre of 'moral parable underlining the ambiguous nature of human progress and of our ultimate lordship over the material domain we have presumed to rule.'[15]

---

[14] Jonathan D. Spence, *The Search for Modern China*. Third edition (New York: W. W. Norton, 2013), p.23.

[15] Charles E. Rosenberg, 'Pathologies of Progress: The Idea of Civilization as Risk,' *Bulletin of the History of Medicine*, vol.72, no.4 (1998): 714–730 (716, 728).

While *Epidemics in Modern Asia* seeks to write disease into Asian history, it does so conscious of the pull that this 'lost world' narrative retains and within the context of three interconnected concerns. First, it explores the interplay of social, cultural, political, and economic factors that have produced epidemic crises. Second, it considers the ways in which epidemics have impacted upon social and political arrangements. And, third, it examines how diseases have been experienced and understood in different Asian settings. Informing these three concerns is an interest in the development of sanitary, hygienic, and medical ideas from the second half of the nineteenth century; the formulation and implementation of expansive public health initiatives premised on prevention at the turn of the nineteenth and twentieth centuries; and the internationalization of health in the mid twentieth century with the creation of the WHO in 1948. The focus is on balancing biophysical and sociopolitical factors, avoiding an over-emphasis on one at the expense of the other.

It is worth stating up-front what the book does not set out to do. It is not a study of the progressive expansion of Western medicine (otherwise known as biomedicine or allopathic medicine) and public health across Asia. Neither does it claim to provide a comprehensive overview of major disease events with their epidemiological histories. The neat chronology of epidemics encountered in many history books suggests a uniform and linear extension of disease through time and across space. It is as if such events unfolded sequentially in defined stages to fill clearly delineated geographic spaces, an idea reinforced in the plotting of disease trajectories on maps. Yet in truth, epidemics and pandemics are far more episodic and ragged phenomena with uncertain beginnings and often indeterminate endings. It is this very amorphousness and unpredictability that renders them so terrifying. When did the third plague pandemic really begin? When did it end? Most pandemics peter out, rather than end abruptly, dying 'ordinarily with a whimper rather than a bang.'[16] The conventional chronology of the third plague pandemic could be pushed back well before the 1850s, just as it could be stretched forward well into the twentieth century. The parenthesized dates that customarily accompany epidemics and pandemics – as they inevitably do here – are no more than provisional markers, not immutable parameters analogous with biographical lifelines. Diseases co-exist, surface and recede, spread and retract in ways far more complex than is often presumed. In this sense, the terms 'event' and 'episode' may be misleading, too, since they imply a self-evident segment of time, whereas we might think of the

---

[16] Charles E. Rosenberg, 'What is an Epidemic?: AIDS in Historical Perspective.' In: *Explaining Epidemics and Other Studies in the History of Medicine* (Cambridge: Cambridge University Press, 1992), pp.278–292 (286).

past 'as an infinity of such moments, each of significance to those who experience it.'[17] Notwithstanding this – and while recognizing that they are the outcome of entangled ecological, social, economic, and political processes – we should remember that epidemics are experienced by those caught up in them as catastrophic ruptures.[18] My purpose in the pages that follow is to capture some of this complexity in a narrative that is nonetheless accessible for those coming at the subject for the first time.

The book is organized thematically, exploring specific moments of crises in relation to five cross-cutting themes: mobility, cities, the environment, war, and globalization. Each chapter adopts a cross-sectional, case study approach, zooming in on a number of epidemics that highlight aspects of these broad social and ecological issues. Cases are considered in relation to specific political transitions over the last 200 years, including the formation and breakup of empires, the evolution of the modern state and nationalism, the advent of Communism, the Cold War, and market liberalization from the late 1970s.

In contrast to existing histories, the book repositions epidemics at the heart of modern Asian history, demonstrating how infectious disease events contributed to the environmental, social, and cultural transformations that marked the onset of modernity. In so doing, the objective is not to reiterate conventional modernization narratives that posit a radical break between traditional practices and the introduction of top-down medical technologies linked to the development of Western-style states and new models of citizenship. Rather, I argue for a more nuanced approach that recognizes continuities and registers change. The book seeks to demonstrate the persistence of older concepts and practices, as well as the often violent resistance to hygienic modernity. Defining societies as 'traditional' or 'modern' reflects the after-drag of a nineteenth-century worldview, wherein Asia was often perceived as culturally stagnant and incapable of reform without the external stimulus of the 'civilized' West.[19] Finally, the book aims to qualify an exclusive focus on the state by exploring the inter-dynamics of popular responses with the knowledge and practices produced by state institutions. Writing a book of this kind inevitably poses many challenges. Not least is the issue of defining the terms: What is an 'epidemic'? How do we define 'modern'? What

[17] Patrick Manning, *Navigating World History: Historians Create a Global Past* (New York and Basingstoke: Palgrave Macmillan, 2003), p.269.

[18] Christos Lynteris, 'Introduction: The Time of Epidemics,' *Cambridge Anthropology*, vol.32, no.1 (2014): 24–31.

[19] Paul A. Cohen, 'Moving Beyond "Tradition and Modernity."' In: *China Unbound: Evolving Perspectives on the Chinese Past* (London and New York: RoutledgeCurzon, 2003), pp.48–84.

do we mean by 'Asia'? In the remainder of the Introduction, I address each of these questions in turn, placing the book's argument in relation to current debates, while drawing out central themes and issues.

Global histories and disease

In arguing for the need to write disease back into history, *Epidemics in Modern Asia* engages with a number of significant currents within contemporary historiography. Since the 1960s and 1970s, 'big' history has sought to view the human past within a wide-ranging ecological and evolutionary timespan. The emphasis has been on environment, populations, and global interconnectedness. In *The Columbian Exchange*, published in 1972, the historian Alfred W. Crosby underlined the biological consequences of 1492. Christopher Columbus's 'discovery' of the Americas initiated a two-way trans-Atlantic movement of organisms: the fateful exchange of pathogens between the Old World and the New resulted in momentous ecological transformations.[20] The French historian Emmanuel Le Roy Ladurie has similarly maintained that the period between the fourteenth and seventeenth centuries represented a new era of global 'microbial unity.' Conquest, trade, and travel expedited the transcontinental dissemination of infections, which played a decisive role in shaping global events. In the words of Le Roy Ladurie, this process marked 'the unification of the world by disease.'[21]

The connection between disease and the movement of human populations viewed within a macro-scale became a key focus in historical scholarship in the 1970s, exemplified by William H. McNeill's *Plagues and Peoples* (1976). The creation of a Mongol Empire that extended from Central Asia to Europe in the thirteenth century enabled multiplying trade networks to develop and thus opened up routes for disease to spread. Ecological and epidemiological balances were upset, intermeshing disease pools. Citing examples from China to the New World, McNeill contends that the diffusion of disease can be linked to a new global connectivity engendered by trade, agriculture, domestication, and war. Accordingly, disease should be regarded as a key determinant of human civilization.[22]

---

[20] Alfred W. Crosby, *The Columbian Exchange: Biological and Cultural Consequences of 1492*. Revised edition (Westport, CT: Praeger, 2003).

[21] Emmanuel Le Roy Ladurie, 'A Concept: The Unification of the Globe by Disease (Fourteenth to Seventeenth Centuries).' In: *The Mind and Method of the Historian*. Translated by Siân and Ben Reynolds (Brighton: Harvester Press, 1981), pp.28–83.

[22] William H. McNeill, *Plagues and Peoples* (London: Penguin, [1976] 1979).

More recently, these insights about the role of disease and environmental factors in patterns of human settlement, development, and conquest have been elaborated in the popular works of Jared Diamond who begins his 1997 book *Guns, Germs and Steel* by asking: 'Why did history unfold differently on different continents?' In addressing this question about the unequal distribution of power, Diamond traces cause and effect to bio-geographical influences. Above all, geographical factors explain the irregular spread of food production and technology – and also, crucially, the evolution of germs.[23] These global histories have thus stressed the significance of infectious disease in the shaping of human societies and cultures. While emphasizing the dynamic and decisive role of the environment in social change, they have accentuated the need to view the past from outside the narrow confines of 'national' history in relation to interregional and transcontinental connections. This is an increasingly important theme in the work of contemporary environmental historians who are concerned with studying the geopolitical importance of disease and examining the extent to which diseases (and immunity to diseases) have tipped the balance of power.[24]

The 'guns, germs, and steel' explanation for European ascendancy has been challenged by some historians who argue that it over-simplifies the multiple and complex contributory causes of change in the past.[25] There are problems, too, with deploying the 'global' as a category for thinking through disease history. Although a long-term approach to the past may avoid the pitfalls of over-specialization, the big view has evident shortcomings, too. In extrapolating epidemics within a macro-framework, historians may lose sight of the specificity of a given place or event. The global may become a way of flattening differences, even while purporting to extend the scope of history from a narrow Eurocentric view to accommodate other places and peoples.[26] Although this book draws connections between places, it also seeks to focus on the differences between them. The aim is to explore the interrelationship between peoples and places across Asia, at the same time as offering an implicit pushback to the universalist claims of global history. As the historian David Ludden has observed, area studies may provide 'a necessary counterweight to the

---

[23] Jared Diamond, *Guns, Germs and Steel: A Short History of Everybody for the Last 13,000 Years.* Revised edition (London: Vintage, 2005), pp.9, 16, 195–214.

[24] J. R. McNeill, *Mosquito Empires: Ecology and War in the Greater Caribbean, 1620–1914* (Cambridge: Cambridge University Press, 2010).

[25] George Raudzens, ed., *Technology, Disease, and Colonial Conquests, Sixteenth to Eighteenth Centuries: Essays Reappraising the Guns and Germs Theories* (Leiden: Brill, 2001).

[26] Sarah Hodges, 'The Global Menace,' *Social History of Medicine*, vol.25, no.3 (2012): 719–728 (725).

decontextualizing force of universal globalism.'[27] Even though global theorists may critique the assumptions within area studies of a world apportioned into distinct culture–language spaces, there is often a presumption in global approaches that globalization entails the erasure of borders and an ineluctable homogenization of cultures.[28] In this book, I argue that studying epidemic histories may provide a way of reflecting on how highly local circumstances interact with global processes.

Anthropological and ethnographic perspectives, in tandem with history, can be helpful in moving beyond a token acknowledgment of context to an engagement with the variables that shape a given community's experience of disease. In recent years, scholars have argued that historical developments in Asia should be reconsidered within their own historical settings and trajectories, and not measured against the putative yardstick of Western progress. Thus, Tony Day has questioned reductive accounts of Southeast Asia that pit the traditional past against the postcolonial present, arguing instead that state formation in the region should be understood as a dynamic and ongoing process. 'Southeast Asian history from early times to the present,' he suggests, might be conceived 'as an overlapping series of localizing, transcultural processes, differentially distributed over the whole region and occurring over many centuries at different rates in different places.' The emphasis, here, is on the 'incongruity' of particular regions: in other words, different places have their own distinct and 'incongruent' histories.[29]

This notion of incongruity may be extended to experiences of sickness and healing. Medical anthropologists and historians have argued that different communities in different places experience and understand the body in different ways. In this sense, the body is not a universal, but is embedded in a dynamic milieu of cultural practices that have their own histories. The historian Shigehisa Kuriyama expresses this idea eloquently when he writes: 'The true structure and workings of the human body are, we casually assume, everywhere the same, a universal reality. But then we look into history, and our sense of reality wavers ... accounts of the body in diverse medical traditions frequently appear to describe mutually alien, almost unrelated worlds.'[30] In gauging the differences

[27] David Ludden, 'Why Area Studies?' In: Ali Mirsepassi, Amrita Basu, and Frederick Weaver, eds., *Localizing Knowledge in a Globalizing World: Recasting the Area Studies Debate* (Syracuse, NY: Syracuse University Press, 2003), pp.131–136 (136).

[28] Pheng Cheah, 'Universal Areas: Asian Studies in a World in Motion,' *Traces*, vol.1, no.1 (2001): 37–70.

[29] Tony Day, *Fluid Iron: State Formation in Southeast Asia* (Honolulu: University of Hawaii Press, 2002), p.32.

[30] Shigehisa Kuriyama, *The Expressiveness of the Body and the Divergence of Greek and Chinese Medicine* (New York: Zone Books, 1999), p.8.

between classical Greek and Chinese medicine, Kuriyama discloses the connections between how bodily processes are experienced and understood, and how notions of personhood are conceived. The differences between Western and Eastern medicine do not simply stem from divergent beliefs, but on a deeper level reflect alternative ways of being in the world. Similarly, anthropologists have shown how modern biomedicine, which assumes a uniformity and neutrality, is itself highly mediated and enmeshed in multiple social and political contexts.[31] Such work provides a persuasive rebuttal both to macro views of the human past, as well as to insistent presentist approaches that contrast contemporary technologies and knowledge to the false and oftentimes delusional claims in history.

What is an epidemic?

This book is entitled *Epidemics in Modern Asia*, but what precisely *is* an epidemic? Today the term 'epidemic' is used widely in the media, often in a non-medical and metaphorical sense to designate the sudden increase of a harmful activity, behavior, or condition. News reports, for example, proclaim 'epidemics' of crime, drug use, and obesity. Etymologically, the term 'epidemic' derives from the Greek *epi* (upon or close to) and *demos* (people) and from at least the beginning of the seventeenth century has been used in English to denote the incidence of a disease in relation to time, space, and persons afflicted. 'Epidemiology' is the investigation of the patterns, causes, and effects of health and disease conditions. According to the *Oxford English Dictionary*, an epidemic is a 'disease prevalent among a people or community at a special time, and produced by some special causes generally not present in the affected locality.' Another broad and influential epidemiological definition of epidemic stresses the notion of expectancy:

The occurrence in a community or region of cases of an illness (or an outbreak) clearly in excess of expectancy. The number of cases indicating presence of an epidemic will vary according to the infectious agent, size and type of population exposed, previous experience or lack of exposure to the diseases, and time and place of occurrence; epidemicity is thus relative to usual frequency of disease in the same area, among the specified population, at the same season of the year.[32]

An epidemic is defined against a variable benchmark of normalcy, even though it may be difficult to retrospectively ascertain a community's

---

[31] Margaret Lock and Vinh-Kim Nguyen, *An Anthropology of Biomedicine: An Introduction* (Chichester and Malden, MA: Wiley-Blackwell, 2010).
[32] Abram S. Benenson, ed., *Control of Communicable Diseases Manual*. Sixteenth edition (Washington, DC: American Public Health Association, 1995), p.535.

expectancy. Given the paucity of data about many diseases in the past, how is it possible to infer with any certainty what the 'usual frequency' of disease occurrence may have been? History and the present exist in a reinforcing loop. While attitudes to epidemics in the present are shaped by past experiences, the interpretations of past disease events are inevitably informed by current concerns. The past and present are in effect read through each other in ways that often pass unnoticed.

Epidemics, understood as the increased incidences of acute infectious diseases, are frequently imagined as exogenous events that act upon the routine functioning of society. However, as we shall see in the course of this book, the distinction between 'endemic' and 'epidemic' disease is often difficult to draw and is largely determined by socio-political factors. As the historian of medicine Roger Cooter has noted, 'what has been perceived as "endemic" in one place has often been seen as "epidemic" in another (or seen as epidemic in the *same* geographical context depending on the political interests of those doing the defining). What determined an "epidemic" in colonial India among the colonizing power, for instance, could be entirely different from what constituted an "epidemic" among the indigenous population.' In summary, Cooter argues that '"epidemics" can be both pathogenically and socio-politically relative.'[33] Moreover, when a disease episode is labeled an epidemic by state and public health authorities, it is given fixed parameters. The emphasis is placed on the numbers of those infected, rather than on the experiences of those who suffer: 'The authoritative and seemingly neutral statistical language of *counting*, so fundamental to the definition of "epidemic," often overwhelms *accounts* of direct and indirect human encounters with epidemics, which are essential elements in much historical and contemporary anthropological research.'[34]

Epidemic or pandemic?

The term 'pandemic' derives from the Greek words *pan* (all) and *demos* (people). There is often confusion about the meaning of 'pandemic' and its use by the media, health agencies, and scientists. This was particularly evident during the H1N1 influenza outbreak

---

[33] Roger Cooter, 'Of War and Epidemics: Unnatural Couplings, Problematic Conceptions,' *Social History of Medicine*, vol.16, no.2 (2003): 283–302 (287–288).

[34] D. Ann Herring and Alan C. Swedlund, 'Plagues and Epidemics in Anthropological Perspective.' In: D. Ann Herring and Alan C. Swedlund, eds., *Plagues and Epidemics: Infected Spaces Past and Present* (Oxford: Berg, 2010), pp.1–19 (4).

('swine flu') in 2009, which the WHO categorized as a phase 6 pandemic. Did the designation 'pandemic' refer to the pathogen's novelty, rapid transmission, geographical distribution, or severity? Historically, the terms 'epidemic' and 'pandemic' have been employed interchangeably and in popular usage have come to refer to 'large-scale occurrences' of infectious and chronic diseases. In this book, pandemic is used to denote the extension of epidemics across borders and often globally. However, the shifting meaning of the term pandemic and the ambiguity about what constitutes 'pandemicity' remind us of the extent to which biomedical and public health terminology remains imprecise and uncodified, reflecting accumulated historical assumptions about disease.

David M. Morens, Gregory K. Folkers, and Anthony S. Fauci, 'What Is a Pandemic?' *Journal of Infectious Diseases*, vol.200, no.7 (2009): 1018–1021 (1019).

Definitions of 'infectious disease' (synonymous with the term 'communicable disease') are also problematic. According to one characterization, an infectious disease is 'an illness due to a specific infectious agent or its toxic products that arises through transmission of such agents or products from an infected person, animal, or reservoir to a susceptible host, either directly or indirectly.'[35] There are a number of issues with this description. For one, distinctions between infection and disease are not always clear-cut or immutable. Scientific consensus about what constitutes an infectious disease may change over time, as a result of innovative diagnostic technologies or breakthroughs that demonstrate a causal relation between a disease hitherto deemed to be chronic and an infectious agent. Beriberi, a disease that was widespread in East Asia and causes paralysis and cardiac and respiratory disorders, was classified as an infectious disease until the Dutch physician Christiaan Eijkman (1858–1930) discovered that the disease was caused by a nutritional deficit in vitamin B1 (thiamine), resulting from consuming de-husked rice.

In fact, the history of beriberi in Japan provides a good example of the socio-political issues at stake in the definition of disease. Known as *kakkebyō* in Japanese, beriberi was a major scourge that undermined the modernizing drive of the Meiji state (1868–1912). Historically, Japanese doctors had considered beriberi an affliction induced by environmental factors, including damp, low-lying ground. There had also been a long

---

[35] Miquel Porta, ed., *A Dictionary of Epidemiology*. Sixth edition (Oxford: Oxford University Press, 2014), p.51.

tradition linking the disease to diet and prescribing barley as an effec-
tual remedy. However, as a 'bacterio-mania' swept through science in the
latter half of the nineteenth century with the ascendancy of bacteriology, the emphasis shifted to identifying a 'germ' as the causal agent of
beriberi.[36] Having invested in a germ-approach to the disease, state officials were reluctant to accept that beriberi might have a different cause,
even with mounting evidence that diet was implicated. The military continued to push for the imposition of sanitary measures to prevent 'contagion.' When doctors did grudgingly concede the link between beriberi
and nutrition, they disguised their volte-face on the germ theory by continuing to pursue laboratory research on the disease's etiology, as if it
was still contentious. The case of beriberi in Japan illustrates how political contexts shape the production of scientific knowledge about disease,
as well as the institutional dynamics that determine policy.[37]

Infectious history: Biology and disease

Research has shown that many chronic diseases, hitherto presumed
to be non-communicable, have infectious origins. The discovery
by Barry Marshall and Robin Warren of the role of the bacterium
Helicobacter pylori in peptic ulcer disease in the 1980s is an example of a disease, once considered non-communicable, that has been
reclassified as an infection. Bacteriology developed from the 1860s,
when it was understood that specific micro-organisms caused specific diseases. Until the 1940s, however, bacteriology was taught as
a subspecialty of medicine and was largely divorced from biology.
Today, developments in molecular genetics have changed how bacteria and other microorganisms are understood. Of the trillions of
cells in the human body, the majority are microbial cells. The role
of this teeming microbial ecology, called the 'microbiome,' was not
fully appreciated until the 1990s, but is now recognized as being
important to human health, playing a key role in the body's physi-
ological processes, such as digestion and immune response.

Joshua Lederberg, 'Infectious History,' *Science*, vol.288, no.5464
(April 14, 2000): 287–293.

---

[36] Edward T. Tibbits, *Medical Fashions in the Nineteenth Century* (London: H. K. Lewis,
1884), pp.54, 38–40.
[37] Alexander R. Bay, *Beriberi in Modern Japan: The Making of a National Disease* (Rochester,
NY: University of Rochester Press, 2012).

How infectious diseases have been understood within biomedicine has also changed over time. Many of the terms and conceptual models used routinely in the epidemiology of infectious disease were not fixed until the late nineteenth and early twentieth centuries. Older, pre-bacteriological meanings were not dispelled, but were overlaid with new ones. Terms such as 'contagion,' 'infection,' and 'immunity' have long histories that predate modern biomedicine. Before the late nineteenth century, for example, 'fever' was an expansive concept that accommodated a welter of undifferentiated conditions. With developments in bacteriology, parasitology, and pathology, 'fever' was progressively disassembled. Disease entities such as malaria and typhus were identified as distinct 'fevers.' In the twentieth century, a further shift occurred as fever came to designate a symptom – an increase in the body's temperature above the norm measured by a thermometer – which indicates an illness. Today, fever is recognized as a crucial part of the body's defense against infection. Tracking the changing meanings of 'fever' demonstrates the complex ways in which past constructions of disease get reconfigured and how, even though former meanings are displaced by advancements in science and medicine, they are never wholly expunged.[38]

While the emphasis in the late nineteenth century on identifying specific disease agents as the causes of specific diseases prompted a move away from earlier approaches, which had emphasized the role of the environment, increasingly the environment is being reintroduced in contemporary medicine and public health, where it is understood to be a key determinant of many infectious diseases. One of the first authoritative reports on emerging infections, published in 1992 under the auspices of the US Academy of Medicine, ascribed disease emergence to economic development and land use, the impact of human interventions on natural and social environments, and the ensuing 'ecological damage' that resulted (Chapter 5).[39] Persistent anxieties about environmental illness suggest the extent to which humans, despite far-ranging technological advances over the last century, remain inescapably part of nature.[40] Although the pathogenesis of many autoimmune diseases is not fully understood, today it is thought that the process may be triggered through a complex interplay between genetics, environmental variables,

---

[38] Christopher Hamlin, *More Than Hot: A Short History of Fever* (Baltimore, MD: Johns Hopkins University Press, 2014), p.4.

[39] 'Executive Summary.' In: Joshua Lederberg, Robert E. Shope, and Stanley C. Oaks, eds., *Emerging Infections: Microbial Threats to Health in the United States* (Washington, DC: National Academy Press, 1992), pp.1–15 (4, 7).

[40] Linda Nash, *Inescapable Ecologies: A History of Environment, Disease, and Knowledge* (Berkeley: University of California Press, 2006).

and infection.[41] The fast growing field of epigenetics, which has developed from the 1990s, studies the role of external factors in determining gene activity, including the cellular processes responsible for disease.

Historians have long debated how we should define disease. A disease may be defined as a collection of physical symptoms experienced as a condition. AIDS and SARS, which are both labeled 'syndromes' (from the Greek word for 'concurrence'), were described as medical conditions before their etiological agents were identified. The English term 'disease' literally means 'dis-ease' or that which is not at ease. Yet although diseases are biological phenomena, they are also invested with cultural values and embedded in social systems. As Rosenberg has remarked: 'In some ways disease does not exist until we have agreed that it does, by perceiving, naming, and responding to it.'[42]

Translating disease

The social, cultural, and political dimensions of disease are perhaps best discernible when different cultures, with distinct practices and beliefs about disease, come into contact. In British India, colonial and indigenous responses to infections, such as smallpox and bubonic plague, revealed the 'continuing and shifting relationship between two different, often antagonistic value-systems.' Western medicine, which could function as a means of social control and serve to legitimate colonial rule, frequently ran up against Indian traditions of healing.[43] It was through this often adversarial encounter with 'scientific medicine' that 'indigenous medicine' was refashioned as an alternative system. Despite claims made about its roots in ancient Indian civilization, it has been argued that Ayurveda was in fact largely re-imagined as a coherent and singular health system from the 1890s, when it came to be integrated into an Indian national movement that opposed British rule.[44]

Recent research has suggested the extent to which the institutions and practices of health in Southeast Asia should be understood in terms of the interaction of local medical traditions with government priorities and

[41] Warwick Anderson and Ian R. Mackay, *Intolerant Bodies: A Short History of Autoimmunity* (Baltimore, MD: Johns Hopkins University Press, 2014), p.143.

[42] Charles E. Rosenberg, 'Framing Disease: Illness, Society, and History.' In: *Explaining Epidemics*, pp.305–318 (305).

[43] David Arnold, 'Cholera and Colonialism in British India,' *Past & Present*, vol.113 (1986): 118–151 (119).

[44] David Hardiman, 'Indian Medical Indigeneity: From Nationalist Assertion to the Global Market,' *Social History*, vol.34, no.3 (2009): 263–283.

international interests.[45] In Cambodia, a French protectorate from 1863 that was later incorporated into French Indochina (1887), colonial health services were compelled to negotiate a multiplicity of Khmer, Cham, and Vietnamese healing traditions. Western biomedicine was not systematically expanded across the country. Instead, French efforts to modernize were frustrated by differences – 'cultural insolubilities' – that challenged the colonial state's authority.[46] As we shall see in Chapter 1, discrepant ideas about disease and health were foregrounded during the plague epidemics in southern China in 1894. While there were differences between Chinese and Western understandings about the disease and how it should be managed, a plurality of beliefs and practices also became apparent within Chinese and Western communities themselves. The plague outbreaks in Canton (today's Guangzhou) and British Hong Kong exposed the complex interactions between the Chinese and the British, state and non-state actors, which led to misunderstandings, often fraught negotiations, and sometimes violent confrontations. Similarly, in Japan well into the twentieth century, modern biomedical conceptions of tuberculosis (TB) interacted with popular interpretations of the disease. In his history of TB in Japan, William Johnston re-examines the circumstances surrounding the Tsuyama massacre in May 1938, when 30 people were killed in the hamlet of Kaio in rural Okayama. The perpetrator of this spree-killing was a young man named Toi Mutsuo who had contracted TB. 'I am dying,' Toi Mutsuo stated in the first of three suicide notes written days before the crime, 'to get revenge on my neighbors for the oppressive hard-heartedness they have towards someone with a disease they believe is incurable.' The Tsuyama massacre draws attention to the gulf that existed in 1930s Japan between persistent cultural attitudes to TB and modern institutions of science and medicine. It reminds us, too, of the violence that may erupt when different ways of understanding disease collide.[47]

While epidemics are biological events, different verbal constructs of a disease reflect the particular perceptions of a given culture. How we name a disease influences how that disease is experienced. Our understanding of risk, too, is dependent on language and styles of communication. Descriptors such as 'contagion' or 'plague' coupled with scientific terminology, such as H5N1 (a strain of type A influenza discussed more

---

[45] Laurence Monnais and Harold J. Cook, eds., *Global Movements, Local Concerns: Medicine and Health in Southeast Asia* (Singapore: NUS Press, 2012).

[46] Sokhieng Au, *Mixed Medicines: Health and Culture in French Colonial Cambodia* (Chicago, IL: University of Chicago Press, 2011), pp.181–191.

[47] William Johnston, *The Modern Epidemic: A History of Tuberculosis in Japan* (Cambridge, MA: Harvard University Press, 1995), pp.109–116 (111).

fully in Chapter 5), convey threats that are at once old and new, familiar but also disturbingly unknown. The challenge of identifying recognized contemporary diseases in the past is compounded by the varying meanings ascribed to specific terms across different cultures. In China, the classical term *huoluan* ('sudden turmoil') was used by writers in the nineteenth century to describe clinical cases characterized by sudden and profuse vomiting and diarrhea. These are symptoms of modern cholera, but they are also symptoms of many other diarrhoeal diseases.[48] Reading back from recent history into the more distant past thus becomes problematic. With what certainty can *huoluan* be conclusively identified as biomedical cholera?

Historians are increasingly challenging diffusionist models of medicine that view modernity in terms of the more or less seamless expansion of Western knowledge and practices across the world in the wake of colonization. Instead, they are exploring the reciprocal processes of translation, mistranslation, and adaptation involved. Rather than viewing Chinese medicine in the twentieth century as the remnant of a pre-modern past, for example, it may be more useful to consider its co-evolution with Western medicine and the modern state. Modern Chinese medicine was produced through a process of cross-fertilization of the old and the new: Chinese medicine was 'neither donkey nor horse,' its mongrel status reflecting modernity's assimilation of the traditional.[49] Western medicine, which was introduced to China by missionaries, was adapted to meet local expectations. Reciprocally, traditional Chinese medicine (TCM) was reconstituted as a modern scientific practice by assimilating Western therapeutic technologies. During the Republican period (1912–1949), for example, reformist Chinese practitioners of acupuncture grafted Western anatomical knowledge onto a traditional Chinese physiology. 'Acupuncture, the icon of Chinese medicine to the twenty-first-century mind,' writes Bridie Andrews, 'is a relatively recent development, at least in the manner it is practised today.'[50]

The translation of health and disease terms into Chinese and Japanese during the late nineteenth and early twentieth centuries also suggests how indigenous terminology was never fully displaced but was implanted into imported categories. The physician Nagayo Sensai (1838–1902) – who had been a member of the Iwakura diplomatic mission to Europe and

[48] Marta E. Hanson, *Speaking of Epidemics in Chinese Medicine: Disease and the Geographic Imagination in Late Imperial China* (Abingdon and New York: Routledge, 2011), p.136.
[49] Sean Hsiang-lin Lei, *Neither Donkey nor Horse: Medicine in the Struggle Over China's Modernity* (Chicago, IL: University of Chicago Press, 2014), pp.15–19.
[50] Bridie Andrews, *The Making of Modern Chinese Medicine, 1850–1960* (Vancouver: UBC Press, 2014), p.197.

the United States between 1871 and 1873 – was struck on his travels by how Western countries were developing comprehensive modern sanitary systems to 'encompass all facets of life.' As the first director of the Sanitary Bureau in 1875, Nagayo was instrumental in promoting Western medicine in Meiji Japan. Indeed, it was he who coined the word for 'hygiene' in Japanese, deliberating in his memoirs on the challenges of translation:

> When writing the draft of the National Medical Code [in 1875], I considered using words that were direct translations from original [Western] words – like *kenkô* [for 'health'] or *hoken* [for 'hygiene']. But these words seemed too blunt and plain, and so I tried to think of other more appropriate terms. Then I recalled the word *eisei* [*weisheng*] from the 'Kosôso hen' [*Gengsang Chu pian*] of Sôshi [*Zhuangzi*]. Of course the meaning of this term in the original text was slightly different [from Western concepts], but the characters appeared elegant and sounded tasteful, and so I chose them to signify the government administration of health protection.[51]

Translation has been crucial to the ways in which diseases have been culturally constructed. In the passage above, Nagayo reveals the importance he attaches to fluency and aesthetics (the elegance of characters) as translation strategies. He reminds us that while translation often purports to transcend linguistic and cultural differences, these differences are in fact re-inscribed in the very process of searching for equivalences. As we shall see in our discussion of cholera in Chapter 1, this is particularly evident in a Japanese context. Practices of translation were central to the formation of the Japanese language, national identity, and social life. While the term 'modern' is often used to label 'Western' aspects of Japanese culture, the Japanese script itself is a complex mediation of Chinese written culture. Rather than thinking of translation as the transference of meaning from a 'source' culture to a 'target' culture, we might re-conceptualize translation as a process of appropriation, where distinctions between 'foreign' and 'native' become blurred. Tracking the translation of disease names between cultures makes visible the complexities of intercultural relations, while revealing the critical stress points – the 'linguistic ligatures' – between past and present, national and supranational, local and global.[52] We are dealing, here, with 'words in motion': with the processes

---

[51] Ruth Rogaski, *Hygienic Modernity: Meanings of Health and Disease in Treaty-Port China* (Berkeley: University of California Press, 2004), p.136; Johnston, *The Modern Epidemic*, p.179.

[52] Indra Levy, 'Introduction: Modern Japan and the Trialectics of Translation.' In: Indra Levy, ed., *Translation in Modern Japan* (Abingdon and New York: Routledge, 2011), pp.1–12 (1, 4, 6).

through which meanings get transferred, and the practical effects that this transference has in the world.[53]

At the same time – and precisely because they embody cultural values – diseases are not all equal: that is to say, some diseases acquire greater prominence than others. In many societies, cholera is more feared than TB, despite the fact that TB 'remains one of the world's deadliest communicable diseases' and was responsible for 1.5 million deaths in 2013 alone.[54] And while TB may have been romanticized in the West, gastrointestinal diseases, such as dysentery, remain far less visible, even though they have been and remain a major cause of mortality. Leprosy, a bacterial disease with low infectivity, has historically provoked anxieties far exceeding the real risks it poses. Although the 1918 influenza killed approximately as many people as the plague in India, it did not elicit the same degree of panic and protest. The impact of a disease rests not simply upon the number of those it afflicts, or on its economic consequences, but also on the assumptions that the disease embodies, and on the symbolic meanings it is invested with by different communities.

Given that our understanding of disease has changed over time and that across different cultures diseases have been defined in very different ways, how can we be certain about the identity of a given disease in the past? Is it valid to retrospectively diagnose diseases in history by bestowing upon them an identity furnished by modern biology? Can we apply present-day diagnostic criteria to the seventeenth-century European 'pox' and define it as syphilis, a disease now known to be caused by a sexually transmitted bacterial infection? Was the medieval Black Death bubonic plague, another disease caused by a bacterium that was discovered in the late nineteenth century? 'Historians and scientists have taken the epidemiology of the modern plague and imposed it on the past,' writes Samuel Cohn, 'ignoring, denying and even changing contemporary testimony, both narrative and quantitative, when it conflicts with notions of how modern bubonic plague should behave.'[55]

Contemporary biotechnologies, such as genomics, are making it possible to identify the biological characteristics of past diseases. The polymerase chain reaction (PCR) process developed in the mid 1980s has enabled scientists to amplify degraded viral DNA extracted from human tissue. It has been possible, for example, to reconstruct the genome of *Yersinia pestis*, the bacterium responsible for plague, by analyzing genetic

---

[53] Carol Gluck and Anna Lowenhaupt Tsing, eds., *Words in Motion: Toward a Global Lexicon* (Durham, NC: Duke University Press, 2009).

[54] Annabel Baddeley, et al., *Global Tuberculosis Report* (Geneva: World Health Organization, 2014), pp.xi, 20.

[55] Samuel Cohn Jr., *The Black Death Transformed: Disease and Culture in Early Renaissance Europe* (Cambridge: Cambridge University Press, 2002), p.2.

material recovered in a fourteenth-century plague pit.[56] However, a tendency persists to read back from the present, making assumptions about how people in the past experienced and understood disease. While recognizing the materiality of disease, this book stresses its historicity and the importance of situating disease in time and place. It argues that disease should 'be understood in context, as a time- and place-specific aggregate of behaviors, practices, ideas, and experiences.'[57]

Epidemics and analogies

Epidemics and pandemics are often compared and contrasted. For example, during the H1N1 swine flu pandemic in 2009, the experience of the 1918–1919 influenza pandemic was often cited. We should be cautious of such analogies, however, and question the basis of the similarities and differences they emphasize. The 1976 influenza epidemic in the United States provides a salutary example of how analogies may promote what the political scientists Richard Neustadt and Ernest May called 'unreasoning.' In January 1976, several US Army recruits at Fort Dix in New Jersey contracted influenza, one of whom subsequently died. The strain of the virus, which caused severe respiratory illness, was thought to be similar to that of the 1918–1919 pandemic, in which over 650,000 Americans died. Panic ensued as the US government anticipated that thousands might die unless there was a robust response. President Gerald Ford rushed a vaccine to market. In the event, only one person died of influenza, while 25 people died from adverse reactions to the vaccine and more than 500 people are believed to have developed Guillain–Barré syndrome (GBS), a condition caused by immunological damage to the nervous system triggered by an infection. The 1976 episode serves as a reminder of the human cost that may result when 'bad' analogies form the basis of policy. Anticipating pandemic threats by drawing on models from the past may constrain thinking, making it more difficult to develop new practices and protocols to meet present and future threats.

Richard E. Neustadt and Ernest R. May, *Thinking in Time: The Uses of History for Decision Makers* (New York: The Free Press, 1986), pp.34–57.

---

[56] Ewen Callaway, 'Plague Genome: The Black Death Decoded,' *Nature*, vol.478, no.7370 (October 27, 2011): 444–446.
[57] Charles E. Rosenberg, 'What is Disease? In Memory of Oswei Temkin,' *Bulletin of the History of Medicine*, vol.77, no.3 (2003): 491–505 (494).

History as crisis

At issue is how we understand 'disease' and, relatedly, how we measure the impact of epidemics on human societies. Is mortality the principal indicator of the significance of an epidemic? Or should the burden of disease be calculated in terms of morbidity? Although quantitative methods and data on mortality and morbidity are obviously crucial, numbers alone may be misleading. While epidemics may produce demographic shocks, inducing fear and panic, they may also have longer-term consequences that are more difficult to assess.

Epidemics often cause compounded crises: traumatic events in which social, economic, and political concerns become entangled. A spike in morbidity and mortality will stretch health systems and impact economic and political systems. Epidemics may produce famines, trigger social unrest, and pose a direct challenge to authority. Or, as in the case of the 1918 influenza pandemic in India (Chapter 5), famines may precipitate or amplify disease events. In mid nineteenth-century Europe, it has been argued that different responses by different social groups to the cholera epidemics revealed latent social tensions, contributing to revolution – although others have taken an opposing view.[58] In the United States, epidemics of diphtheria and TB incited little concern in the nineteenth century, despite their high mortality. In contrast, Asiatic cholera and yellow fever provoked widespread panic. 'Since most societies tend to operate on a crisis basis,' John Duffy has observed, 'the diseases which were most effective in precipitating social change were those with the greatest shock value.'[59]

Calling a disease outbreak an 'epidemic' conveys urgency and 'mobilizes social action and consumer behavior.' It suggests an imminent threat and is likely to elicit a visceral response.[60] Epidemic crises may create the space for health agencies to extend their authority by exploiting this urgency. In the Philippines under US rule, epidemics – and in particular an epidemic of cholera between 1902 and 1904 – became an opportunity for the colonial state to consolidate and further its control over the local population (Chapter 4). State responses to emergency situations may have unforeseen consequences. The moral authority of a government

[58] Richard J. Evans, 'Epidemics and Revolutions: Cholera in Nineteenth-Century Europe,' *Past & Present*, vol.120 (1988): 123–146.
[59] John Duffy, 'Social Impact of Disease in the Late 19th Century.' In: Judith Walzer Leavitt and Ronald L. Numbers, eds., *Sickness and Health in America: Readings in the History of Medicine and Public Health* (Madison: University of Wisconsin Press, 1997), pp.418–425 (422).
[60] Charles E. Rosenberg, 'Siting Epidemic Disease: 3 Centuries of American History,' *Journal of Infectious Diseases*, vol.197 (2008): S4–S6 (S6).

may be undermined as a result of its handling of an epidemic. Similarly, the imposition of sanitary cordons and quarantines may have counter-vailing effects, arousing opposition and setting off violent protest. Colonial over-reactions to the plague pandemic in India during the late 1890s provoked other, unanticipated social and political crises. In this case, draconian sanitary interventions helped to aggravate smoldering resentments and fanned the flames of an anti-colonial, nationalist movement (Chapter 2).

Is there a danger of focusing disproportionately on epidemic crises simply because they are more conspicuous in the sources than less spectacular but equally debilitating diseases?[61] Do histories of epidemics perpetuate the view of disease as anomalous and exceptional? These are legitimate concerns since more people succumbed to the 'normal' flu than died from, say, an emerging infection such as SARS, even though coverage of SARS in 2003 far exceeded the reporting of seasonal flu. Besides, what precisely do we mean by crisis? In its most general sense, a crisis refers to a critical moment: a make-or-break event. The word's origin is in fact medical, signifying a sudden change or a turning point in a disease. Describing a situation as a 'crisis' determines how it is viewed, investing the situation with heightened significance and prompting a more intense response. In this way, crises may open up possibilities for certain individuals, groups, or institutions. For example, journalists may find it easier to place stories about an epidemic rather than a routine disease; funding for basic microbiological research may be more readily obtainable in the face of an outbreak; and politicians may use the shock of a crisis to push through unpopular policies.

Crises have often served as justifications for state interventions, and they have played a critical role in shaping modern political institutions: in the re-planning of cities, as a rationale for sanitary measures and infra-structural reform, and as an impetus for new legislation. Analyzing how certain events come to be viewed as crises may also shed light on the way that notions of normalcy are constructed; indeed, both notions – normalcy and crisis – are interdependent, the one evoked in defining the other. They are also contingent terms, since a crisis for some may be normalcy for others.[62] In the aftermath of the 1817 cholera epidemics in India, some colonial commentators spoke of devastation, while others saw nothing exceptional. Thus, R. H. Kennedy, a medical officer in the Bombay Presidency, did not perceive any 'peculiar malignity' and noted

[61] Norman G. Owen, 'Toward a History of Health in Southeast Asia.' In: Norman Owen, ed., *Death and Disease in Southeast Asia: Explorations in Social, Medical and Demographic History* (Singapore: Oxford University Press, 1987), pp.3–30 (6–7).

[62] Janet Roitman, *Anti-Crisis* (Durham, NC: Duke University Press, 2014).

that the cholera epidemic did not present '[a] more distressing image of desolation to our view than what we are in the habit of beholding with philosophic calmness, and ranking among the ordinary casualties of Indian life.'[63]

Although there is certainly a risk that concentrating on crises may skew our understanding of history, studying moments of contestation may be useful if they reveal underlying processes, anxieties, and assumptions, which remain hidden in 'normal' times. In the 1960s, social historians argued that epidemics provided a window onto class structure and social attitudes, gender history and subaltern experience. Tracking shifting attitudes to epidemics of cholera across time could function as a way of disclosing cultural change. Successive outbreaks of cholera in the United States could provide 'a tool for social and economic analysis' and offer 'a natural sampling device for the social historian.'[64] In the words of the historian Roderick McGrew: 'An epidemic intensifies certain behavior patterns, but those patterns, instead of being aberrations, betray deeply rooted and continuing social imbalances.'[65] Others have argued, however, that this emphasis on the revelatory potential of crises may over-simplify the relation between epidemics and social movements.[66] Of course, the idea that epidemics offer a unique optic onto society is hardly new and was articulated by many sanitarians in the nineteenth century. Epidemics revealed to them the disconcerting squalor of the industrial slum, prompting the compilation of sanitary reports, which served to catalyze reform.

While recognizing the many issues that a crisis approach to history entails, in this book I argue that focusing on moments of situated disruption may help to demonstrate the ways that disease and health are contested on the ground.[67] The book offers a counter-argument to those global histories that stress transnational flows and tend to ignore situated agency. Crises may serve, in other words, as a counterpoint to de-territorialized global approaches, reminding us of the importance of difference, disconnection, and violence in the making of the modern world.

---

[63] Arnold, 'Cholera and Colonialism in British India,' p.122.

[64] Charles E. Rosenberg, 'Cholera in Nineteenth-Century Europe: A Tool for Social and Economic Analysis,' *Comparative Studies in Society and History*, vol.8, no.4 (1966): 452–463; *The Cholera Years: The United States in 1832, 1849, and 1866* (Chicago, IL: University of Chicago Press, 1962), p.4.

[65] R. E. McGrew, 'The First Cholera Epidemic and Social History,' *Bulletin of the History of Medicine*, vol.34 (1960): 61–73 (71).

[66] Hamlin, *Cholera*, pp.11–13.

[67] Warwick Anderson, 'Making Global Health History: The Postcolonial Worldliness of Biomedicine,' *Social History of Medicine*, vol.27, no.2 (2014): 372–384 (377–378).

Defining the 'modern'

The scope of this book extends roughly from 1800 to the present, a period of modernization in Asia. Modernization and modernity are particularly elusive terms to define. Historians have tended to characterize them in relation to rationalizing processes linked to the development of a capitalistic economic system, industrialization, wage labor, the institutions of the nation-state, and the rise of secularism. Defined in these terms, modernity is closely linked to the advent of the Western nation-state and its bureaucratic appurtenances, and to its global extension through the establishment of empire. As we shall see, much of Asia was carved up by European imperial powers from the late fifteenth century, when the Portuguese, Spanish, and Dutch founded colonies there. While the Dutch held Indonesia until 1942, the British dominated India and Malaya (today's Peninsular Malaysia), the French created the colonial federation of Indochina, the United States took over the Philippines from the Spanish at the end of the nineteenth century, and Japan controlled Taiwan from 1895 and then Korea from 1910 to 1945. Colonial states mobilized new technologies to rule the peoples of the lands they acquired. It has been claimed that these technological systems functioned as 'tools of empire.'[68]

There are problems with this interpretation of colonial modernity in Asia, since it assumes, a priori, that certain political formations, such as empire, are uniquely Western. However, as the historian John Darwin has suggested, empire might in fact be considered 'the default mode of state organization.'[69] Second, this approach over-emphasizes the transformative capacity and authority of state institutions and their agents. The colonial archives – bulging with statistical reports, government edicts, and dispatches – are misleading in this respect. While they may suggest colonial confidence and power, this impression belies the vulnerability and unease that many colonials felt surrounded by non-Europeans in an alien and often hostile environment. As Ann Laura Stoler has remarked in relation to the archives of the Dutch East Indies: 'Grids of intelligibility were fashioned from uncertain knowledge; disquiet and anxieties registered the uncommon sense of events and things; epistemic uncertainties repeatedly unsettled the imperial conceit that all was in order.'[70]

---

[68] Daniel R. Headrick, *The Tools of Empire: Technology and European Imperialism in the Nineteenth Century* (New York: Oxford University Press, 1981).

[69] John Darwin, *Unfinished Empire: The Global Expansion of Britain* (London: Allen and Lane, 2012), p.7.

[70] Ann Laura Stoler, *Along the Archival Grain: Epistemic Anxieties and Colonial Common Sense* (Princeton, NJ: Princeton University Press, 2009), p.1.

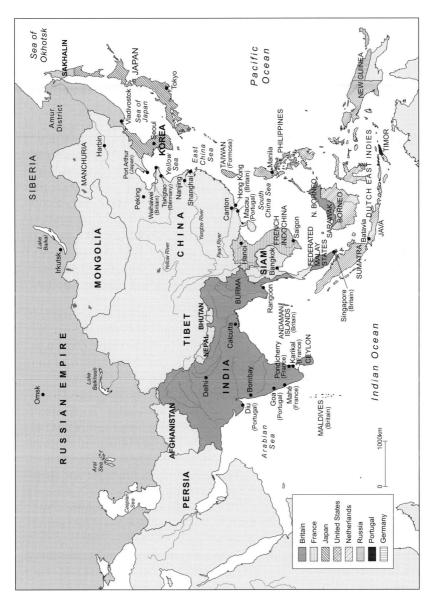

Map 0.2. Empires in Asia (1914)

Epidemics and colonial sovereignty

By the end of the nineteenth century, much of Asia had been divided up amongst Western powers. Map 0.2 shows different imperial possessions as greyscale blocks, with the discrete sovereignty of different colonial states demarcated by borders. Such cartographic representations, however, obscure the ambiguities that characterized many colonial jurisdictions. While much of upland Southeast Asia effectively eluded state control, elsewhere colonial states governed through complex arrangements with indigenous authorities. In India, for example, the British promoted paramountcy, a system whereby the rulers of princely states retained the right to manage their own affairs under British 'protection' (Chapter 4). Other zones, although lying outside the formal jurisdiction of the colonial state, remained imperial 'spheres of influence.' Examining epidemics in history can serve to highlight the unevenness of imperial sovereignty; the degree to which imperial formations 'are not securely bounded and are not firmly entrenched, neither regular nor well regulated.' Epidemics reveal territorial ambiguities and the porosity of borders, the limits of state power, and the importance of local identities.

Ann Laura Stoler, 'On Degrees of Imperial Sovereignty,' *Public Culture*, vol.18, no.1 (2006): 125–146 (135).

A related issue is the degree to which Western technologies and know-how displaced other practices and systems of knowledge. For example, we may dispute the claim that from the mid nineteenth century people became increasingly technologized, 'fitting into and effortlessly moving through new technological networks.'[71] Underlying such assertions of unobstructed mobility lie assumptions about the consistency and seamlessness of networks and their uniform distribution across vastly different terrains. Metropolitan projections of a technologically infused world were not descriptions of the world as it was, but rather blueprints for how the world ought to be.

Additionally, the extent to which colonial powers actually subjugated Asia is itself debatable. Although European empires may have laid claim to vast territories, 'the nature of such claims was tempered by control that

---

[71] Morris Low, 'Introduction.' In: Morris Low, ed., *Building a Modern Japan: Science, Technology, and Medicine in the Meiji Era and Beyond* (New York and Basingstoke: Palgrave Macmillan, 2005), pp.1–10 (1).

was exercised mainly over narrow bands, or corridors, and over enclaves and irregular zones around them.' As Lauren Benton has argued, European empires have tended to be understood in terms of bounded territorial sovereignty, and are typically pictured on maps as monochrome blocks, rather than as variegated, uneven spaces. 'Territorial control was, in many places, an incidental aim of imperial expansion,' she observes, 'politically fragmented; legally differentiated; and encased in irregular, porous, and sometimes undefined borders.'[72]

While indigenous populations are often viewed as a background for European actions, Europeans did not supplant the indigenous cultures they colonized. Southeast Asia's mountainous and forested inland terrain made much of it inaccessible to them. A fragmented coastline with innumerable islands posed further obstacles to state control. Much of Indonesia, which consists of over 17,000 islands spread out between the Indian Ocean and the Pacific Ocean – from Sumatra to New Guinea – did not fall under effective Dutch rule until the end of the nineteenth and the beginning of the twentieth centuries, and even then the colonial grip was weak. Similarly, swathes of British Burma (also known today as Myanmar) and Malaya remained all but nominally governed. Although the Spanish dominated the lowlands of the Philippines, they exerted little control over the rest of the land. The fragmented nature of the archipelago, consisting of over 7,000 islands stretching some 1,500 miles from the Sulu Islands towards Taiwan, as well as the inaccessibility of the highlands, militated against centralized governance. The impact of European colonization across Asia was thus decidedly uneven, and the reach of the colonial state's authority often restricted. Its rule was frequently overstretched and could easily taper off into non-existence. As the anthropologist James C. Scott has observed, viewing Asian history solely through the prism of the modern state leaves out vast tracts of Asia where communities successfully confounded the 'internal colonialism' of state-making.[73]

Yet, while conceding the limits of Western colonial control in Asia, it would be disingenuous to minimize the importance of Western domination. Contemporary state borders have been largely determined by imperial powers, as have the names of postcolonial nation-states. The 'Philippines,' named by Ruy López de Villalobos in 1543 after Philip, Prince of Asturias – who subsequently became King Philip II of Spain – encapsulates the country's colonial history, reflecting 'the partly Hispanic roots of

---

[72] Lauren Benton, *A Search for Sovereignty: Law and Geography in European Empires, 1400–1900* (Cambridge: Cambridge University Press, 2010), pp.1–39 (2).
[73] James C. Scott, *The Art of Not Being Governed: An Anarchist History of Upland Southeast Asia* (New Haven, CT: Yale University Press, 2009).

Filipino nationhood.'[74] Spanish rule may have been patchy and in many areas nominal, but it did nonetheless connect the scattered islands of the archipelago. Similarly, in other parts of Asia – as we shall see in our discussions of China and Japan later in this book – the extension of European power, particularly in the nineteenth century, was to have crucial political, economic, and social consequences for development.

By the same token, modern biomedicine and public health have been profoundly shaped by the colonial past. 'We need to recognize,' writes Warwick Anderson, 'that the basic language of Western medicine, with its claims to universalism and modernity, has always used, as it still does, the vocabulary of empire.'[75] The effects and often violent after-effects of colonialism are inevitably a major focus of this book, which explores the impact of colonialism on places and peoples across Asia, uncovering empire's ruins on the material environment, as well as its accumulated legacy on bodies and minds.[76] Rather than understanding modernity in Asia as the progressive and even diffusion of Western technologies across the region – technologies linked to state-making activities – the book considers modernity in relation to cross-cutting themes of mobility, urbanization, the environment, war, and globalization. The aim is not to underplay the significance of colonialism or to suggest that technologies did not fundamentally change societies. Instead, it is to suggest a more complex interplay between colonial and indigenous communities, as well as the varied ways in which technologies were produced and used.

Asia as method

So far we have explored definitions of 'epidemic' and 'modernity,' and we have identified some of the challenges that these terms pose for historians. Given this is a book about Asia, the question arises as to what precisely 'Asia' means. Although Asia may be understood as the eastern part of the continental Eurasian landmass, which extends from the Atlantic to the Pacific Oceans, it also includes numerous island chains, such as Indonesia, the Philippines, and Japan. There are problems with the division of the world into continents, as if continents were self-contained geological and cultural spaces. Continents (like nation-states) 'become reified

---

[74] Luis H. Francia, *A History of the Philippines: From Indios Bravos to Filipinos* (New York: The Overlook Press, [2010] 2014), pp.9–13 (11).

[75] Warwick Anderson, 'Where is the Postcolonial History of Medicine?' *Bulletin of the History of Medicine*, vol.72, no.3 (1998): 522–530 (529).

[76] Ann Laura Stoler, 'Introduction: "The Rot Remains": From Ruins to Ruination.' In: Ann Laura Stoler, ed., *Imperial Debris: On Ruins and Ruination* (Durham, NC: Duke University Press, 2013), pp.1–35.

as natural and fundamental building blocks of global geography, rather than being recognized as the constructed, contingent, and often imposed political–geographical units that they are.' The boundaries defining 'Asia' have shifted historically, as have the terms 'East' and 'Orient.' In this sense, Asia is a 'metageographical' construct that perpetuates a form of environmental determinism.[77]

Defined as the place that is not Europe, Asia reflects a fundamentally biased view of the world. As the Chinese literary scholar Wang Hui has argued, 'Asia' is in fact a European notion fashioned in the writings of Montesquieu, Adam Smith, Hegel, and Karl Marx where it functioned as an oppositional category crucial to the construction of Europe's own identity. Recycled into Chinese, Japanese, and other 'Asian' traditions, the term has now become fraught with contradictions. It is, writes Wang, 'at the same time colonialist and anti-colonialist, conservative and revolutionary, nationalist and internationalist, originating in Europe and shaping Europe's image of itself, closely related to visions of both nation-state and empire, a notion of non-European civilization, and a geographic category established through geopolitical relations.'[78]

Over the last 200 years, there has been debate in many 'Asian' countries about the meaning of 'Asia.' For example, in China and Japan, Asia has tended to be defined in opposition to Western imperialism and attempts by colonial powers to subjugate the non-Western world. An emphasis on the primacy of the nation-state has sat uneasily, here, beside a pan-Asian discourse that aims 'to create a radically politicized cultural regional concept.' At the beginning of the twentieth century, intellectuals in many Asian countries espoused a cosmopolitan vision, which celebrated cultural commonalities and diversities, and opposed imperialist and state-centric views of Asia.[79]

More recently, other definitions of sub-regions within Asia have been critiqued. The term 'Southeast Asia,' for example, does not describe an area that is geographically distinct, but rather connotes a territorial aggregate that gained currency from the mid twentieth century. 'Southeast Asia' is largely an external view, since Asians themselves have not historically defined themselves in such terms. The Chinese notion of *Nanyang* ('Southern Ocean') refers not so much to a discrete region as to the ethnic Chinese migrant communities in maritime Southeast Asia: Malaysia,

---

[77] Martin W. Lewis and Kären E. Wigen, *The Myth of Continents: A Critique of Metageography* (Berkeley: University of California Press, 1997), pp.8, 42.

[78] Wang Hui, 'The Politics of Imagining Asia: A Genealogical Analysis,' *Inter-Asia Cultural Studies*, vol.8 (2007): 1–33 (27).

[79] Rebecca E. Karl, 'China in the World at the Beginning of the Twentieth Century,' *American Historical Review*, vol.103, no.4 (1998): 1096–1118.

Singapore, the Philippines, Thailand, Indonesia, and Vietnam.[80] Indeed, the notion of Southeast Asia as a distinct geopolitical space gained credence largely as a result of the Pacific campaigns during the Second World War, and subsequently Cold War conflicts, notably in Vietnam and Cambodia. For the purposes of its operations, WHO divides Asia into the 'South-East Asia Region' extending from the Indian subcontinent through Burma to Indonesia, and the 'Western Pacific Region' that encompasses China, Japan, and Australasia. More recently, geopolitical and economic shifts have given rise to a new interest in the Pacific Rim as a region. Yet as an analytical unit, the Pacific Rim tends to exclude complexity and too often fails to recognize 'that the people who inhabit the lands fronting the Pacific are not equal participants in the activities that structure the region and in the discourse surrounding it.'[81]

Mapping the nation, imagining disease

The political scientist Benedict Anderson has argued that in the nineteenth and twentieth centuries, vernacular languages – disseminated through the printing press and promoted through state institutions of education – created a new spatio-temporal consciousness called the 'nation.' The historian Thongchai Winichakul has similarly argued that maps and mapping provided a powerful means of imagining the nation. In Siam (Thailand), indigenous sacral conceptions of space were eclipsed in the nineteenth century by a modern geography that emphasized boundaries, territorial sovereignty, and margins. According to Winichakul, mapping operated in conjunction with the military and 'both anticipated and executed what Siam should be.' If nineteenth-century mapping was central to the construction of national space, it also played a key role in shaping how epidemic diseases were imagined. It could be argued that both phenomena – nation and disease – have been intimately connected. As spatial events, epidemics made visible the sovereign territories they threatened, revealing the extent to which 'a map was a model for, rather than a model of, what it purported to represent.'

Thongchai Winichakul, *Siam Mapped: A History of the Geo-Body of a Nation* (Honolulu: University of Hawaii Press, 1994), pp.x, 15, 130.

---

[80] Donald K. Emmerson, 'Southeast Asia': What's in a Name?' *Journal of Southeast Asian Studies*, vol.15, no.1 (1984): 1–21.

[81] Ravi Palat, 'Reinscribing the Globe: Imaginative Geographies of the Pacific Rim,' *Bulletin of Concerned Asian Scholars*, vol.29, no.1 (1997): 61–69 (69).

'Asia' is hardly adequate as a unifying term to denote such a varied region that straddles an expansive continent and myriad islands. At the most, it can merely serve as an oppositional label to 'Europe.' What does Iran have in common with Thailand, China, or Japan? To suggest a parity between these countries involves agglomerating unlike categories and suppressing critical differences. Even within Asia, countries such as China are too diverse to make any simple categorization meaningful. On the one hand, emphasizing regional commonalities undermines the distinctiveness and specificity of particular societies and cultures, which are lumped together as 'Asian.' On the other hand, it serves to cut off those societies and cultures from a broader, global history. Conceptualizing 'East Asia' and achieving consensus over regional identity and history continues to pose challenges for 'East Asians' themselves, while the identification of East Asia with China has tended to reflect a Sinocentric viewpoint.[82]

In this book, Asia is understood, not as a clearly bounded region, but as a dynamic arena of interaction, characterized at once by diversity and by historic interconnections and continuities: from Pakistan, the Bay of Bengal, and the Andaman Sea in the West to the Sea of Japan and Siberia in the East.[83] The aim is to rethink Asia in relation to the experiences of communicable disease, rather than to posit a distinct geographical or political entity called 'Asia.' In this sense, following the Taiwanese cultural theorist Kuan-Hsing Chen, we might say that the term Asia functions as a 'method' for interrogating nationalist histories and challenging 'the old binary opposition between East and West, which erases Asia's rich multiplicity and heterogeneity.'[84] Accordingly, Asia might be regarded as a strategic device that is 'good to think with and think from, rather than a fixed, hegemonic geographical region or essential civilizational entity.'[85] As the editors of the volume *Asia Inside Out* observe: 'Instead of viewing regions, cultures, and peoples as physically bounded units occupying continents and polities, we need to focus on multilayered, interactive processes that embrace both land and sea routes and incorporate political dynamics of empires, nation-states, neoliberal

---

[82] Sun Ge, 'The Predicament of Compiling Textbooks on the History of East Asia.' In: Gotelind Müller, ed., *Designing History in East Asian Textbooks: Identity Politics and Transnational Aspirations* (London and New York: Routledge, 2011), pp.9–11.

[83] K. N. Chaudhuri, *Asia Before Europe: Economy and Civilisation of the Indian Ocean from the Rise of Islam to 1750* (Cambridge: Cambridge University Press, 1990), p.11.

[84] Kuan-Hsing Chen, *Asia as Method: Toward Deimperialization* (Durham, NC: Duke University Press, 2010), p.215.

[85] Warwick Anderson, 'Asia as Method in Science and Technology Studies,' *East Asian Science, Technology and Society*, vol.6 (2012): 445–451 (448).

markets, and postsocialist global engagements at relevant historical junctures.'[86]

Inevitably, the book reflects my own interests as a historian. The focus thus tends to be more on East Asia and China, than on South Asia. But the choice about what to include has also been determined by other practical considerations. While the secondary literature on India is vast and generally accessible, material about epidemics in East Asia is much less readily available. The aim of *Epidemics in Modern Asia* is consequently to bring a new focus on East Asia, while connecting this with research on South Asia, and presenting case studies of epidemic episodes that exemplify the major themes and issues under discussion.

Archives of disease

What sources can we draw on to study epidemics in history? The availability of data on epidemics varies greatly over time. Aside from written records, archaeology may yield information on the diseases of the past, while DNA sequencing technologies are increasingly important in demonstrating our genetic links to epidemics in the distant past, as well as in helping to corroborate the identity of pathogens from retrieved tissue samples.[87] Material culture may also be useful for studying epidemics in history: cemeteries, hospitals, laboratories, and quarantines may furnish insights into how diseases have been experienced, understood, and managed.

From the late nineteenth century, data on epidemic disease were increasingly systematized in countries such as the United States and Britain. Records were kept of so-called 'notifiable diseases' that were considered to pose particular risks to the population. In the context of Asia, epidemic crises are written about in numerous colonial sources: government reports, official correspondence, and public health treatises. The historian may draw, for example, on the colonial records of the British, French, Spanish, and Dutch in Southeast Asia, the Imperial Maritime Customs Service (IMCS) reports in China, and Japanese government and colonial archives. However, these archives give only a partial view of the past. The records may represent the viewpoints of those caught up

---

[86] Peter C. Perdue, Helen F. Siu, and Eric Tagliacozzo, 'Introduction: Structuring Moments in Asian Connections.' In: Eric Tagliacozzo, Helen F. Siu, and Peter C. Perdue, eds., *Asia Inside Out: Changing Times* (Cambridge, MA: Harvard University Press, 2015), pp.1–22 (6).

[87] Robert Peckham, 'Ghosts in the Body: Infections, Genes, and the Re-enchantment of Biology.' In: Olu Jenzen and Sally R. Munt, eds., *The Ashgate Research Companion to Paranormal Cultures* (Farnham and Burlington, VT: Ashgate, 2013), pp.95–106.

in moments of crises, who therefore lack a critical vantage. The information included in the records tends to be based on assumptions about the nature of the disease and its victims, reflecting preconceptions and prejudices. Material in national and colonial archives inevitably emphasizes the role of the state in producing knowledge about and formulating policy to manage infectious disease. As we have seen, however, epidemic disease is a transnational phenomenon that crosses borders.

The vast majority of this state-sponsored archival material was written by men and inevitably reflects a gender bias. There is thus a need to reconfigure Asian history in order to accommodate women's perspectives, and particularly rural women who have often been doubly excluded from political representation. The historian of modern China, Gail Hershatter, for example, has sought to retrieve this 'missing history' by giving voices to rural women who lived through the revolutionary decades of the 1950s and 1960s in the PRC, a period that saw radical land reform and collectivization (Chapter 3). In a series of interviews with elderly women from Shaanxi province, Hershatter underscores the importance of personal recollections – of memory, rather than an exclusive reliance on the recorded facts contained in state sources – for understanding the past and women's place in it.[88]

An interest in the history of disease in Southeast Asia is growing, as evidenced in college courses on the topic, news stories, films, and academic articles. Yet for all that, research remains disparate. Fragmentary evidence for disease in much of Southeast Asia has led to extrapolations and retrospective readings. Even in China there is a lack of reliable demographic data. While the Nationalist government made some attempt to retain records from 1928, military conflict and social turmoil (1927–1936, 1946–1950) severely disrupted government activities. The historian also needs to be cautious when dealing with what records do survive. A case in point is TB in Japan, where many patients refused to consult doctors who were known to diagnose the disease. An association with TB might lead to the families of those infected being ostracized. As a consequence, TB was intentionally misdiagnosed as catarrh or pneumonia, which were more culturally neutral. This has consequently led to the consistent underestimation of mortality from TB during the late nineteenth century and on into the early twentieth century.[89]

Epidemics in Modern Asia draws on a wide range of primary and secondary sources, including government documents, medical reports,

---

[88] Gail Hershatter, *The Gender of Memory: Rural Women and China's Collective Past* (Berkeley: University of California Press, 2011).

[89] Johnston, *The Modern Epidemic*, pp.55–56.

ethnographic literature, and fiction. Historians are required to read across media in order to understand the past. As we shall see in Chapter 1 in our discussion of cholera epidemics in Japan, accounts of natural disasters in the nineteenth century often collated different forms of testimonial evidence to create a 'disaster collage.' Fictional material blended with the non-fictional, stylized illustrations co-existed with documentary texts, including official reports, promulgations, letters, and other miscellanea.[90]

Aside from traditional archival material, the book also makes use of press reports and the testimony of writers who recorded their experiences in memoirs, as well as documentary films and movies. Professional and personal accounts can give important insights into epidemic crises. For example, the description of the Manchurian pneumonic plague epidemic in 1910 by the Cambridge-trained Chinese physician Wu Lien-teh, offers fascinating glimpses into how the disease was experienced by a physician 'on the ground' (Chapter 4). It also suggests the extent to which Wu was responsible for crafting what was to become the dominant narrative of China's modernization through medicine and public health. Similarly, documentaries and fictional accounts exploring the HIV/AIDS crisis help us to understand how epidemics are lived, and remind us that behind the grand narratives of 'epidemics' there are multiple individual stories. Thus, Ruby Yang's documentary *The Blood of Yingzhou District* (2006) or Yan Lianke's semi-fictional novel *Dream of Ding Village* (2006) highlight the social, cultural, and political contexts of the HIV blood contamination scandal in China during the 1980s and 1990s, which left hundreds of thousands of farmers infected as a result of negligent practices in provincial blood collection programs (Chapter 5). This diversity of material enables a multi-dimensional understanding of epidemics and demonstrates the diverse responses they have elicited from the state, supranational organizations, and individual citizens.

A key focus of this book is on the congeries of ideas and images that shape how people understand disease. Over the last decade, videos and photographic images have also influenced how epidemics are reported and experienced. New digital technologies now allow for information to be uploaded to social media websites such as Facebook, YouTube, Baidu, and Weibo using digital cameras, mobile phones, or other smart devices. Noticeboards, discussion forums, chat rooms, livecasts, and blogs function as focal sites where views are exchanged, information imparted, and narratives about epidemics constructed. Today, the global media play an

---

[90] Stephan Köhn, 'Between Fiction and Non-fiction: Documentary Literature in the Late Edo Period.' In: Susanne Formanek and Sepp Linhart, eds., *Written Texts–Visual Texts: Woodblock-Printed Media in Early Modern Japan* (Amsterdam: Hotei, 2005), pp.283–310 (288).

important role in producing and promoting discourses about disease, often generating panic about epidemics in places where there may be no infection. The Internet makes distant events proximate, transforming remote actors into central ones. National disease surveillance authorities no longer have a monopoly on information, but compete with other private or non-governmental organizations. With increased access to the Internet, the public may view news sites and consult outbreak reporting systems, such as HealthMap/ProMED. Near real-time surveillance systems, including the Global Public Health Intelligence Network (GPHIN) developed by Health Canada, make use of search engines to monitor for epidemics, trawling the websites of news agencies, as well as local and national newspapers. Given their dependency on media sources, however, these Web-based systems are invariably slanted towards regions with more developed media networks, or countries where the dissemination of information may be less impeded.[91] Today, the historian of epidemics must contend with the big data of this rapidly expanding archive, conscious of the biases that are embedded in these new digital technologies.

Organization of the book

Each chapter explores a theme by considering three or four case studies. These are framed by an introduction and a conclusion draws out the main issues. The book eschews a narrow, chronological approach. Instead, it tracks continuities and discontinuities between different places at different times. As noted earlier, the themes (mobility, cities, the environment, war, globalization) are not treated as taken-for-granted categories, but rather they are approached as questions. The purpose, in other words, is to interrogate key themes in Asian history through epidemic histories.

Chapter 1 investigates mobility across and within Asia during the nineteenth century. Here, the focus is on specific epidemics in relation to the traffic of pathogens, people, and trade. Epidemics are understood as moments when networks – biological, social, political, and economic – converge and collide. The changing scale, rate, and speed of mobility during the nineteenth century prompted states to adopt novel strategies for preventing, managing, and controlling trade, migrant populations, and epidemic diseases. These state-sponsored regulations aimed at dealing with accelerated global flows led to resistance and conflict. The concept of 'mobility' is expanded in Chapter 1 to include the diffusion of ideas

---

[91] Nigel H. Collier, 'A Review of Web-based Epidemic Detection.' In: Sara E. Davies and Jeremy R. Youde, eds., *The Politics of Surveillance and Response to Disease Outbreaks: The New Frontier for States and Non-state Actors* (Farnham and Burlington, VT: Ashgate, 2015), pp.85–105.

about diseases and the transfer of technologies for their management. If diseases were imported through pathways of trade, so too was knowledge about these diseases and the language used to describe them. The aim in Chapter 1 is to examine the operations of different kinds of intertwined mobility: from microbial traffic to the process of meaning-making in language.

Chapter 2 considers urbanization and its effects in relation to epidemics. How did cities create conditions for disease to spread? To what extent were colonial urban planning and municipal politics shaped by racial ideologies that located infectious disease in native bodies and the spaces they inhabited? This chapter considers cities as concentrated spaces that make population surveillance and the regulation of human activities feasible. It also examines the connections between infectious disease and new forms of urban technical and managerial expertise. Underlying these specific concerns is a broad, overarching question: What is a city? In addressing this question, attention is paid to the different forces that have driven urbanization – and also promoted disease – military power, trade, and bureaucracy.

Environmental changes caused by intensified land clearance, infrastructural development (the construction of dams, roads, and railways), urbanization, and increasing energy use, have had a major impact on human health. Chapter 3 shifts the emphasis onto epidemics and the environment. It begins by interrogating the notion of the 'environment' in relation to the correlate terms 'nature,' 'biosphere,' and 'ecosystem.' Epidemics are viewed as episodes that foreground the convergence of human and natural ecologies. The focus is on addressing the following questions: To what extent should epidemics be understood as the outcome of environmental crises? What countervailing effects have been produced by attempts to intervene with the environment to mitigate disease threats? How have evolving conceptions of disease shaped environmental change? And finally: What role does politics play in how human–environment relations are framed?

In Chapter 4, the linkages between human conflict and epidemics are investigated. The nineteenth and twentieth centuries saw the proliferation of conflict across many regions of Asia: first, as imperial powers sought to expand their dominions in wars of conquest; second, in conflicts that arose from imperial rivalries; and third, in national struggles for independence that followed the breakup of empire. These conflicts were crucial in creating the ground for infectious disease emergence, while epidemics played a critical part in determining the nature and outcome of these conflicts. The chapter considers the different species of violence that are accommodated by the term 'war': from military campaigns to civil wars, and insurgency struggles where a geopolitics of terror has become entangled with an epidemiology of infection. It also reflects on the ways in which the specter of a pending war, along with recent histories of military conflict, may determine responses to ongoing and future epidemics.

Chapter 5 examines how globalization is driving infectious disease across Southeast and East Asia. It tracks the social and environmental transformations wrought by capital expansion and market liberalization, with a particular focus on the role of agribusiness in the emergence of viral infections. The emphasis is on showing how epidemic crises are produced under certain conditions: namely, when highly local circumstances intermesh with global forces. Meanwhile, however, responses to pandemic threats often assume a world that is naturally segmented into nations and states, reducing our capacity to manage borderless infections.

In adopting a comparative and transdisciplinary approach in this book, I have inevitably had to impinge on numerous fields far removed from my own expertise. Although portions of the material covered will be more or less familiar to some readers, other material will be less familiar. The purpose in writing *Epidemics in Modern Asia* has been, not only to ask new questions and address new issues, but to encourage fresh perspectives on old questions, reassessing modern Asia as a space of interaction through contagious histories.

1   Mobility

In the nineteenth century, concerns about intensifying interregional and global mobility prompted impassioned debates in many countries about where, how, and by whom the boundaries were to be drawn that demarcated the individual from the state, the nation from the world. This chapter examines these debates in a number of sites across Asia, specifically in the context of epidemics and the entanglement of different kinds of circulation that they brought into view: the traffic of disease, the transference of people, goods, and capital, and the dissemination of knowledge and technical expertise. In what ways did epidemics foreground economic and social networks? How were different species of mobility encouraged, regulated, or prevented? What kinds of violence did epidemics induce, particularly in relation to conflicts over freedom, power, and sovereignty?

It is, perhaps, too easy to think of mobility solely in relation to trade, migration, and the spread of disease – in other words, as an outward diffusion or expansion that impacts upon a more-or-less static 'target' society. According to this view, mobility is conceived as an exceptional process, in contrast to the fixed locations from which – and to which – the person or thing is moving. Mobility has tended to be understood 'through the same analytical lens' of global flows, with the mobile contrasted to the static.[1] It has also been associated with the transition from a world where modernizing institutions were able to fix identities and relations, to one that is increasingly mobile and therefore hard to order. The argument has been made that global capitalism, coupled with new information technologies, has produced an unsettling new fluidity: 'liquid modernity.' Modern life is characterized by a fundamental inconstancy – by 'fragility, temporariness, vulnerability and inclination to constant change.'[2]

Studying epidemic episodes in the past may help us to rethink this binary between mobility and fixity, localization and transnational

---

[1] Nina Glick Schiller and Noel B. Salazar, 'Regimes of Mobility Across the Globe,' *Journal of Ethnic and Migration Studies*, vol.39, no.2 (2013): 183–200 (184).

[2] Zygmunt Bauman, *Liquid Modernity* (Cambridge and Malden, MA: Polity Press, [2000] 2012), p.viii.

connection, past and present. As the anthropologist James Clifford has suggested, we might begin to re-conceptualize mobility by reflecting on the processes of human movement or travel inherent in culture. 'Practices of displacement,' Clifford proposes, may be thought of 'as *constitutive* of cultural meanings rather than as their simple transfer or extension.'[3] In each of the three cases presented in this chapter, I elaborate on this insight by exploring epidemics in relation to different kinds and scales of mobility. The argument developed is that epidemics should be understood not simply as the spread of an externally originating disease, but in terms of dynamic interactions and displacements taking place within and between cultures. These interchanges, driven by the onset of capitalism and imperialism, can be re-conceptualized as mutual processes of cross-cultural translation, wherein the foreign and the native are co-produced. Translation, here, encompasses processes of material, technological, and symbolic exchange: in other words, mobility extends from the circulation of disease to the ways in which concepts about disease migrate between cultures and get reinterpreted within local systems.[4]

The first of the three cases involves an outbreak of cholera in colonial Manila in 1820, which provoked a massacre of Chinese and Western foreigners by local Filipinos. These conjoined events – epidemic and massacre – are explored in relation to economic, social, and political shifts taking place after 1815, specifically in the wake of political reform and the end of the Manila galleon trade, which saw the progressive opening up of Manila to global commerce. What light can this epidemic violence shed on networks of trade and circuits of migration across Asia that were being remodeled at the beginning of the nineteenth century? How did these contextual factors drive the epidemic itself?

The second case concerns the importation of cholera to Japan after 1858. It examines how disease became embroiled in intensifying debates about the 'opening up' of the country to foreign trade and the establishment of extraterritorial treaty ports during the final years of the Tokugawa period (1603–1868) and beyond. Foreigners were closely associated with the disease, which was imagined as a toxic Western import. Japanese nationhood was, in part, articulated in relation to the dangers posed by foreign incursions and the transplantation of modern ways. If external pressures undermined the Tokugawa regime, concurrently, 'they strengthened an emerging national consciousness among a growing body

---

[3] James Clifford, *Routes: Travel and Translation in the Late Twentieth Century* (Cambridge, MA: Harvard University Press, 1997), p.3.

[4] Lydia H. Liu, 'Introduction.' In: Lydia H. Liu, ed., *Tokens of Exchange: The Problem of Translation in Global Circulations* (Durham, NC: Duke University Press, 1999), pp.1–12.

of political actors.'[5] The focus in this section is thus on the contradictions that cholera exposed: while Japanese nationalism normalized stasis, pitting a rooted native culture against perilous foreign ideologies of free trade, it was precisely this alien threat that provided the stimulus for Japan's modernization and its adoption of Western hygienic modernity. During the Meiji period – so called after the name assumed by the emperor on his coronation in 1868 – disease surveillance was instituted through the establishment of a medical police that monitored the movement of citizens. As Akihito Suzuki and Mika Suzuki have observed, 'the Meiji government forged its modern state medicine and public health policies largely through its response to cholera from the 1870s to the 1890s. Epidemics of cholera, as in many other countries, were a crucible for the modernisation of medicine in general and public health in particular.'[6] In tracking these connections, the aim in this section is to show how cholera in Japan was central to debates about the state's accountability to its citizens, about the nature of modernity, and the demarcation of private and public spheres. Epidemics also revealed contradictions that underlay the vision of a liberal world order: the need for the free and safe movement of people, goods, and ideas necessitated systems of surveillance, coercion, and confinement.[7] Meanwhile, attempts to regulate such movement – by defining and fixing relations – often had an obverse effect. As we shall see in our discussion of prostitution in Chapter 2, modernization created conditions for new kinds of mobility. In his account of late modernity, the sociologist Zygmunt Bauman sums up this countervailing process when he asserts, 'it was the quest for the solidity of things and states that most often triggered, kept in motion and guided their liquefaction; liquidity was not an adversary, but an effect of that quest for solidity.'[8]

The final case investigates the multiple factors driving bubonic plague in China. It considers the expansion of the opium trade in the eighteenth century and developments on the Qing Empire's southwestern frontier, as well as the profound social upheavals – including the Taiping Rebellion (1850–1864) – which resulted in the redirection of traffic and mass population displacements. How did these movements determine the epidemiology of the plague? Finally, and relatedly, outbreaks of plague in Canton

[5] Andrew Gordon, *A Modern History of Japan: From Tokugawa Times to the Present* (Oxford: Oxford University Press, 2003), p.48.

[6] Akihito Suzuki and Mika Suzuki, 'Cholera, Consumer, and Citizenship: Modernisations of Medicine in Japan.' In: Hormoz Ebrahimnejad, ed., *The Development of Modern Medicine in Non-Western Countries: Historical Perspectives* (London: Routledge, 2009), pp.184–203 (186).

[7] Hamlin, *Cholera*, p.5.   [8] Bauman, *Liquid Modernity*, p.ix.

and Hong Kong in 1894 are examined in relation to interregional and transnational pathways of commerce. This section also reflects on Hong Kong as a 'space of flow' and reconsiders the violence that resulted from the British colonial government's efforts to impede the movement of Chinese residents out of the colony on the grounds of disease prevention.[9] Epidemics are explored in terms of the convergence and divergence of different networks: biological, social, political, and economic.

Migration in Asia

Today, across the world, people are on the move. This process of migration has been particularly conspicuous in Asia from the 1970s, when demand for migrant labor grew rapidly in response to trade liberalization, the reorganization of production, and inflows of international capital. By one estimate, there are over 30 million migrant workers across the region, including contract laborers in the Middle East, and those working in the high-growth economies of Southeast Asia. East Asia and the Pacific region have an emigrant population of over 20 million, with migrant workers accounting for 20 percent or more of the labor force in countries such as Malaysia and Singapore.[10] In the PRC, internal rural to city migration is taking place on a colossal scale: out of Shanghai's population of 22 million, eight million are migrants.[11] The 2010 census revealed that 20 percent of the PRC's population had lived in a different place six months prior to the census. As we shall see in our discussion of globalization in Chapter 5, this large-scale migration is the result of China's structural reforms and market liberalization from the late 1970s and 1980s, which precipitated the development of a booming export economy. Men and women from the countryside have left their villages – 'gone out' in the words of migrant workers themselves – to power the assembly lines in southern Chinese cities such as Dongguan and Shenzhen.[12] Remittances sent home have been crucial to China's rural economy, as they have been in many countries across Asia. Of course, we should be wary of pitting a mobile present against a static past. Internal migration on a mass scale had occurred in China long before the late twentieth century. There are

---

[9] Elizabeth Sinn, 'Lesson in Openness: Creating a Space of Flow in Hong Kong.' In: Helen F. Siu and Agnes S. Ku, eds., *Hong Kong Mobile: Making a Global Population* (Hong Kong: Hong Kong University Press, 2008), pp.13–43.

[10] Ahmad Ahsan, et al., *International Migration and Development in East Asia and the Pacific* (Washington, DC: World Bank, 2014), p.10.

[11] Weiping Wu and Piper Gaubatz, *The Chinese City* (Abingdon and New York: Routledge, 2013), p.275.

[12] Leslie T. Chang, *Factory Girls: Voices from the Heart of Modern China* (London: Picador, 2009), p.13.

antecedents in the inter-provincial migration of workers to the coastal areas and to Manchuria during the late Qing and Republican periods, for example. In the course of the Civil War (1927–1950) and during the Japanese invasion and occupation (1931, 1937–1945), many people were uprooted. After the Communist state was established in 1949, millions were forcefully moved in a process that has left deep scars.[13]

Similarly, although transnational migration has accelerated as a result of cheaper travel, economic conditions, labor surpluses, political circumstances, and regional conflicts, it is important not to overlook earlier diasporic networks and population movements. Migration, in this sense, is nothing new. For centuries, Chinese merchants traded textiles, cotton, rice, opium, timber, and many other commodities along the coasts of Southeast Asia.[14] Traders from Asia plied the Silk Route, navigating the Indian Ocean and China Seas. The sea was a means of connection, linking dispersed littoral societies and riparian communities through ties of trade, culture, and religion.[15] After the establishment of Islam in the seventh century and the growth of Muslim communities in Southeast Asia from the twelfth and thirteenth centuries, the *hajj* drew Muslim pilgrims to Arabia from across the region.

In the early modern period, however, there was a quickening and expansion of migration linked, in part, to new networks of maritime trade created by distending European empires. From the middle of the nineteenth century, multiple factors including technological innovations in transport and transoceanic travel, upheavals in India and China, capitalist production and the growth of a labor market, as well as the consolidation of imperial power, served as further catalysts for migration. As Christopher Bayly has observed, 'contemporary changes were so rapid and interacted with each other so profoundly, that this period could reasonably be described as the "birth of the modern world."'[16] Between the 1840s and the Second World War, around 20 million Chinese and 30 million Indians migrated to Southeast Asia, and to territories around

---

[13] Diana Lary, 'The Static Decades: Inter-Provincial Migration in Pre-Reform China.' In: Frank N. Pieke and Hein Mallee, eds., *Internal and International Migration: Chinese Perspectives* (Richmond: Curzon, 1999), pp.29–48.

[14] Eric Tagliacozzo and Wen-Chin Chang, 'The Arc of Historical Commercial Relations between China and Southeast Asia.' In: Eric Tagliacozzo and Wen-Chin Chang, eds., *Chinese Circulations: Capital, Commodities, and Networks in Southeast Asia* (Durham, NC: Duke University Press, 2011), pp.1–17.

[15] Sunil S. Amrith, *Migration and Diaspora in Modern Asia* (Cambridge: Cambridge University Press, 2011), p.1.

[16] C. A. Bayly, *The Birth of the Modern World, 1780–1914: Global Connections and Comparisons* (Oxford: Blackwell, 2004), p.11.

the Indian and Pacific Oceans – including to the Americas.[17] They moved to service the needs of expanding cities, working on the docks, in industry, and on plantations (Chapter 3). Coolie labor was also crucial in Japan's imperial expansion, while during the early twentieth century thousands of sojourners moved within the Qing Empire from the northern coastal provinces of Shandong and Hebei to Manchuria, returning home for the Chinese New Year celebrations (Chapter 4).[18]

Unsettling labor: Coolies

In 1807, the British Parliament passed the Abolition of the Slave Trade Act, which was followed by further legislation in 1833 extending the clampdown on slavery across the Empire. From the 1830s, the traffic of indentured laborers from India and China was encouraged to service the needs of expanding colonial industries. The term 'coolie' was used in the nineteenth and early twentieth centuries to describe these contracted laborers who migrated to work on sugar, cotton, and rubber plantations, in mines, as well as in railway construction and other labor-intensive industries. Use of the word 'coolie' is recorded in the sixteenth century and its origins are often traced back to two Tamil and Gujarati terms. The Tamil word *kuli* means payment for menial work, while the Gujarati term *Kuli* is the name of a lowly Gujarati tribe whose members were involved in ostensibly nefarious activities. The English term 'coolie' thus conjoined the concept of payment with the devious person of the *Kuli*. As Jan Breman and E. Valentine Daniel have suggested, the designation 'coolie' implied both mobility and immobility. On the one hand, coolies were perceived as unskilled migrant laborers, adrift from their places of origin. Their vagrant status made them 'unsettling' to colonial authorities. On the other hand, coolies were viewed as 'unable and/or unwilling to move to new work places' – a reluctance that 'made it necessary for colonial capitalism to detach them from their home milieu by buying them out.' Contradictory attitudes towards the coolie informed colonial responses. While 'the immobility of peasant-coolies called for unsettling by the

---

[17] Adam McKeown, 'Global Migration, 1846–1970,' *Journal of World History*, vol.15, no.2 (2004): 155–189 (157).

[18] Thomas R. Gottschang and Diana Lary, *Swallows and Settlers: The Great Migration from North China to Manchuria* (Ann Arbor: University of Michigan Center for Chinese Studies, 2000).

good graces of capitalism,' this dislocation and 'the potential capriciousness of their mobility called for settling by a series of labour regimes.'

Jan Breman and E. Valentine Daniel, 'Conclusion: The Making of a Coolie.' In: E. Valentine Daniel, Henry Bernstein, and Tom Brass, eds., *Plantations, Proletarians and Peasants in Colonial Asia* (London: Frank Cass, 1992), pp.268–295 (282).

Population movements had health consequences for migrants and their host communities. Today, migration is understood to be an important determinant of global health and development, particularly in terms of acute or chronic infectious disease burden. The outcome of mobility may, of course, be favorable as well as adverse for health, and the literature on migration has emphasized the consequences for health of mobile individuals and populations crossing the 'prevalence gap' between locations characterized by different health risks.[19]

Disease followed European advances, spreading through proliferating imperial networks. The first cholera pandemic from 1817 and the third plague pandemic in the late nineteenth and early twentieth centuries were diffused along expanding pathways of trade and migration. Pilgrimages, particularly Muslims traveling west from South and Southeast Asia to the Middle East, also contributed to the interregional dispersal of diseases such as cholera and plague. In the Spring of 1865, an epidemic of cholera in Mecca killed an estimated 15,000 pilgrims. The disease was likely brought there on two ships from Singapore, ferrying Malaysian, Javanese, and Indian pilgrims. An expansion of steamer traffic from the mid-century and the inauguration of the Suez Canal in 1869 further increased the risks of disease spreading globally.[20]

The nineteenth century saw a massive migration of labor across Asia, which was also crucial in the circulation of infections. Migrants were vulnerable to disease during their journey: from their arrival in crowded port cities where they took ship to their disembarkation in unfamiliar and often hostile surroundings, where endemic diseases posed a threat. Congested cities provided a breeding ground for infections, facilitating disease transmission, while new environments posed risks to those with little or

[19] Douglas W. MacPherson and Brian D. Gushulak, 'Human Mobility and Population Health: New Approaches in a Globalizing World,' *Perspectives in Biology and Medicine*, vol.44, no.3 (2001): 390–401 (394).
[20] LaVerne Kuhnke, *Lives at Risk: Public Health in Nineteenth-Century Egypt* (Berkeley: University of California Press, 1990), pp.65–68.

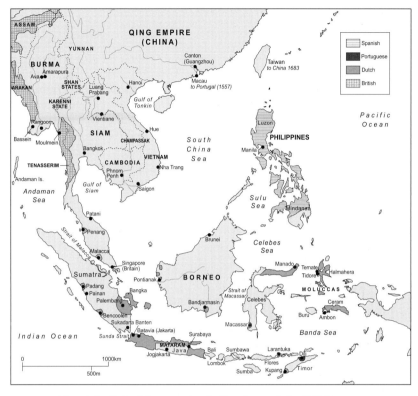

Map 1.1. Colonial expansion in Southeast Asia (1826)

European empires in Southeast Asia

Europeans in Asia exploited pre-existing trade networks that linked China with Southeast Asia. Textiles, rice, spices, opium, timber, and many other commodities had been traded across the region for centuries. However, European colonists also introduced new notions of sovereignty and territorial power, which profoundly changed the future of Asia. The Portuguese were the first Europeans to establish a string of trading bases along India's southwest coast in the early sixteenth century in an effort to dominate the lucrative spice trade to Europe, and the southern Malay entrepôt of Melaka was captured by them in 1511. The Spanish, too, had ambitions in Asia. In 1542, Ruy López de Villalobos named the Philippines in honor of Philip, heir to the Spanish throne. A formal process of colonization began when Miguel López de Legazpi was appointed governor general of the Spanish East Indies in 1565 and founded a settlement on the island of Cebu. For 300 years, silver from New Spain (Mexico) reached the Philippines through the Manila galleon trade, while in exchange porcelain, silk, ivory, spices, and other exotic goods were shipped through the Philippines to Mexico and Europe. Meanwhile, the Dutch United East India Company (*Vereenigde Oostindische Compagnie* or VOC) established an emporium in Batavia (Jakarta) on the island of Java in 1619 (Map 1.1). Granted a royal charter by Queen Elizabeth in 1600, the English East India Company (EIC) dominated trade in the Indian subcontinent and established bases in Southeast Asia. In 1819, Sir Thomas Stamford Raffles founded Singapore as an EIC trading gateway after signing a treaty with Sultan Hussein Shah of Johor and Temenggong Abdul Rahman, with the British acquiring sovereignty in 1824. Burma was secured the same year after the seizure of Rangoon (Yangon) by a British seaborne expedition during the First Anglo-Burmese War (1824–1826), while Malacca (Melaka) on the Malay peninsula was transferred to British administration as a result of the Anglo-Dutch Treaty, which partitioned the East Indian Archipelago (Indonesia).

Milton Osborne, *Southeast Asia: An Introductory History*. Revised edition (Crows Nest, NSW: Allen & Unwin, 2013), pp.70–92.

no immunity to novel pathogens. In the 1880s and 1890s, south Indian migrants who crossed the Bay of Bengal to work on plantation estates in Malaya were especially susceptible to malaria, which was endemic in the region (Chapter 3).[21]

An awareness of the health threats posed by multiplying interregional and global connections, as well as the destabilizing economic consequences of epidemics, led to increasingly coordinated state efforts from the mid nineteenth century to control the movement of people and commodities with the imposition of quarantine measures.[22] Such procedures were not only adopted to stem the flow of infected migrants, but also to check the importation of infected cargo, since maritime health authorities

---

[21] Sunil S. Amrith, 'Migration and Health in Southeast Asian History,' *Lancet*, vol.384, no.9954 (November 1, 2014): 1569–1570.

[22] Mark Harrison, *Contagion: How Commerce Has Spread Disease* (New Haven, CT: Yale University Press, 2012).

'were positively preoccupied with cargo, wherever it came from.'[23] During the plague pandemic in the 1890s, the British implemented more stringent and systematic preventive processes under pressure from rival powers that threatened to impose an embargo on goods from British India. Measures included proscribing the pilgrimage to Mecca, setting up inspection and quarantine stations on the Gulf of Suez, and instituting a more rigorous inspection system in ports. Although piecemeal and often half-heartedly applied, these imperial efforts to establish a more coherent transnational disease surveillance capacity anticipated the formation of global agencies such as the WHO in the twentieth century.[24]

Globalization tends to be thought about in relation to cross-border flows, but we might think of globalization instead 'as consisting of systemic processes of closure and containment' (Chapter 5). In the second half of the nineteenth century, states actively sought to constrain internal and trans-border movement. This impetus to regulate mobility was predicated 'on a pervasive paradigm of suspicion,' wherein the perceived threat posed by migrants converged with anxieties about disease and potential disorder.[25] The aim was to create a functional 'membrane' so that deleterious circulations could be sifted out from other indispensable flows.[26]

A world in motion: Cholera in Manila

In 1817, an epidemic of cholera broke out in Bengal in the Ganges Delta. Cholera is an acute diarrheal infection most commonly brought on by ingesting food or drinking water contaminated with the bacterium *Vibrio cholerae*. It was not until 1883, however, that the German physician and bacteriologist Robert Koch (1843–1910) isolated the causal agent in India, following his earlier research during an epidemic in Egypt. The disease's relatively short incubation period and high death rate made it particularly feared, as did its acute symptoms: diarrhea and vomiting, with sufferers acquiring a distinctive gray-blue complexion from dehydration, dying within days.[27]

It is likely that cholera had long been endemic in India and Southeast Asia, although the causes of the disease's new, explosive virulence

---

[23] David S. Barnes, 'Cargo, "Infection," and the Logic of Quarantine in the Nineteenth Century,' *Bulletin of the History of Medicine*, vol.88, no.1 (2014): 75–101 (76).

[24] David Arnold, 'The Indian Ocean as a Disease Zone,' *South Asia: Journal of South Asian Studies*, vol.14, no.2 (1991): 1–21 (18).

[25] Ronen Shamir, 'Without Borders? Notes on Globalization as a Mobility Regime,' *Sociological Theory*, vol.23, no.2 (2005): 197–217.

[26] Valeska Huber, *Channeling Mobilities: Migration and Globalization in the Suez Canal Region and Beyond, 1869–1914* (Cambridge: Cambridge University Press, 2013), p.242.

[27] Robert Pollitzer, *Cholera* (Geneva: World Health Organization, 1959), pp.19–20.

continue to be debated. Descriptions of cholera appear in the work of Jacob Bontius (1592–1631), a physician of the VOC in Batavia in 1629, but there the disease is not characterized by the same degree of lethality with which it later came to be associated. In 1817, there were many views about its origins. A prevalent belief held that it was caused by 'miasmas' or toxic emanations from the ground. Some conjectured, however, that it had been caused by poisonous discharges from the eruption of Mount Tambora on the island of Sumbawa, Indonesia, in 1815 – the largest recorded volcanic eruption in human history.[28] The 1817 pandemic is often described as the first of six cholera pandemics, although there is controversy over the bounding of these pandemics.[29] The notion of clearly delineated and successive pandemic 'waves' has been challenged since in many regions, including Japan, cholera remained endemic with periodic outbreaks (Figure 1.1).[30]

The pandemic occurred against the backdrop of major geopolitical shifts, notably the ascendancy of the British in South and Southeast Asia. Conflicts in Europe from the mid eighteenth century had ramifications in Asia. The Seven Years' War (1754–1763) involved European powers in a struggle over colonial possessions in North America, Central America, West Africa, India, and the Philippines. The British briefly occupied Manila, the capital of the Spanish Philippines, between 1762 and 1764. Subsequently, the Napoleonic Wars (1803–1815) and the defeat of Napoleon by combined Prussian and British forces had significant repercussions in South and Southeast Asia. The EIC was able to extend its influence across the subcontinent at the expense of the French, moving in to quash Indian resistance. Infection proceeded along developing imperial circuits and its diffusion coincided with this expansion of British influence in Asia.

In late September 1820, an outbreak of cholera occurred in Manila, affecting Filipino villages along the Pasig River, especially in Tondo, to the northwest of the city. Disease followed a devastating typhoon, which compounded the crisis. To stem the epidemic, Spanish authorities sought to prevent villagers from using river water. A hastily assembled public relief committee was established. Although there are no reliable statistical data, contemporary accounts suggest that mortality was in the thousands. Streets were described as being full of carts conveying the dead, while those unaffected by the disease were overwhelmed and unable to tend to

---

[28] Gillen D'Arcy Wood, *Tambora: The Eruption that Changed the World* (Princeton, NJ: Princeton University Press, 2014), pp.72–96.

[29] Hamlin, *Cholera*, p.4.

[30] William Johnston, 'Epidemics Past and Science Present: An Approach to Cholera in Nineteenth-Century Japan,' *Harvard Asia Quarterly*, vol.14, no.4 (2012): 28–35.

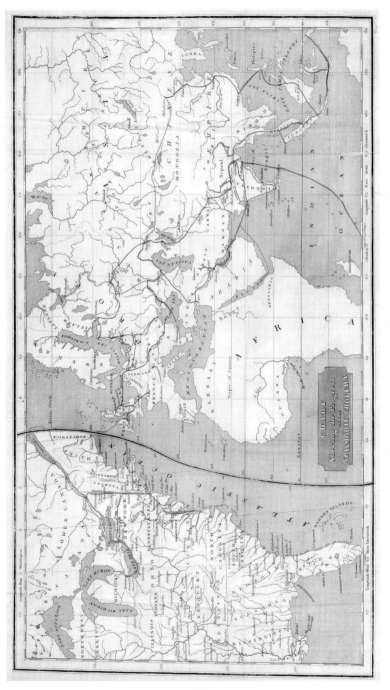

Figure 1.1. Amariah Brigham, 'Chart Shewing the Progress of the Spasmodic Cholera.' Frontispiece in: *A Treatise on Epidemic Cholera; Including an Historical Account of Its Origin and Progress, to the Present Period* (Hartford, CT: H. and F. J. Huntington, 1832). Courtesy: Historical Maps Collection, University of Princeton.

Mapping the progress of cholera

Maps have played an important role in defining epidemics and pandemics as spatial phenomena. As we saw in the Introduction ('Zoonoses: Global hotspots'), they provide a means of visualizing the connections between different disease locales at different times. Although purporting to represent impartial views of the world, maps such as Figure 1.1 from *A Treatise on Epidemic Cholera* by the American physician Amariah Brigham (1798–1849), embed power relations. Note, for example, how the map pivots on Europe – and, in particular, Britain – the center of world power. Published in 1832, Brigham's map shows the cholera's global diffusion from Bengal. Cities are linked by a red line, indicating the main pathways of the disease's spread. Cholera appears to have followed an overland route across northern India to Afghanistan and Russia. It was also disseminated via an expanding transoceanic maritime traffic from India, and by 1819 it had reached Ceylon (Sri Lanka). Over the next few years, the disease was to diffuse along trading routes to Mauritius and East Africa and throughout Asia to China, Korea, and Japan. Epidemics impacted port cities across Southeast Asia. From Bengal, cholera reached Penang, spreading across the Malay peninsula where – according to John Crawfurd (1783–1868), a Scottish physician and employee of the EIC – it 'committed dreadful ravages in Siam and the neighbouring countries,' killing an estimated 100,000 people. In Bangkok, King Rama II issued a decree that limited movement, directing people off the roads and away from market places. As a Thai chronicler noted: 'The whole populace was forbidden to travel and to kill animals . . . All people had to stay at home unless there was a compelling reason for them to go out.' In the capital, a ceremony for warding off evil forces was ordered with the chanting of sutras, the firing of cannon around the city, and a procession of Buddhist monks carrying relics. By April 1821, cholera had reached Java's north coast, where it was purportedly carried by junks from Semarang. News of the disease's inexorable progress caused people to flee, and villages were left deserted when cholera was rumored to be on its way. Some 125,000 may have perished on Java in 1821.

Tom Koch, *Disease Maps: Epidemics on the Ground* (Chicago, IL: University of Chicago Press, 2011), pp.112–114.

B. J. Terwiel, 'Asiatic Cholera in Siam: Its First Occurrence and the 1820 Epidemic.' In: Norman G. Owen, ed., *Death and Disease in Southeast Asia: Explorations in Social, Medical and Demographic History* (Singapore: Oxford University Press, 1987), pp.142–161 (150–151).

the sick or inter the dead.[31] The Frenchman Paul de la Gironière left a highly dramatized version of the epidemic in his memoirs:

Within a few days of its first appearance the epidemic spread rapidly; the Indians succumbed by thousands; at all hours of the day and of the night streets were crowded with the dead-carts. Next to the fright occasioned by the epidemic, quickly succeeded rage and despair.

Rumors began to circulate amongst the *Indios* (a disparaging term for native Filipinos) of a plot to exterminate local people. It was alleged that foreigners had poisoned wells and contaminated the Pasig: 'The Indians said, one to another, that the strangers poisoned the rivers and the fountains, in order to destroy the native population and possess themselves of the Philippines.'[32] On the morning of October 9, an armed mob, several thousand strong, hunted down and attacked foreigners. Spanish troops failed to crush the uprising, which killed over 100 persons: 14 Britons and Americans, 12 French, two Dutch, and 85 Chinese who were accused of conspiring with the foreigners (Figure 1.2).

'In the Philippine Islands,' noted one British observer, 'the malady was marked by one of those terrific outbursts of barbarian despair which have more than once signaled the progress of this pestilence.' Writing to a friend in Penang, J. W. Campbell, commander of *HMS Dauntless*, observed that on his arrival in Manila, 'I perceived even before I landed that some dreadful catastrophe had marked its progress with desolation and had produced stagnation in the Commercial operations on the River and in the port.' And from Canton in December 1820, the Protestant missionary Robert Morrison (1782–1834) commented in a letter to a relative: 'There has been a very shocking massacre of from thirty to forty Europeans of different nations of Europe, and of about eighty Chinese, at Manilla [sic]. The perpetrators of this cruel act were the native Manilla people. The pretext was a supposition that foreigners had introduced the disease called cholera morbus, which had prevailed extensively, and was very fatal.'[33]

Established as the capital of the Spanish Philippines by de Legazpi in 1571, Manila was a way station for trade with Asia and had long served as a trans-shipment hub in the Manila–Acapulco galleon trade. Silver crossed the Pacific from the Americas, while silk, ivory, porcelain, spice,

[31] José P. Bantug, *A Short History of Medicine in the Philippines During the Spanish Regime, 1565–1898* (Quezon City: Colegio Médico-Farmacéutico de Filipinas, 1953), pp.29–30.

[32] Paul P. de la Gironière, *Twenty Years in the Philippines* (New York: Harper & Brothers, 1854), p.20.

[33] Eliza A. Morrison, *Memoirs of the Life and Labours of Robert Morrison*, 2 vols. (London: Longman, Orme, Brown, Green and Longmans, 1839), II, p.37.

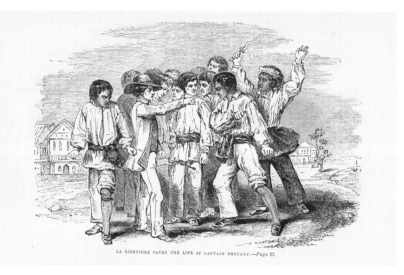

LA GIRONIERE SAVES THE LIFE OF CAPTAIN DROUANT.—*Page 22.*

Figure 1.2. 'Dr. Gironière Saves the Life of Captain Drouant.' In: Paul P. de la Gironière, *Twenty Years in the Philippines* (New York: Harper & Brothers, 1854), p.22.

Epidemic and massacre

The physician Paul de la Gironière (1797–1862) described events during the 1820 epidemic and massacre in Manila in his memoirs, *Twenty Years in the Philippines*, originally published in French in 1853. The son of an aristocrat ruined by the French Revolution, de la Gironière had arrived in the Philippines shortly before the epidemic. Subsequently, he established an estate at Jalajala in the province of Rizal to the east of Manila, where he raised cattle and cultivated sugarcane, coffee, and rice. His account of the massacre is highly subjective and provides a one-dimensional portrayal of the local inhabitants, who are invariably viewed as 'scoundrels': impulsive, quick to anger, and violent by nature. Figure 1.2, reproduced from de la Gironière's memoirs, shows the physician wielding a cane as he bravely faces down a menacing group of *Indios*, one of whom brandishes a dagger with an undulating blade, known as a *kris* or *keris*. Given the lack of 'native' sources, historians are often reliant on colonial versions of events or on memoirs such as those by de la Gironière. These writings, however, give only partial views and are shaped by prevailing racial assumptions. A major challenge for historians is finding ways of accessing the world of native peoples.

and other commodities from Asia were shipped to Acapulco in western Mexico and thence overland to Veracruz in the east for shipment to Spain.[34] This exclusive dependency on external trade resulted in a lack of internal investment and it was not until the second half of the eighteenth century, when demand for Chinese silk fell in relation to English and Indian cotton, that attempts were made to develop local exports. In 1789, restrictions were lifted on the shipment of Asian goods by foreign ships. Previously, only the Chinese had been permitted to trade between Manila and the rest of Asia. As a result, the port boomed and the city's population expanded. Trading ships from North America and Europe made regular calls, and 1809 saw the establishment of the first English commercial house there.[35] The galleon trade finally came to an end in 1815, with resultant economic and social transformations. In 1834, the Royal Philippine Company was dissolved and Manila was formally opened to world trade.

The Spanish merchants in Manila, who had formerly controlled the galleon trade, found it difficult to compete with European traders on these new terms and soon lost their commercial monopoly, lobbying the colonial administration for greater regulation of foreign traders. Manila's progressive opening to foreign commerce brought about other changes in agricultural practices and land ownership. Enterprising natives and *mestizos*, acting as middlemen for foreign traders, amassed substantial estates. Conversely, many small cultivators lost their lands, becoming sharecroppers. Cholera thus arrived just as the Philippine port was opening to world trade with consequential shifts occurring within Philippine society.[36] The effects of these adjustments were evident in the local reactions to the 1820 epidemic. Disease served to underscore and exacerbate pre-existing grievances and tensions.

According to one account, cholera had been brought to Manila from Calcutta by the *Merope*, an infected ship of the EIC sailing under the command of 25-year-old Captain David Nicoll, who was stabbed in the back during the massacre. Some commentators suggested that the violence was the result of a misunderstanding. Others noted that the Spanish governor general, Mariano Fernandez de Folgueras (1766–1823), distrusted his officers, the majority of whom were Mexicans. At the time,

---

[34] Arturo Giraldez, *The Age of Trade: The Manila Galleons and the Dawn of the Global Economy* (Lanham, MD: Rowman & Littlefield, 2015).

[35] Manuel A. Caoili, *The Origins of Metropolitan Manila: A Political and Social Analysis* (Quezon City: New Day Publishers, 1988), p.39.

[36] Jeyamalar Kathirithamby-Wells, 'The Age of Transition: The Mid-Eighteenth to the Early Nineteenth Centuries.' In: Nicholas Tarling, ed., *The Cambridge History of Southeast Asia. Vol.1: From Early Times to c.1800* (Cambridge: Cambridge University Press, 1993), pp.572–620 (608–612).

Mexico was engaged in a war of independence with Spain, which was to come to an end in August 1821, when the country's sovereignty was finally recognized in the Treaty of Córdoba.[37] Still others, however, maintained that it was Spaniards who had purposefully incited the mob. The Irish-born American trader Peter Dobell (1772–1852), the first imperial Russian consul in Manila, who had arrived with his wife and daughter in March 1820, noted that while the Spanish were suspicious of the foreign traders, there was mutual 'jealousy and envy' amongst the different nationalities competing to establish bases in the Philippines. Dobell linked the massacre to the new Spanish constitution of 1812, which had given 'extensive privileges & liberal encouragement to foreigners, who might think proper to settle in the Philippines,' while 'rendering the natives as free & equal, in rights, &c., as their former masters.'[38]

Another witness, Charles Louis Benoit, a surgeon on a French vessel, presented a paper on the Manila epidemic at the University of Montpellier in 1827, in which he attributed the slaughter to a residual antipathy towards foreigners that could be traced back to the British occupation of Manila and Cavite during the Seven Years' War. The cholera outbreak, he declared 'was the signal for the barbarous massacre committed with impunity on the persons of the foreigners and of a few Chinese who, because of the war of the year 1762, were looked upon with disfavor by the priests and by a large part of the population.'[39]

The raising of the mob was also attributed to native suspicions of foreign scientific practices. According to Benoit, who was himself to die during a cholera epidemic in the 1880s, the government set up stalls in the streets to dispense brandy and 'quinine' (presumably some infusion of ground *cinchona* bark, since it was only in 1820 that the alkaloid quinine was first isolated and extracted from the bark in a purified form) – concoctions that were 'a thousand times more pernicious than the disease that they were intended to guard against.'[40] Victor Godefroy, a French physician, was waylaid by a mob in the neighborhood of Santa Cruz 'while administering medicine to an Indian suffering from the effects of the Epidemical complaint, and after being beat and cut in the most barbarous way, he was taken to the Police Office where he was put in the stocks.'[41] His brother, Félix-François Godefroy, a naturalist sent to

[37] Bantug, *A Short History of Medicine in the Philippines*, p.30.

[38] 'Peter Dobell on the Massacre of Foreigners in Manila, 1820,' *Bulletin of the New York Public Library*, vol.7 (1903): 198–200 (199).

[39] Dean C. Worcester, *A History of Asiatic Cholera in the Philippine Islands: With an Appendix* (Manila: Bureau of Printing, 1909), p.179.

[40] Bantug, *A Short History of Medicine in the Philippines*, p.30.

[41] *The Calcutta Annual Register for the Year 1821* (Calcutta: Government Gazette Press, 1823), pp.256–258 (257).

gather specimens in a scientific mission under the auspices of Duke Élie Decazes (1780–1860), was less fortunate. Having arrived some seven weeks previously, he was staying in a hotel close to the San Fernando Bridge in Binondo, the commercial heart of the city. As Dobell observed: 'In the French ships, had arrived a naturalist sent out by the government to make collections, & some persons, who intended to remain in the Philippines to cultivate sugar, cotton &c &c.' Godefroy's collection of 'serpents and other venomous reptiles' gave credence to local suspicions of the foreigners' malevolent intent.[42] According to Dobell, among the naturalist's possessions was 'a quantity of Peruvian bark' (in other words *cinchona*). Godefroy was cut down while seeking refuge in the house of another Frenchman.

On October 20, de Folgueras promulgated a decree 'to the natives of the Filipinas Islands, and especially to those in the district of Tondo,' in which he censured 'certain malicious persons' for inciting 'a general frenzy' against foreigners.[43] As Filomeno Aguilar has observed, although 'only obliquely criticized in the decree, members of the friar community, according to later accounts, were deemed responsible for the macabre episode.'[44] There had been longstanding tension between the religious orders and the civil administration. Given the small number of peninsular and Mexican Spaniards in the archipelago, as well as the geographical distance from Madrid, the colonial state was obliged to depend on the religious orders to administer the colony. Missions and parishes doubled as administrative centers, contributing to the increasing wealth and influence of the friar curates. Governors regularly complained of clerical abuses and appealed to Madrid with little effect.

It was not the Europeans, however, but the Chinese who bore the brunt of local Filipino hostility and were, by all accounts, the chief victims of the Manila massacre. The links between southern China and maritime Southeast Asia were longstanding and many settlements across the region had significant Chinese populations comprised of merchants and artisans who monopolized enterprise and industry, 'filling the commercial space between ruler and ruled' (Chapter 2). From the second half of the sixteenth century, Chinatowns began to develop in port cities and the Chinese were increasingly categorized as a distinct ethnic group: they were known as *sangleys*, a word that likely derives from the Hokkien dialect of

---

[42] 'Massacre at Manilla,' *The Annual Register, or a View of the History, Politics, and Literature of the Year 1821* (London: Baldwin, Cradock, and Joy, 1822), pp.314–324 (322).

[43] Emma Helen Blair and James Alexander Robertson, eds., *The Philippine Islands, 1493–1898*, 55 vols. (Cleveland, OH: Arthur H. Clark Co., 1907), LI, pp.43–44.

[44] Filomeno V. Aguilar, *Clash of Spirits: The History of Power and Sugar Planter Hegemony on a Visayan Island* (Honolulu: Hawaii University Press, 1998), pp.16–26.

coastal southeast China and means 'trader.'[45] In the Spanish Philippines, the prominence of the *sangleys* and their strategic position as intermediaries between Western and native economies made them particular targets for aggrieved sections of the native and Spanish communities. The colonial regime remained deeply distrustful of the Chinese, who were periodically persecuted and faced with expulsion. In 1766, for example, they had been expelled from the Philippines in retribution for collaborating with the British during the occupation of Manila and Cavite, an event alluded to by Benoit in his explanation for the violence against them in 1820.[46] In addition to the Chinese, there was a thriving *mestizo* community (persons of mixed Chinese and Filipino ancestry). The *mestizos* were formally recognized as a distinct class in the mid eighteenth century, when they began to assume a more pivotal role in economic development as middlemen, buyers, and suppliers – as well as landowners.[47]

What light do these disquieting events in Manila in 1820 throw upon this crucial moment in Southeast Asian history? Above all, they suggest that highly local circumstances need to be understood within interregional and global contexts. The violence triggered by the cholera outbreak brought to visibility the motile world of early nineteenth-century Southeast Asia. To be sure, as we have already noted, the expansion of European power in Asia was dependent upon pre-existing Asian networks. Well before the European advance, commodities from across Asia had flowed through global circuits of exchange.[48] These networks did not cease. Long after the arrival of Europeans and the introduction of clippers and later steamships, the Chinese junk trade remained an important dimension of Southeast Asia's economic life. Yet the epidemic in Manila also underscored a new world produced by the expansion of empire, the 'opening up' of global trade, and the increasing entanglement of native and Western economies. Linked to this was the diffusion of ideas about property, race, and sovereignty. Filipino, Chinese, Indian, Persian, Armenian, French, Dutch, German, Danish, British, Portuguese, American, and Spanish individuals and communities interacted in new ways. The foreigners in Manila included missionaries, planters, sailors, soldiers, traders, diplomats, surgeons, explorers, and naturalists. We learn, for example, of a French agriculturalist, Mr. D'Arbelles, who had

---

[45] Anthony Reid, *Imperial Alchemy: Nationalism and Political Identity in Southeast Asia* (Cambridge: Cambridge University Press, 2010), pp.54–56.

[46] Edgar Wickberg, *The Chinese in Philippine Life, 1850–1898*. Revised edition (Quezon City: Ateneo de Manila University, [1965] 2000), pp.3–43.

[47] E. Wickberg, 'The Chinese Mestizo in Philippine History,' *Journal of Southeast Asian History*, vo.5, no.1 (1964): 62–100 (71).

[48] Sunil S. Amrith, *Crossing the Bay of Bengal: The Furies of Nature and the Fortunes of Migrants* (Cambridge, MA: Harvard University Press, 2013), p.61.

moved to the Philippines from the Isle de France by way of Calcutta; of a German tavern keeper, Mr. Hantleman; and of Mr. Baptist from Madras, who worked as a translator of Spanish and English.[49] The epidemic revealed a city in motion, defined by crisscrossing relations of class, race, and occupation. This was a world comprised of those on official business and those promoting private ventures; of the permanently settled and those just passing through. It was also a world of rivalry that could darken quickly into violence; a place where different regimes of value collided, sometimes fatally. The epidemic was both the outcome of global processes – of expanding empire and shifting geopolitics – even as it was shaped by highly specific economic, social, and political circumstances.

passive

The prevalence of cholera in the Philippines after 1820 has been much debated. Outbreaks occurred in the 1840s and 1860s. Although we know little about their impact, the disease in the 1860s appears to have diffused more widely through the archipelago. Some commentators have suggested that outbreaks of cholera recurred annually after 1820. As we shall see in our discussion of the Philippine–US War in Chapter 4, however, particular social and political configurations were crucial in determining the shape and scope of future epidemics there.

Epidemics and the paradigm of pervasive suspicion in Japan

Cholera was spread southeastward from Bengal by the movement of troops and trade. As a port city, Manila was a critical conjuncture, where epidemiological pathways converged. The 1820 epidemic in the Philippines revealed a society experiencing the pressures of economic, political, and social change. It was, so to speak, a society in motion. The epidemic massacre in Manila should be understood, not as the reaction to an exogenous force (cholera), but as the point where various kinds of mobility slammed into each other. The next section explores this idea of epidemic friction further, demonstrating how cholera in Japan became bound up in debates and conflicts about Japan's 'opening up' to the world. There, too, although in very different ways, cholera epidemics were symptoms and catalysts for change. The country's 'invasion' by disease was associated with Western attempts to force trading concessions on Japan: cholera, sovereignty, modern preventive technologies, and economic circulations became interlinked.

---

[49] *The Calcutta Annual Register for the Year 1821*, pp.256–258.

By 1822, cholera had dispersed to East Asia, reaching Nagasaki on Kyushu, the southernmost of Japan's four main islands. It is likely that the disease had been imported through trade from India via Southeast Asia and China. Possibly it had come directly from Batavia, albeit some commentators insisted that the disease had been introduced from the Korean peninsula by way of Tsushima and the port city of Shimonoseki. There may well have been several points of entry.[50] Although it then spread to Osaka and Kyoto on Honshu, it does not appear to have reached Edo (today's Tokyo), the largest city in Asia with a population of almost one million.[51] Contemporary observers noted the virulence of the disease and its gruesome symptoms:

In Osaka today, enormous numbers of people are dying from a severe epidemic. There are funeral rites for two and three hundred persons every day. The disease begins with diarrhea, and the stomach is severely distorted and twisted out of shape. Abdominal pains, vomiting, and cramps in the arms and legs soon follow. In this disease, after one or two diarrhetic movements, the arms and legs turn cold, and the vital pulse disappears.[52]

In Japan, the new epidemic disease was commonly called *korori* (meaning 'sudden death'), 'a native term used to depict any sudden, catastrophic illness.'[53] In its Japanized version it was also known as *korera*, and in popular culture it was represented as a hybrid beast with the ideograph for 'tiger' (*ko*) affixed to the characters for 'wolf' (*ro*) and 'badger' or 'raccoon dog' (*ri*), a monstrous combination that evoked the swift, ferocious, cunning, and mercurial nature of the disease.

Thirty-six years after this initial epidemic, cholera returned to Japan, this time purportedly reintroduced to the country from Shanghai through the port city of Nagasaki by the US battleship *Mississippi*. From Nagasaki, where it raged through the summer of 1858, cholera spread eastward to Osaka and from there to Edo, extending as far north as Hokodate on the southeast coast of Hokkaido. Estimates of mortality vary greatly, but according to one source some 200,000 people died during the epidemic, with Edo particularly hit.[54] Not surprisingly, given the numbers

[50] Ann Bowman Jannetta, *Epidemics and Mortality in Early Modern Japan* (Princeton, NJ: Princeton University Press, 1987), pp.158–159.

[51] Johnston, 'Epidemics Past and Science Present,' pp.28–29; Louis Cullen, 'Tokugawa Population: The Archival Issues,' *Japan Review*, vol.18 (2006): 129–180 (152).

[52] Tetsuo Najita, 'Ambiguous Encounters: Ogata Kōan and International Studies in Late Tokugawa Osaka.' In: James L. McClain and Wakita Osamu, eds., *Osaka: The Merchants' Capital of Early Modern Japan* (Ithaca, NY: Cornell University Press, 1999), pp.213–242 (232).

[53] Jannetta, *Epidemics and Mortality*, pp.47–49.

[54] Bettina Gramlich-Oka, 'The Body Economic: Japan's Cholera Epidemic of 1858 in Popular Discourse,' *East Asian Science, Technology, and Medicine*, vol.30 (2009): 32–73 (35); Johnston, 'Epidemics Past, and Science Present,' p.30.

affected, the epidemic was widely reported in popular broadsides known as *kawaraban* (a word that literally means 'tile-block printing'). These were 'quickly produced, inexpensive woodblock prints featuring various types of texts, illustrations, and even maps of disaster areas and the like.'[55] Contemporary accounts of the 1858 epidemic convey the prevalent fear and panic induced by the disease. The writer Hata Ginkei (1796–1870) in his work *Dreams Along the Street* (1858), which was dedicated to those who died during the epidemic, describes various popular superstitions about cholera, including how the disease was brought on by a comet, how villages were saved by local deities, and how a talisman-carrying ferryman prevented cholera demons from crossing a river.[56] The satirical writer and journalist Kanagaki Robun (1829–1894) – the pen name of Nozaki Bunzō – also published a description of the epidemic entitled *Reports about the Cholera Epidemic of 1858*, essentially a collation of official notices, rumors, pamphlets, and illustrated broadsheet stories. Assuming the voice of a fictional narrator called Kinton Dōjin, Robun records the panicked responses and social turmoil produced by the epidemic (Figure 1.3).[57]

Coffins were stacked in the streets and funeral processions were a common sight. The air was infused with smoke from overflowing crematoria and the wafting stench of decomposing bodies. During the epidemic, people participated in so-called 'cholera festivals' to ward off the disease, rituals that incorporated elements from earlier 'smallpox festivals' staged to appease the smallpox deity (*kami*). Red smallpox prints (*hōsō-e*) were produced as amulets, since the deity was thought to favor the color red.[58] It has been argued that smallpox served as the prototypical disease in Japan, shaping responses to subsequent epidemics, including those of cholera. Smallpox had been introduced to Japan by the eighth century, when the first recorded epidemic occurred, killing perhaps a third of the population with a particularly high mortality amongst children. As Akihito Suzuki has observed, 'the epidemiological profile of the disease moulded and conditioned people's response to epidemic diseases in general. Centuries of smallpox epidemics had formed the basis, from which had developed anti-cholera measures and other public health policies in modern Japan.'[59] Although the cause of cholera was ascribed to miasma

---

[55] Gerald Groemer, 'Singing the News: *Yomiuri* in Japan During the Edo and Meiji Periods,' *Harvard Journal of Asiatic Studies*, vol.54, no.1 (1994): 233–261 (235).

[56] Johnston, 'Epidemics Past, and Science Present,' p.31.

[57] Gramlich-Oka, 'The Body Economic,' pp.37–41.

[58] Hartmut O. Rottermund, 'Demonic Affliction or Contagious Disease? Changing Perceptions of Smallpox in the Late Edo Period,' *Japanese Journal of Religious Studies*, vol.28, nos.3/4 (2001): 373–398.

[59] Akihito Suzuki, 'Smallpox and the Epidemiological Heritage of Modern Japan: Towards a Total History,' *Medical History*, vol.55, no.3 (2011): 313–318 (314).

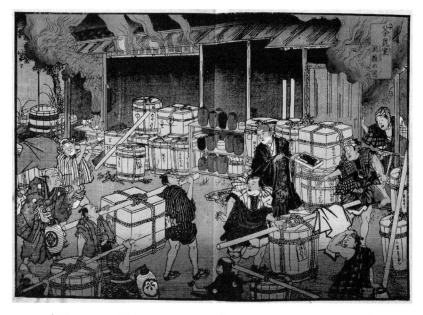

Figure 1.3. 'Edo crematory during the cholera epidemic of 1858.' In: Kinton Dōjin [Kanagaki Robun], *Ansei Umanoaki Korori Ryūkō Ki* (Edo: Tenjudō, 1858). Courtesy: Special Collections, Waseda University Library.

Deadly labor: Picturing cholera

Japanese *ukiyo-e* ('pictures of the floating world') provide insights into how disease and health were understood and experienced in nineteenth-century Japan. Although this genre of illustration developed out of the milieus of pleasure quarters in cities – the so-called 'floating world' of brothels, restaurants, and theaters – prints were also produced dealing with natural disasters, including the treatment and prevention of diseases such as smallpox, measles, and cholera. Figure 1.3 from Kanagaki Robun's account of the cholera epidemic, which was published under the pseudonym Kinton Dōjin, depicts a crematorium in Edo. Workers toil by the light of lanterns, carrying corpses in numbered boxes for incineration in a giant furnace. Smoke from joss sticks drifts from a shrine.

or harmful exhalations, many believed that the disease was the work of malignant spirits. Exorcising ceremonies were performed, involving beating drums and firing guns. Shrines produced papier-mâché talismans to ward off the disease. Coming after the destruction caused by the 1855 Edo earthquake, some viewed the epidemic as a divine portent and retribution for what they perceived as Japan's inexorable moral decline.

The cholera outbreak of 1858 aggravated old divisions and brought to light new ones. It occurred at a moment of crisis in Japan, which marked the end of the Tokugawa or Edo period (1603–1868). From the seventeenth century, Japan had been ruled by military commanders, or *shoguns*, of the Tokugawa family, who had imposed a rule of virtual isolation on the country, known as *sakoku* (meaning literally 'locked country'). A series of edicts placed restrictions on foreign traders and missionaries and eventually excluded them altogether. The exceptions were the Chinese and the Dutch, who from 1641 were confined to the manmade island of Deshima in the Bay of Nagasaki, originally constructed for the Portuguese. There were also restrictions on the Japanese, who were forbidden from traveling overseas, a policy of isolation that lasted more than two centuries.[60]

Increasingly, however, Western powers – and in particular the United States – began to apply pressure on Japan to open up. In China, Britain had forced the Qing dynasty to accede to demands for further British trading rights after victory in the two Opium Wars of 1839–1842 and 1856–1860. In 1842, under the terms of the Treaty of Nanking (Nanjing), Britain was ceded the island of Hong Kong and five 'treaty ports' were established – in effect, Western extraterritorial enclaves in China. There, the British (with other nationalities) acquired trading 'concessions' or 'settlements' in the port cities, giving them degrees of independence under the jurisdiction of foreign consuls. A second group of treaty ports was established after 1860, serving as 'a vehicle for Western interests in trade, diplomacy and evangelism.'[61] Extraterritoriality has often been presented as a Western imposition that overrode indigenous legal traditions. However, such a view discounts 'the legacy of pluralism' that characterized China and Japan, where different laws and courts existed for different ethnic, social, and professional groups, and where indigenous traditions mediated new Western extraterritorial communities.[62]

---

[60] J. E. Hoare, *Japan's Treaty Ports and Foreign Settlement: The Uninvited Guests, 1858–1899* (Folkstone: Japan Library, 1994).
[61] Frances Wood, *No Dogs and Not Many Chinese: Treaty Port Life in China, 1843–1943* (London: John Murray, 1998), p.1.
[62] Pär Kristoffer Cassel, *Grounds of Judgment: Extraterritoriality and Imperial Power in Nineteenth-Century China and Japan* (Oxford: Oxford University Press, 2012).

US demands on Japan reflected the United States' growing importance as a Pacific power. In 1848, the United States had gained control of California following the Mexican–American War (1846–1848). US clippers passed Japan on their route to Canton, while whalers operated in Japanese waters. By the mid-century, the rise of steam-powered vessels necessitated strategically located coaling stations. In 1853, Commodore Matthew C. Perry (1794–1858) of the US Navy had threatened the Japanese government with a squadron of warships, insisting that Japan open to trade. The following year, the Treaty of Kanagawa (Yokohama) was signed, allowing the establishment of a US consulate in Japan and permitting US traders to operate from the ports of Shimoda and Hakodate. Significantly, on July 29, 1858, a few weeks before the cholera outbreak, the US–Japanese Treaty of Amity and Commerce was concluded on board the US warship *Powhatan* in Edo Bay, marking what was to be the first of the 'unequal treaties.' Other treaties were swiftly concluded with Holland, Russia, Britain, and France. Treaty ports, similar to those in China, were established at Osaka, Kanagawa, Nagasaki, Niigata, and Hyōgo (Kobe). This pattern of 'informal imperialism' through the institution of extraterritorial treaty ports and fixed trade tariffs had been completed by 1869 and was to remain in force until 1899.[63]

There was intense debate in Japan about the merits of seclusion and the risks of acceding to Western demands. These occurred against a backdrop of political crisis set off by the death of the young shogun Tokugawa Iesada (1824–1858), possibly from cholera. To many Japanese commentators, the second ongoing Opium War (also known as the 'Arrow War') reinforced the dangers faced by Japan from belligerent Western powers. Those who advocated opening up argued that concessions were unavoidable. Disapproval of foreign incursions into Japan overlapped with mounting opposition to the shogunate's authority. An anti-Tokugawa movement formed with a simple credo: 'Revere the Emperor and Expel the Barbarians.'[64] To avert an anti-foreign backlash, the shogunate sought to de-couple associations of cholera with foreigners by employing terms for gastrointestinal disease, rather than the foreign word *korera*.[65]

---

[63] Harald Fuess, 'Informal Imperialism and the 1879 Hesperia Incident: Containing Cholera and Challenging Extraterritoriality in Japan,' *Japan Review*, vol.27 (2014): 103–140 (105).

[64] Brett L. Walker, *A Concise History of Japan* (Cambridge: Cambridge University Press, 2015), p.145.

[65] Gramlich-Oka, 'The Body Economic,' p.45.

From the outset, however, responsibility for the epidemic was laid on the unwelcome foreigners, and conspiracies about the origins of the disease abounded. As one Japanese observer noted in 1858: 'When the English sailors land, they look for a well and check the quality of the water. The people from that area spread the wild rumor that the Englishmen are poisoning wells.' Other rumors circulated about foreigners willfully contaminating the sea and local fish stocks, which led to the boycotting of fishmongers and a surge in demand for other non-seafood, such as vegetables and poultry.[66]

Reports persisted that cholera was the 'Englishman's poison,' imported to Japan in much the same way that opium was alleged to have been brought into China as a stratagem for subjugating the Qing Empire.[67] The naval engineer and statesman Katsu Kaishū (1823–1899), who was in Nagasaki in 1858, commented on a widely held conviction that 'officers from British ships had come ashore and sought out wells and poisoned the water within them,' thereby causing the epidemic. Johannes Pompe van Meerdervoort (1829–1908), a Dutch physician who had been invited by the Tokugawa *bakufu* (administration or government of the shogunate) to teach Western medicine at the Kaigun Denshujo Naval Academy, likewise noted the hostility to foreigners, adding that there was 'a feeling of being in a state of war.' As cholera swept through Nagasaki, the Japanese 'began to say that the cause of the disease was that Japan had been opened by the foreign countries, and soon they even regarded foreigners like myself as the enemies.'[68]

The epidemic became entangled with domestic and international politics. Like Pompe van Meerdervoort, Matsumoto Jun (1832–1907), who served as personal physician to the last shogun, Tokugawa Yoshinobu (1837–1913), dealt with the cholera epidemic at some length in his memoirs and commented: 'At the time the theory of 'expel the barbarians' was very popular, so to take the corpse of a Japanese, even that of a criminal, and give it to a foreigner so that he can divide the entrails and cut up the eyes was something of consequence to the honor (*taimen*) of the nation (*kokka*).' Japanese corpses are explicitly equated, here, with 'Japan.' The violent penetration of the Japanese body is analogized with a foreign assault akin to the country's invasion by a foreign-imported disease from Shanghai and India. Although the shogunate had minimal

---

[66] Gramlich-Oka, 'The Body Economic,' p.45.

[67] Najita, 'Ambiguous Encounters.' In: McClain and Osamu, eds., *Osaka*, p.233.

[68] Susan L. Burns, 'Constructing the National Body: Public Health and the Nation in Meiji Japan.' In: Timothy Brook and André Schmid, eds., *Nation Work: Asian Elites and National Identities* (Ann Arbor: University of Michigan Press, 2000), pp.17–50 (21–22).

involvement in managing the epidemic, by the final years of the Tokugawa era, 'the body was being refigured as the object of social and political concern.'[69] As Michael Bourdaghs has observed of this period, 'the state of individual human bodies was repeatedly linked to the well-being of the nation as a whole.'[70]

Sickness was implicitly equated with the political instability set in motion by cholera and foreign intervention. Correspondingly, disease was associated with economic disruption. Defending and regulating the body, ensuring its restoration to health, became a political imperative that extended from the individual body of the citizen to that of the nation. At the same time, this matrix of health, disease, political order, and economic vigor was cast in terms of flows and obstruction: Japan's 'opening up' to Western trade and the country's exposure to toxic foreign ways; the transmission of disease and counter-efforts to halt infective circulations; as well as the ramifications for health of blocking vital economic exchanges. Such equations drew upon and reconfigured prevalent views from the Edo period that attributed pathology to hindered flow. Disease was associated with unhealthy accumulations: ideas of harmful bodily torpor recapitulated the dangers of economic inertia. 'The diseases of the body,' Kuriyama notes in his reflections on popular Japanese prints that depict a deadly measles epidemic in the early 1860s, 'are almost secondary by-products of the primary problem of a diseased society; the physical pathology of stagnant flow is the corporeal translation of the social sin of indolence.'[71]

With the restoration of the Meiji Emperor in 1868, there was increasing focus on reforming Japan's 'national body politic' (*kokutai*). 'Hygiene,' or *eisei*, became a key word of the era and cholera was known as 'the mother of hygiene,' since it was in response to the cholera epidemics that *eisei* was developed. In 1869, Iwasa Jun (1836–1912) and Sagara Chian (1836–1906) were delegated with the task of establishing a modern medical system. Prussia, in particular, presented a model of nation-building that could be emulated. The pace of institutional change quickened after 1877, when cholera struck again just as the new Meiji government confronted the Satsuma Rebellion, an uprising of disgruntled

---

[69] Burns, 'Constructing the National Body.' In: Brook and Schmid, eds., *Nation Work*, pp.23–24.

[70] Michael Bourdaghs, 'The Disease of Nationalism, the Empire of Hygiene,' *Positions: East Asia Cultures Critique*, vol.6, no.3 (1998): 637–673 (643).

[71] Shigehisa Kuriyama, 'Fukushin: Some Observations on Economic Development and the Imagination of the Body in Japanese Medicine of the Edo Period.' In: Yōzaburō Shirahata and W. J. Boot, eds., *Two Faces of the Early Modern World: The Netherlands and Japan in the 17th and 18th Centuries* (Kyoto: International Research Center for Japanese Studies, 2001), pp.47–58 (52).

samurai. Indeed, it is likely that troops returning to the cities from the Rebellion helped to spread the disease. The case of the *Hesperia* in 1879 – a German merchant ship that broke Japanese quarantine regulations and entered the port of Yokohama illegally – reignited debates about the dangers posed to Japan by Western extraterritoriality.[72]

A Bureau of Hygiene was founded within the Home Ministry in 1875, with a remit to oversee medical and sanitary issues. During the 1877 cholera outbreak, quarantine and isolation procedures were rigorously implemented, public gatherings prohibited, and restrictions enforced on the passage of people and goods from infected areas. Local sanitary committees were established and sanitary officers appointed. Police enforced in-house quarantine, daubing the doors of cholera-affected houses with the characters '*Cholera Here.*' In this way, disease became a highly visible 'public affair, publicized in the newspapers in dramatic accounts of police roundups of those who tried to escape quarantine.' The encroachment by government into the hitherto private realm of health was unprecedented, reaching 'a degree previously only experienced by those suspected of serious crimes.'[73]

The US physician Duane B. Simmons (1834–1889), chairman of the Yokohama Foreign Board of Health who worked at the city's Juzen Hospital, noted of the 1877 epidemic in Yokohama: 'A special police force was detailed, and physicians with necessary medicines were placed in attendance at the several police stations, where it was ordered that all new cases of cholera should be reported. Notices were posted on the main entrance of the residence of affected persons, announcing the existence of the disease on the premises.' Carbolic acid, or phenol, was used to disinfect property, while the 'matting, bedding and clothing of those attacked' were destroyed and the bodies of the dead cremated. Summing up, Simmons commented that the response to the 1877 epidemic, which he had helped to orchestrate, marked 'the first attempt made by the Japanese government to combat the scourge by scientific measures.'[74] Ironically, although the introduction of cholera into Japan had been widely associated with foreigners, Westerners in the treaty ports were at the forefront of the battle against the disease. Prints of the 1877 epidemic depict jets of phenol being discharged from cannon against a sword-wielding demon, while a 'prevention squad,' clad in Western-style military uniform, launches a regimented anti-cholera offensive.

[72] Fuess, 'Informal Imperialism and the 1879 Hesperia Incident.'
[73] Rogaski, *Hygienic Modernity*, pp.151–152.
[74] D. B. Simmons, 'Cholera Epidemics in Japan.' In: *China: Imperial Maritime Customs, Series 2, Medical Reports for the Half-Year Ended 30th September 1879*, no.18 (Shanghai: Statistical Department of the Inspectorate General, 1880), pp.1–30 (10).

Not surprisingly, intrusive government actions were resented and generated considerable public opposition. The forceful removal of cholera patients into isolation sparked rumors of sinister plots, as well as reports about the nefarious carryings-on of malevolent doctors. Hospitals were viewed as alien spaces by many Japanese, who were also suspicious of Western medicine. Police and physicians were attacked and, in some vicinities, full-blown rioting took place. Speaking in 1906 before a meeting of local officials, Nagayo Sensai observed that it was as a result of the work of the Bureau of Health during the cholera epidemics in the late 1870s 'that society began to have a little awareness of the necessity for hygiene.'[75]

By the 1880s, in part as a result of the experience of cholera, a functioning public health system was in place with a Central Sanitary Board and a Sanitary Bureau, along with a sanitary police force, as well as a network of local hygiene associations. Hygiene became a state-driven ideology that sought to inculcate in citizens a consciousness of their own bodies. Indeed, the disciplinary connotations of hygiene are intimated in the Japanese word *eisei*, which ultimately derives from a Chinese character meaning 'to police or patrol an area.'[76] Textbooks emphasized the importance of home hygiene, while hygiene was progressively incorporated into education from the 1890s, as the Bureau turned its attention to enforcing its practices in schools. The aim, in short, was to create new Japanese subjects who would learn to police their own bodies.[77] The break with the past, which this system represented, has perhaps been over-emphasized, and the earlier influences of Western medicine in Japan overlooked. Medical modernization has also tended to be viewed solely as the initiative of the centralizing state.[78] However, the role of the state in defining how sickness and health were understood, and the intrusive measures to which the body were subject, were in fact strongly contested as the case of cholera demonstrates.

So far in this section, I have suggested that cholera epidemics in Japan foregrounded complex external and internal processes. While they need to be viewed in a geopolitical context, nineteenth-century cholera epidemics should also be understood in relation to the shifting relationship between the state, public authorities, and the individual in Japanese society. Arguments about Japan's 'opening up' to global markets under the

---

[75] Burns, 'Constructing the National Body.' In: Brook and Schmid, eds., *Nation Work*, p.27.

[76] Johnston, *The Modern Epidemic*, p.179.

[77] Sabine Frühstück, *Colonizing Sex: Sexology and Social Control in Modern Japan* (Berkeley: California University Press, 2003), p.50.

[78] Suzuki and Suzuki, 'Cholera, Consumer, and Citizenship.' In: Ebrahimnejad, ed., *The Development of Modern Medicine in Non-Western Countries*, p.185.

pressure of Western powers, or the exclusive focus on the spread of disease, often ignore these multiple, dynamic contexts. Disease amplified tensions and conflicts within Japanese society: it served as a trigger for change, even as it revealed changes that had begun long before the epidemics struck.

Here, we might return to the idea of Japan as a culture of translation discussed briefly in the Introduction. We have already seen how 'cholera' was translated through the language of the monstrous and pictured as a hybrid monster – part tiger, wolf, and badger. Instead of viewing Meiji hygienic discourse as entailing the subjugation of traditional values, we might reconsider the relationship between modernity and tradition as one of mutual translation: imported ideas were reconfigured as they interacted with inherited beliefs and values.[79] One example of this process is the emphasis in popular responses to the cholera on the importance of a dietary regime. In addition to *korori/korera*, the term *kakuran* was also employed to describe cholera. This was the translation of a disease category within Chinese medicine that referred to a condition caused by excessive eating and drinking, which led to a corresponding cooling of the stomach. In seeking to ward off disease, people took advantage of a consumer market economy to buy 'healthy' food to assuage the symptoms of *kakuran*. The development of a market system and a consumer culture, as well as the commercialization of health-seeking behavior, were enabled by advances in communication, which underpinned Edo's position as a domestic consumer hub.[80]

The cholera epidemics thus reveal continuities between early Edo, traditional *yōjō* (a regimen for nurturing a healthy life), Western medicine, and popular culture – continuities that are often ignored in histories that emphasize rupture and dissent. From this perspective, at least, it becomes evident that the Meiji promotion of a hygienic and healthy 'national body' did not entail the wholesale removal of traditional beliefs and values, but their re-inscription into the modernization process itself. As Miri Nakamura has noted in her discussion of the writing of Izumi Kyōka (1873–1939), and specifically in relation to his tale *The Holy Man of Mount Kōya* (1900), Western knowledge of hygiene was translated into the language of the supernatural, with disease located in the hybrid bodies of monstrous women. The supernatural was not an anti-modern, irrational force, but operated in complicity with a modern hygienic discourse. Such work

---

79 Miri Nakamura, 'Monstrous Language: The Translation of Hygienic Discourse in Izumi Kyōka's *The Holy Man of Mount Kōya*.' In: Indra Levy, ed., *Translation in Modern Japan*, pp.165–185.

80 Suzuki and Suzuki, 'Cholera, Consumer, and Citizenship.' In: Ebrahimnejad, ed., *The Development of Modern Medicine in Non-Western Countries*, pp.190–191, 197, 199.

reminds us that Meiji modernity should not be construed as a simple imitation of its Western counterpart, but as a more complex formation, where 'foreign' and 'native' elements comingled.[81]

Nonetheless, as we have seen, hygiene as a form of disciplinary practice was critical in forging the Japanese nation. It also became central to Japan's subsequent imperial expansion in Taiwan, Korea, and Manchuria (Chapters 3 and 4). In 1905, Korea was compelled to agree to the setting up of a Japanese protectorate, leading to the country's full annexation in 1910. Epidemic preventive measures – namely the control of infection by civil and military policing – became a key component of colonial governance. It was the pro-Japanese Gabo Reform government (1894–1896), and not the Japanese colonial government, that first sought to establish a sanitary police system in Korea. However, under Japanese rule, the police assumed control of quarantines and acquired intrusive powers of surveillance over the daily life of Koreans. Army and naval doctors were appointed as directors of provincial hospitals, while the emphasis was on identifying and isolating disease carriers, rather than promoting prevention and treatment. By 1911, the sanitizing system was wholly in place with the police deputed to oversee sanitation work.[82]

Trade and plague in China: From Yunnan to Hong Kong

The previous two cases have focused on cholera, which caused mass mortality across much of Asia during the nineteenth century, impacting upon the development of emergent institutions of public health. 'It is in the magnitude of the *reaction* to it,' writes Hamlin, 'that cholera stands out as the signal disease of the nineteenth century.'[83] The first nine international sanitary conferences between 1851 and 1894 were convened expressly to decide on global measures to prevent cholera's spread through the movement of goods and people from Asia, with cholera at the forefront of international debates about quarantine.

In the final decade of the nineteenth century, bubonic plague was to rehearse many of the same issues as cholera. How far could the state legitimately intercede in the private lives of its subjects? To what extent was it possible to sift out damaging circulations from healthy flows? Beyond this was the question of where the disease came from and how, given its

[81] Nakamura, 'Monstrous Language.' In: Levy, ed., *Translation in Modern Japan*, pp.180–181.

[82] Park Yunjae, 'Sanitizing Korea: Anti-Cholera Activities of the Police in Early Colonial Korea,' *Seoul Journal of Korean Studies*, vol.23, no.2 (2010): 151–171 (151).

[83] Hamlin, *Cholera*, p.4.

obscure etiology, it could be stopped. Bubonic plague is a disease now known to be caused by the zoonotic bacteria *Yersinia pestis*, transmitted by the bite of infected fleas that are hosted by rodents, notably rats. In some cases, bubonic plague results in distinctive swollen lymph nodes or 'buboes' appearing in the armpits and groin areas of those infected. Bubonic plague is one of three forms of plague infection, the others being septicemic plague and pneumonic plague (Chapter 4). Even after the plague bacillus was discovered in June 1894 in Hong Kong by the Swiss-born but naturalized Frenchman Alexandre Yersin (1863–1943) and the Japanese bacteriologist Kitasato Shibasaburō (1853–1931), however, its route of transmission was unknown (Figure 1.4).[84] It was not until 1898 that Paul-Louis Simond (1858–1947) discovered the disease's vector – rat fleas – in India.

Like cholera, plague dispersed through expanding pathways of trade. From inland China it diffused to the Pearl River Delta. Once it reached Hong Kong in early 1894, it was shipped to port cities across the globe: Hong Kong, Bombay, Alexandria, Porto, Buenos Aires, Rio de Janeiro, Honolulu, San Francisco, Sydney, and Cape Town.[85] Its dissemination highlighted the extent of global interconnectivity by the end of the century, as well as the role that new modes of travel, such as steamships and railways, played in the global propulsion of infection. Millions were to die: by one count as many as 11 million in India alone.

As we saw in the discussion of the 'unequal treaties' imposed upon Japan, by the mid nineteenth century East Asian countries were facing increasing pressure to open up to Western trade. The justification for this enforced accession was the manifest benefits that progress, under-girded by free trade, would bring to the recipient country. Lord Macart-ney, dispatched from Britain to the Qing court on an official mission in 1793, had famously likened China to a floundering boat, which had somehow contrived to stay afloat, but which would soon, on account of its decrepit condition, be 'dashed to pieces on the shore.'[86] Closed and stagnant, the dynamism of Western trade would be its salvation. Qing China was viewed as a nation in terminal decline, earning it the sobri-quet the 'sick man of Asia' in debates about the need for reform and modernization during the final years of the nineteenth century.

---

[84] L. Fabian Hirst, *The Conquest of Plague: A Study of the Evolution of Epidemiology* (Oxford: Clarendon Press, 1953), p.107.

[85] Myron Echenberg, *Plague Ports: The Global Urban Impact of Bubonic Plague, 1894–1901* (New York: New York University Press, 2010).

[86] J. L. Cranmer-Byng, ed., *An Embassy to China: Being the Journal Kept by Lord Macartney During His Embassy to the Emperor Ch'ien-lung, 1793–1794* (London: Longmans, 1962), p.213.

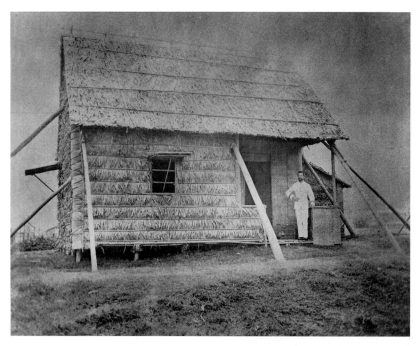

Figure 1.4. 'Alexandre Yersin in front of his matshed, Hong Kong (1894).' Courtesy: Institut Pasteur, Paris.

Matshed laboratory: Identifying the plague

The physician and microbiologist Alexandre Yersin was a keen amateur photographer, who took numerous pictures of native people and villages during his travels through Central Vietnam and Cambodia between 1890 and 1894. Several of his photographs of Hong Kong taken during the plague survive. Yersin was dispatched to the British crown colony by the French colonial authorities, who were anxious about the disease spreading to Indochina (Chapter 2). Yersin met with a decidedly lukewarm reception in Hong Kong and there was intense rivalry between Yersin and Kitasato in the race to identify the plague 'germ.' While the Japanese scientist and his team worked in the Kennedy Town Hospital, Yersin had a makeshift laboratory constructed where he pursued experimental work (note the caged white rabbit by Yersin's feet in Figure 1.4). In June 1894, Yersin discovered the bacillus and his seminal paper on the bubonic plague was published in the *Annales de l'Institut Pasteur*. From 1967, the plague bacillus has been known after him as *Yersinia pestis*.

Robert Peckham, 'Matshed Laboratory: Colonies, Cultures, and Bacteriology.' In: Robert Peckham and David M. Pomfret, eds., *Imperial Contagions: Medicine, Hygiene, and Cultures of Planning in Asia* (Hong Kong: Hong Kong University Press, 2013), pp.123–147.

The Qing, originally from Manchuria (Chapter 4), had overthrown the previous Han-Chinese Ming dynasty in 1644, consolidating their power with the conquest of Taiwan in 1683. At its height, Qing China was a vast multiethnic empire. Although there were signs of new stresses in the eighteenth century, the reign of Emperor Qianlong (1711–1799) saw the integration of extensive territory into the Chinese state. China roughly doubled in size, a strategic new frontier was established in the West, and from the mid eighteenth century the growth of cities encouraged long-distance trade. These economic and social developments created an environment that facilitated the spread of infectious disease, and in particular the diffusion of plague from the province of Yunnan in the southwest of the country that borders on present-day Burma, Laos, and Vietnam.[87]

While some scholars have insisted that the plague was never truly endemic in Yunnan, and that the infection had come overland via caravans from Central Asia, others have maintained that plague was indeed endemic in Yunnan in species of native rodents, including the yellow-chested rat. Although the identification of earlier epidemics with plague remains largely conjectural, there is some evidence to suggest that the plague was implicated. According to one report, the scholar and statesman Hong Liangji (1746–1809) had noted the association of a plague-like infectious disease with rats in Yunnan in the eighteenth century:

Shi Tau-Nan, the son of Shi Fan, now the Governor of Wang-Kiang, was notorious for his [poetic] gift, and was only thirty-six years old when he died... Then, in Cháu-Chau [in Yunnan] it happened that in daytime strange rats appeared in the houses, and lying down on the ground, perished with blood-spitting. There was not a man who escaped the instantaneous death after being infected with the miasma. Tau-Nan composed thereon a poem, entitled 'Death of Rats,' the masterpiece of his; and a few days after, he himself died from this queer rat epidemic.[88]

---

[87] Carol Benedict, *Bubonic Plague in Nineteenth-Century China* (Stanford, CA: Stanford University Press, 1996), pp.49–99.

[88] Kumagusu Minakata, 'Plague in China,' *Nature*, vol.59 (February 16, 1899): 370.

The historian Carol Benedict has argued that the plague was a consequence of development; rather than proof of decay, it was a sign of economic vigor. In the first half of the nineteenth century, commercial traffic between Yunnan and Lingnan – a region that comprises the provinces of Guangxi and Guangdong – intensified as a result of the domestic opium trade. Yunnan became progressively integrated into a larger economy to the extent that by 1850, when plague broke out, the disease was able to spread quickly from Kunming, Dali, and Mengzi to towns along major trade routes. In other words, the appearance of plague in Yunnan and its spread to the southeastern littoral were directly connected with movements of populations and goods that signaled frontier expansion.[89]

Conflicts within China were also to determine the disease's epidemiology. The Emperor Qianlong's military campaigns in Central Asia, Burma, and Vietnam took place in an unsettling domestic context of indigenous rebellions, which began to occur in different parts of the Chinese Empire. These tensions were to persist under Qianlong's successors. Particularly from the 1850s, as Benedict has suggested, social unrest and conflict deflected the pathways of the Yunnan opium trade to Beihai and the Leizhou peninsula in southern Guangdong. The Panthay Rebellion (1856–1873), a revolt of the Muslim Hui people against the Qing, resulted in large numbers of refugees. Soldiers were reported to have perished from the plague amongst the imperial forces fighting in the campaign against the leader of the rebellion, Du Wenxiu, in 1867.[90] Traveling through Yunnan during the insurrection as a member of a French diplomatic mission, the customs administrator Émile Rocher (1846–1924) drew a map of the plague's progression across the province, noting connections between the conditions in besieged cities and the intensified movement around the province, which allowed plague to disperse more widely. Rocher hypothesized that the disease had originally been introduced from Burma, or possibly by pilgrims returning from Mecca.[91]

The Taiping Rebellion (1850–1864) – in effect a full-scale civil war – also disrupted trade and created critical diversions. This anti-dynastic rebellion was led by Hong Xiuquan (1814–1864), who believed himself to be Jesus's younger brother and proclaimed himself 'King of the Heavenly Kingdom of Great Peace' (*Taiping*). Hong gathered 20,000 followers and in 1851 they marched from the province of Guangxi northeast to Wuchang on the Yangtze River (Chang Jiang), before pushing on to

[89] Benedict, *Bubonic Plague*, pp.49–99.
[90] David G. Atwill, *The Chinese Sultanate: Islam, Ethnicity and the Panthay Rebellion in Southwest China, 1856–1873* (Stanford, CA: Stanford University Press, 2005), p.172.
[91] Émile Rocher, 'Notes sur la peste au Yün-nan.' In: *La province chinoise de Yün-Nan*, 2 vols. (Paris: Leroux, 1879–1880), II, pp.279–280.

Nanjing, where the Taiping established a government.[92] The Rebellion, which took a decade for the Qing to crush and led to at least 20 million deaths, dislocated agriculture and trade, fueling the mass flight of civilians. Pestilence, including cholera and plague, flourished under such conditions. As the scholar Yu Yue (1821–1907) reportedly observed:

In the early days of the reign of T'ung Chih [Tongzhi Emperor], Yunnan was thrown into a confused state by the Taiping rebellion, and this was followed by a plague epidemic. Immediately preceding the epidemic there was found a great number of dead rats in walls and ceilings. Human beings breathing the odour of putrefaction from the dead rats invariably fell sick.[93]

Compounding this was the disturbance caused by the two Opium Wars, and the establishment of new treaty ports, which reconfigured the routes of internal trade. Throughout the 1840s, commerce along the Xi, a tributary of the Pearl River in Guangdong – the main conduit between Canton and Yunnan – and the Xun River in Guangxi was interrupted, 'first by bandits and secret-society activity and then by rebellion and open revolt as Taiping forces clashed with Qing imperial troops.' To bypass these trouble spots, traders used alternative routes across Yunnan, with Beihai near the Leizhou peninsula increasingly serving as a transit hub for their operations. 'Between 1850 and 1870,' notes Benedict, 'the triangular zone stretching from southeastern Yunnan through Tonkin to Beihai and the Leizhou peninsula was one in which the level of human movement was unusually high for a peripheral subregion.' Significantly, 'this is an ecological area where the yellow-chested rat thrives.' Plague in China was thus linked, not only to interregional trade, but to complex environmental and epidemiological factors, as well.[94]

The officers of the Imperial Maritime Customs Service (IMCS) were briefed to track epidemics, recording their absence or presence, causes, courses, and fatality. They plotted the plague's progress through southern China, cross-referencing previous IMCS reports, along with a wide array of other texts, including travel literature and historical records. Clinical and microscopic observations were intermixed with notes on the squalid living conditions of the Chinese and assessments of local traditions, superstitions, rumors, and hearsay. In 1882, Dr. J. H. Lowry, a medical officer working at Pakhoi (Beihai), recorded an outbreak there, observing that 'in nearly every house where the disease broke out the rats

[92] Stephen R. Platt, *Autumn in the Heavenly Kingdom: China, the West, and the Epic Story of the Taiping Civil War* (New York: Alfred A. Knopf, 2012), pp.305–307.
[93] Wu Lien-teh, et al., *Plague: A Manual for Medical and Public Health Workers* (Shanghai: Weishengshu National Quarantine Service, 1936), p.13.
[94] Benedict, *Bubonic Plague*, pp.56, 71.

had been coming out of their holes and dying on the floors.'[95] A few years later, A. P. Happer, commissioner of customs in Mengzi, southeast Yunnan, reported the plague's appearance, which he described as 'a kind of malignant fever' that caused 'a hard swelling to the neck, in the armpits, or in the groin.' The death of numerous rats was a harbinger of the epidemic, while cattle also appeared affected. 'Surrounded by such distressing signs,' he observed, 'it is no wonder that inhabitants of hamlets often desert their houses and belongings *en masse*, to seek immunity on the mountain side.'[96] In 1890, again in Pakhoi, Dr. A. Sharpe Deane noted the receipt of a letter from Lunchow (Longzhou) in Guangxi with news that there had been an outbreak there, and that the disease had most likely spread southwest from Bose and Nanning. By the 1890s, plague had reached the Pearl River Delta. In February 1894, there was an outbreak in Canton, a city of over 1.5 million inhabitants. Mortality figures are impossible to determine with any accuracy, given the absence of official records, with estimates ranging from 40,000 to 100,000 people killed in a matter of months.[97]

Epidemic control and the Imperial Maritime Customs Service

The IMCS was established in Shanghai in 1854 during the Taiping Rebellion, when the central Qing administration was overstretched and unable to collect tax. Although formally controlled by the Qing government, the senior echelons of the IMCS were staffed by foreign nationals and predominantly by British personnel. The Service's principal task was collecting customs duties, but its responsibilities soon extended well beyond this to include the postal administration and the management of designated treaty ports. The IMCS also promoted Western science, medicine, and technology in China. More specifically, it established a rudimentary public health

---

[95] J. H. Lowry, 'Notes on an Epidemic Disease Observed in Pakhoi in 1882.' In: *China: Imperial Maritime Customs, Series 2, Medical Reports for the Half-Year Ended 30th September 1882*, no.24 (Shanghai: Statistical Department of the Inspectorate General, 1883), pp.31–38 (33).

[96] A. P. Happer, 'Mêngtzŭ Trade Report for the Year 1889.' In: *China: Imperial Maritime Customs: Returns of Trade and Trade Reports for the Year 1889* (Shanghai: Statistical Department of the Inspectorate General, 1890), pp.533–551 (539–540).

[97] W. J. Simpson, *A Treatise on Plague: Dealing with the Historical, Epidemiological, Clinical, Therapeutic and Preventive Aspects of the Disease* (Cambridge: Cambridge University Press, 1905), p.64.

network with the appointment of medical officers who wrote regular reports on the health conditions in different treaty ports. These reports remain important documents for historians of medicine in China, shedding light on local epidemics, their spread, and evolving approaches to prevention and management. In 1870, Sir Robert Hart, who served as the inspector general of the IMCS from 1863 until his death in 1911, noted:

> It has been suggested to me that it would be well to take advantage of the circumstances in which the Customs Establishment is placed, to procure information with regard to disease amongst foreigners and natives in China; and I have, in consequence, come to the resolution of publishing half-yearly, in collected form, all that may be obtainable.

The Scottish parasitologist Patrick Manson (1844–1922) worked as a medical officer for the IMCS in Amoy (Xiamen) from 1871 to 1883, where he demonstrated that the mosquito was the host of the parasitic filarial worm that causes lymphatic filariasis, or elephantiasis. At the turn of the century, there were thousands of employees working for the IMCS in a network of customs stations and sub-branches across China. After the establishment of the Republic of China in 1912, the IMCS became known as the Chinese Maritime Customs Service.

C. A. Gordon, *An Epitome of the Reports of the Medical Officers to the Chinese Imperial Maritime Customs Service, from 1871 to 1882* (London: Baillière, Tindall, and Cox, 1884), p.xiii.

In Canton, the plague was attributed to a number of causes. While it was ascribed to miasma, it was also widely believed to be divine punishment for human transgressions. There were street processions and elaborate exorcism rituals were performed to appease the gods. Gongs were beaten and firecrackers were lit to ward off the plague demons. Since there was little tradition of quarantine in China, the Qing government's response was limited to a number of basic sanitary measures. In an official directive promulgated in April 1894, streets were ordered to be cleaned and refuse disposed of in the Pearl River. Night-soil was to be collected in covered buckets by 10 o'clock in the morning. The clothes of plague victims were to be incinerated, fishing and the slaughter of pigs were forbidden. Rewards were offered for the collection of dead rats, which were to be discarded outside the city. An illustrated Shanghai newspaper published in 1894 describes one such rat catching initiative in Guangdong, noting the futility of attempting to halt the epidemic by catching and killing rats. So-called 'benevolent societies' or philanthropic organizations (*shantang*), funded by Cantonese merchants, played a more central role through their charitable relief, including tending to the sick in hospices and providing free coffins for the poor.

Plague brought to the fore tensions between Chinese and foreigners. John Kerr (1824–1901), an American physician and Presbyterian missionary to China who witnessed the plague, declared that in contrast to colonial Hong Kong, where modern scientific methods were applied, in Canton 'Chinese medicine and Chinese superstitions had full and unrestricted sway.' Despite contrasting the responses to the epidemic in both cities, however, Kerr conceded that the disease had apparently disappeared in Canton at the same time as it had in Hong Kong.[98] Both port cities, lying some 90 miles apart, or six hours by steamer, were closely connected with 11,000 passengers moving back and forth each week. At the beginning of March, an estimated 40,000 'of the lowest class of coolies' had traveled from Canton to Hong Kong to celebrate the Lunar New Year. On May 10, after a meeting of the Sanitary Board, the emergency provisions of the Public Health Ordinance (1887) were invoked and the British crown colony was declared an infected port.

By the late nineteenth century, Hong Kong was a global hub, touted as the third-largest port of the British Empire. It was an entrepôt for the trans-shipment of goods between Europe, India, Southeast Asia, as well as regional riverine and sea trade between north and south China. Although the British had intended Hong Kong to serve as a gateway into China, in the event the traffic also worked in reverse: the new colony became a thoroughfare for Chinese migrants. With the Gold Rush from the late 1840s, the port had become the leading Pacific gateway for Chinese 'gold mountain seekers' (*gam san haak*) heading for the West Coast United States and Australia.[99] In 1900, 82,456 ships with an aggregate registered tonnage of 18,445,133, carrying over two million passengers, entered and cleared the port.[100] Intensifying cross-border traffic produced anxieties about the state's capacity to manage a fluid Chinese population. At the same time, the imposition of restrictions on the free movements of goods and people was rejected by colonial officials as undermining the very conditions that contributed to the colony's success as a world

---

[98] John Kerr, 'The Bubonic Plague,' *Chinese Medical Missionary Journal*, vol.13, no.4 (1894): 178–180 (179).

[99] Elizabeth Sinn, *Pacific Crossing: California Gold, Chinese Migration, and the Making of Hong Kong* (Hong Kong: Hong Kong University Press, 2013).

[100] 'Despatch by His Excellency the Governor on the Blue Book for 1900,' *Hongkong Sessional Papers 1901*, no.41, pp.743–746 (743).

port: namely, unhampered flow and openness. The plague outbreak in 1894 was to accentuate this tension.

Although the causal agent of the plague was discovered in Hong Kong in June 1894, the disease's mode of transmission remained unknown. The plague was widely viewed as a contagious 'filth disease,' linked to the unsanitary living conditions of the Chinese. As Dr. James A. Lowson, acting superintendent of the Government Civil Hospital, remarked in his medical report on the plague, the squalid state of the poor Chinese district of Taipingshan made it particularly vulnerable to disease: 'I am bound to admit that, if ever any place was ripe for such an epidemic, certain parts of Hongkong [sic] in May 1894 were in a condition for it to spread like wildfire.'[101] Government measures focused on sanitary interventions aimed at cleansing the Chinese districts of the colony. The Sanitary Board was strengthened with the setting up of a Permanent Committee to direct operations. By-laws were passed and confirmed by the Executive and Legislative Councils that boosted the Committee's powers significantly. Volunteers were dispatched to assist in house-to-house inspections of Chinese dwellings, and to disinfect and whitewash affected properties. Those suspected of suffering from the disease were moved to improvised isolation hospitals, including a floating hospital hulk, *Hygeia*, which had previously been used for smallpox patients (Figure 1.5).

As news of the epidemic spread, fearful Chinese residents fled the colony. In a report to the Colonial Office, Governor Sir William Robinson (1836–1912) described the Chinese abandonment of Hong Kong *en masse*: 'Compradores, contractors, shroffs, tradesmen, domestic servants and coolies all joined together in a general exodus altogether numbering some 100,000 persons.' Shops were closed, once crowded streets were deserted, and the colony's sugar refineries had ceased operation: 'No more melancholy sight than that presented by the city of Victoria at this period can well be imagined.'[102] As the *Times* of London reported: 'Half native population [of] Hongkong left, numbering 100,000. Leaving by thousands daily; 1,500 deaths; several Europeans seized; one died. Labour market paralyzed. Deaths nearly hundred daily. Government anticipates failure of opium revenue; proposes taking over and destroying all unhealthy native quarters.'[103] In an effort to prevent the disease from

---

[101] James A. Lowson, 'The Epidemic of Bubonic Plague in Hongkong, 1894,' *Hongkong Government Gazette* (April 13, 1895), pp.369–422 (371).

[102] 'Sir William Robinson to Mr. Chamberlain'(July 10, 1895). In: *British Parliamentary Papers: China 26: Correspondence, Annual Reports, Conventions, and Other Papers Relating to the Affairs of Hong Kong, 1882–1899* (Shannon: Irish University Press, 1971), pp.429–454 (434).

[103] 'News in Brief,' *Times* [of London] (June 13, 1894), p.5.

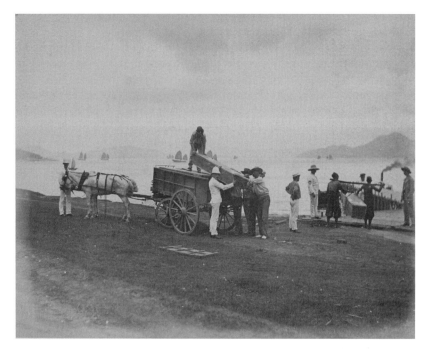

Figure 1.5. D. K. Griffith, 'Removal of the dead to steam-launches for burial at Sandy Bay (1894).' Courtesy: Bernard Quaritch (Private Collection).

D. K. Griffith's 'plague scenes'

The third plague pandemic in the 1890s coincided with a period of technological advance. Although descriptions of the plague as the 'black death' emphasized the disease's antiquity, this was the first pandemic to be concertedly photographed. From the 1860s, photography had been used as an educational and diagnostic tool in Western medical institutions in China. While photomicrography enabled the representation of the plague bacillus in scientific journals, photography was also deployed to capture plague scenes. Figure 1.5 is a photograph by the commercial photographer David Knox Griffith (1841–1897), who was based in Shanghai in the 1870s and, from the 1880s, worked in Hong Kong. Griffith's 'plague scenes' were produced in 1894 and widely circulated in the metropolitan press, including in publications such as the *Illustrated*

London News and the *Graphic*. These are some of the most enduring images of the plague in Hong Kong. Griffith was to remark on Chinese 'hostility to photographic manipulations' on the grounds that for the Chinese, 'the photographic image is the soul of the original,' presaging the subject's death. 'In my own case,' he observed, 'I have had my chair torn to pieces on the road, my coolies beaten, and my camera broken.' Despite such claims of local antipathy to photography, Griffith himself had been employed in the Hong Kong studio of Lai Afong (ca.1839–1911), one of the most influential Chinese photographers active from the 1850s to the end of the century.

D. K. Griffith, 'A Celestial Studio,' *Photographic News*, vol.19, no.873 (May 28, 1875): 259–261.

dispersing, the government clamped down on the movement of the Chinese community. The kin of those who had died attempted to evade these quarantine restrictions in order to repatriate the bodies of their relatives for proper burial in China, as opposed to their unceremonious disposal by colonial officials in a plague pit. As the *Hongkong Telegraph* declared, 'though the Chinese may perhaps be allowed to kill themselves with their epidemic, they must not and shall not be allowed to kill us all.'[104]

Many Chinese resented the government's intrusive sanitary measures and were deeply suspicious of Western medical institutions, which undermined Chinese precepts. In Canton, rumors circulated of Western doctors gouging out the eyes of children to make plague medicines, and placards were displayed 'accusing the Government of every kind of atrocity and inciting the people to take vengeance on the foreigners.' Indignant Chinese accounts of incarceration on the hulk *Hygeia* and rumors of gruesome Western medical procedures provide another perspective on the plague.

A Chinese view of the plague

While historians have explored the racial prejudices that informed harsh colonial responses to the plague, there remains a tendency to view the 1894 outbreak in triumphalist terms as the victory of modern science over native superstitions. Despite breakthroughs

[104] 'Sanitation Among Chinese,' *Hongkong Telegraph* (May 22, 1894), p.2.

in bacteriology, however, the etiology and transmission pathways of the plague remained obscure and there was little that Western medicine could do to treat the disease. As the passage below indicates, from a Chinese viewpoint, the prospect of enforced isolation on the hulk *Hygeia* was terrifying:

> As for Hongkong, the plague there is being dealt with solely by the foreign officials. A friend who arrived at Canton from that island yesterday, spoke of the enormous number of fatalities there, and the foreign methods of dealing with the plague, which appear to us ridiculous enough: He said that when a person is stricken with the plague at Hongkong the foreign officials take them to the floating hospital moored in the mid-stream. First they make the patient swallow 12 oz. of brandy, mixed with some kind of liquid medicine. Then they put six pounds of ice on top of the patient's head, while the chest, hands and feet are also loaded with a pound of ice each. In this manner not one person out of ten manages to leave that floating hospital alive. Searchers are also sent during the day time into the various dwelling-houses and if they happen to see some one in a recumbent position or taking a nap, down he is pounced upon as having been plague-stricken, and the unlucky person is forcibly taken to the floating hospital where with the remedies above mentioned his life is soon taken away. In this way numberless persons have met an undeserved fate.
>
> [Translated from a Cantonese newspaper] *North China Herald* (June 15, 1894) p.946.

There was increasing resistance to house-to-house visitations; plague cases went unreported and patients were concealed from the authorities. When 300 volunteers from the Shropshire Light Infantry and detachments from the Royal Engineers and Royal Artillery were brought in to help with the disinfection and clearance work, opposition from the Chinese intensified. As Governor Robinson observed in a dispatch to London: 'Complaints were made that the privacy of women's apartments was being invaded, that women and children were being "frightened out of their wits" by the daily visits of the Military and Police, and then it began to be rumoured that the "Foreigners" had unspeakable designs on the women and children.'[105] In a letter to the London newspaper from Kowloon, one colonial resident observed that the panic amongst the Chinese population was not so much due to fear of the plague as to dread of the Western doctor:

---

[105] 'Sir William Robinson to the Marquess of Ripon' (June 20, 1894). In: *British Parliamentary Papers*, pp.411–446.

The Chinese mind is steeped in the most soul-destroying superstition. The dread *feng shui*, the spirits of their ancestors, the myriads of demons that throng the air, are to them active principles, and as virulent as they are active. They know every European can cast spells over them, can, with an outward show of benefit, destroy their health, and they are sure we have deliberately caused this plague, for they see it passes the European by and slays the Chinaman.[106]

During the crisis, the Tung Wah Hospital Committee assumed a critical role, striving to mediate between the Chinese community and the government. Opened in 1872, the Tung Wah Hospital was a *shantang* that provided free Chinese medical assistance to the poor, along with other educational and social welfare services. The Committee also functioned as an informal lobby group for the Chinese community. A meeting of the Tung Wah Committee on May 20, which was attended by the superintendent of police and the colonial surgeon, was interrupted by an angry mob. The superintendent of police was stoned when he attempted to leave the building and his sedan chair was overturned, resulting in a detachment of mounted Sikhs called in to restore order.[107]

Under these fraught circumstances, the government agreed not to force patients onto the hospital hulk. A makeshift plague hospital was established at the 'Glass Works' building in Kennedy Town, where Chinese patients would be overseen by the Tung Wah. Nonetheless, the government continued to refuse to allow plague victims to leave the colony and the gunboat *HMS Tweed* was positioned off Taipingshan. Negotiations began now that involved Li Hanzhang, the Qing-appointed governor in Canton and finally, on June 9, Governor Robinson backed down and reluctantly allowed Chinese patients to return to China, even though the decision was opposed by the Permanent Committee of the Sanitary Board. Above all, Robinson was concerned about the impact that further conflict would have on the colony's trade, which was already appreciably affected. The governor's compromise did not diffuse tensions, however. Emergency by-laws continued to incite opposition as anti-foreign placards reappeared in Canton and a cleanup operation was undertaken with some 350 dwellings 'condemned as unfit for habitation' and about 7,000 Chinese 'dislodged from the infected houses.'[108]

Tensions mounted further at the end of June, when the colonial authorities discovered that a Chinese hospital had opened at Lai-chi-kok, across the border in mainland China, on the Kowloon peninsula. Unreported

---

[106] *Times* [of London] (August 28, 1894), p.6.
[107] Elizabeth Sinn, *Power and Charity: A Chinese Merchant Elite in Colonial Hong Kong.* Revised edition (Hong Kong: Hong Kong University Press, 2003), pp.159–183 (166).
[108] 'Sir William Robinson to the Marquess of Ripon' (June 20, 1894). In: *British Parliamentary Papers*, p.413.

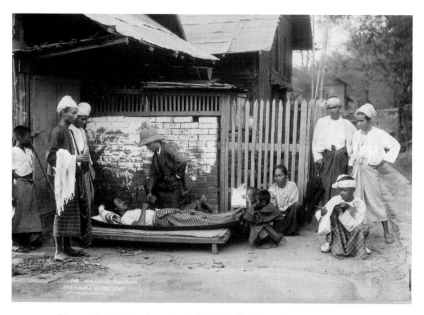

Figure 1.6. Criouleansky & Marshall, 'The plague in Mandalay: Examining a patient (1906).' Courtesy: Wellcome Library, London.

Colonial governance and epidemic photography

Colonial plague photography rarely conveys crisis, but rather focuses on public health procedures, accentuating the role of colonial personnel in managing disease: through campaigns of inoculation, house inspection, the erection of quarantines, or the cremation of plague victims. These largely static and orchestrated scenes convey authority and suggest the smooth operations of a colonial bureaucracy. In this way, plague photography performs an ideological function and promotes the idea of colonial governance as benevolent, impartial, and rational. The picture reproduced here (Figure 1.6) was taken in Burma during a plague outbreak in 1906 in which there were 8,657 recorded deaths. This period saw the development of the colony's public health service. Aside from these plague scenes, the commercial firm Criouleansky & Marshall specialized in portraits of colonial elites and local dignitaries, as well as 'ethnographic' tourist photography and postcards depicting tribal hill people, Shan chiefs, native women in traditional garb, and Buddhist monks.

Judith L. Richell, *Disease and Demography in Colonial Burma* (Singapore: NUS Press, 2006), p.185.

plague patients were being ferried there from Hong Kong without official clearance but with the assistance of the Tung Wah Committee. Differences became apparent between the governor and the Permanent Committee of the Sanitary Board; between the dictates of trade and the priorities of public health. Pressed upon by members of the Hong Kong General Chamber of Commerce, who were anxious not to disrupt the colony's trade any further, the governor consented to Chinese patients being moved and even arranged for two junks to collect them from the Kennedy Town Wharf. However, the Permanent Committee of the Sanitary Board vehemently opposed this decision on the grounds that moving the sick would jeopardize the health of the colony through reinfection and undermine Board's work and authority. The controversy was played out publicly in the pages of the colony's newspapers as governor and Sanitary Board openly squabbled. In the event, the conveyance of patients to Lai-chi-kok was suspended and a patrol dispatched to prevent the sick from crossing the harbor. Yet this decision was reversed again when the Permanent Committee finally agreed to allow plague sufferers to travel. By this time, however, the plague was subsiding. On September 3, the government issued a proclamation declaring that Hong Kong was no longer an infected port, even though the disease was to recur with varying levels of intensity in succeeding years.[109]

The conflicts triggered by the plague epidemic in Hong Kong and Canton underscored differences of attitude and belief. They also highlighted the perceived threat posed to the colonial state by a highly mobile native population. For the governor, the priority was keeping the colony's commercial lifeline open; for the Sanitary Board, it was ensuring the containment of disease. The challenge for colonial officials, in other words, was preventing certain kinds of injurious circulation, which were inimical to order (plague, panic, and rumor), while allowing other kinds of vital flows upon which the colony depended for its existence as a port city founded on trade.

Conclusion: Synchronic networks

The case studies presented in this chapter – cholera in colonial Manila and Japan, and bubonic plague in China and colonial Hong Kong – have underlined the extent to which epidemic crises were the product both of internal causes and of broader, intersecting global transformations during the nineteenth century: shifting economic and military power, the rise of the nation-state, nationalism, and empire. The aim has been to

---

[109] 'Proclamation,' *Hongkong Government Gazette Extraordinary* (September 3, 1894).

purposefully stretch the notion of mobility in order to rethink economic, social, and political relations. While mobility includes physical travel and modes of communication, the concept may also be extended to encompass other mobile situations. We might think of the violent 'mobs' in Manila, Nagasaki, Canton, and Hong Kong, for example, as forms of the mobile: 'The mob is seen as disorderly precisely because it is mobile, not fully fixed within boundaries and therefore needs to be tracked and socially regulated.'[110] In other words, I have argued that epidemics should be viewed in relation to different kinds and scales of mobility, and that mobility might be reconsidered as a process intrinsic to society; not solely as a horizontal movement across space but in terms of mobile economic, social, and political interrelations. The focus has been on tracking the connections between mobility and change, modernity, regional networks, and global connectivity.

Each of the epidemics considered in this chapter was linked to new pathways of trade and movements of people, as well as to increasingly concerted efforts to manage these streams with border controls and law enforcement measures. While mobility created frictions between native populations and foreigners, it also opened up divisions within local communities: between race and class, colonial and subaltern, and between different groups that held different beliefs about the cause of disease and its mode of transmission. The epidemic in Manila in 1820 revealed a world in motion. It was both a new world, produced by novel political and economic forces, and a world shaped by historical influences. Different regimes of mobility instigated contact and conflict. Cholera and massacre brought into view the range of intersecting migratory traffic: traders, soldiers, naturalists, and laborers. The epidemic made visible and inflamed latent tensions between rulers and the ruled, the Spanish and their Western rivals, the Chinese and the *Indios*, civil authority and the Church. It is only through an approach to Asian history that explores the synchronism of such networks that we can cut through the weight of accumulated regional, colonial, and national histories to grasp these interconnections.[111]

The outbreak of cholera in Japan in 1858, allegedly brought to Nagasaki by a US battleship, was connected to concerns and debates about the dangers of acceding to foreign demands for extraterritorial rights. If *korera* was associated with foreigners, the imposition of public health measures to restrict movement was influenced by Western hygiene

---

[110] John Urry, *Mobilities* (Cambridge: Polity, 2007), p.8.
[111] Denys Lombard, 'Networks and Synchronisms in Southeast Asian History,' *Journal of Southeast Asian Studies*, vol.26, no.1 (1995): 10–16.

tenets. Cholera helped to shape the apparatuses of government after the Meiji Restoration: from border control strategies geared to regulating the entry of infected persons and goods into Japan, epidemic control was progressively integrated into routine domestic policing, with the object of monitoring the movement of Japanese citizens. Nowhere was this paradigm of pervasive suspicion more conspicuous than in Japan's colonies, where border technologies operated as a means of disease surveillance and social discipline (Chapter 3).

In China, bubonic plague was spread by developing trade paths, the displacement of local populations, and troop movements. In 1894, Hong Kong's nodal position served to diffuse disease through Asia, in particular to India. Intensified circulations with larger and speedier ships increased the risk of the disease's spread. The plague in the British crown colony highlighted the social and cultural contexts of mobility. While the repatriation of the Chinese dead and those infected was vehemently opposed by colonial authorities, this attempt to impose stasis was viewed as overbearing and resisted by the Chinese. The conflicts triggered by the plague in Hong Kong exposed different cultural attitudes and beliefs. For colonial agents, the epidemic reinforced the threat posed to colonial society by a migrant Chinese population. The priority was to prevent certain forms of detrimental transmission, which endangered the colony – the diffusion of disease and the spreading of false rumors – while allowing other kinds of wholesome movement.[112]

Although the ostensible object of isolation was the removal of infected persons to safeguard the colony's collective health, the rationale for constraining movement was often formulated in terms shaped by previous debates about the hazards posed by illicit Chinese fluidity. In 1894, as they confronted the plague, agents of the colonial state – having consistently argued against the imposition of quarantine on the grounds of its cost and impracticability – found themselves in an untenable situation. The dictates of commerce, bacteriology, medicine, and sanitarian science – with their different scales and categories of mobility – collided. In this world of competing mobilities, how was it practically possible to produce an integrated system that functioned like a sifter, separating benign flows from malignant ones?

An important theme in this chapter has been the appropriation and reverse appropriation of knowledge viewed in the context of transnational exchanges. Epidemics might be understood as complex cultural conjunctures, which involve translations and mistranslations. They might

---

[112] Robert Peckham, 'Infective Economies: Empire, Panic and the Business of Disease,' *Journal of Imperial and Commonwealth History*, vol.41, no.2 (2013): 211–237.

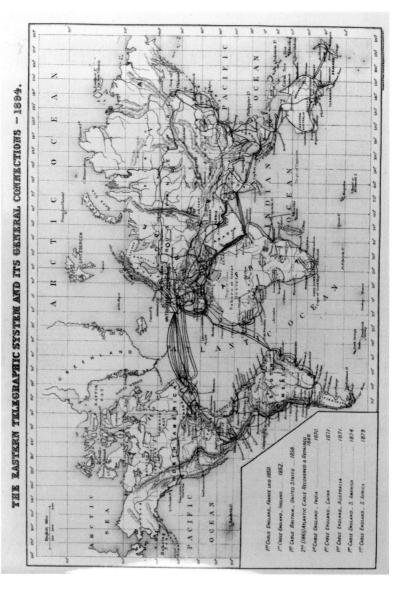

Figure 1.7. 'The Eastern Telegraphic System and Its General Connections, 1894.' © Cable & Wireless Communications 2015, by kind permission of the Telegraph Museum Porthcurno.

Telegraphic surveillance

By the late nineteenth century, telegraphic cables connected mainland China to Hong Kong, Indochina, the Philippines, and India, promoting new forms of connectedness (Figure 1.7). News could be relayed across Asia in minutes, rather than weeks. This new connectivity arguably extended the reach of London over the colonies, eroding the power of local authorities. However, in the face of a crisis, local officials could also use the telegraph to mitigate their responsibility. The telegraph had consequences for disease surveillance, as well: information about disease now traveled faster than the disease itself, thus buying time for authorities to gird themselves for imminent outbreaks. By the same token, local crises could tip more easily into cross-regional and global panics as news stories moved through the cables, sparking fears of approaching epidemics. Messages were expensive to send; given payment was per word, a compressed style of telegraphic communication developed.

Robert Peckham, 'Panic Encabled: Epidemics and the Telegraphic World.' In: Robert Peckham, ed., *Empires of Panic: Epidemics and Colonial Anxieties* (Hong Kong: Hong Kong University Press, 2015), pp.131–154.

be viewed, from this perspective, within the context of the 'wider global world of intercultural import–export.'[113] Medical practitioners and scientists followed the routes of disease, as well. Knowledge traveled along the pathways of trade and migration: from 'quinine' in Manila to hygienic public health practices in Japan and China. This knowledge was introduced to societies with their own momentum, however, and was not simply imposed from without. While Japanese notions of 'hygiene' and 'hygienic citizenship' certainly reflected Western influences, older beliefs and cultural processes – in this case the dietary regime – were also recast to shape modern ways. Hygienic notions co-existed with other translated notions of disease, such as the idea of *kakuran*, an importation from Chinese medicine. Beliefs were thus not clear-cut but rather multilayered and equivocal: there were numerous and often conflicting explanations of disease. In China, classical medical interpretations and folklore about plague's ghostly origins and the practice of exorcism overlapped with cleanup operations. The British, too, in colonial Hong Kong

[113] Clifford, *Routes*, p.23.

veered between environmental preoccupations and germ theory. In short, this is not a story that can be told according to an impact–response model, where projectile epidemics hit against and shattered inert 'traditional' societies. Rather, we might think of epidemics as triggering opposition and violence, even as they reveal entanglements and mutual dependencies.

2 Cities

How has urbanization influenced the diffusion of disease? To what extent
have epidemics shaped urban space and determined how cities are experienced? This chapter addresses these interrelated questions by considering
epidemics in relation to a number of cities. Each of the four cities considered here – Batavia, Hanoi, Singapore, and Bombay – are colonial cities,
in as much as their development took place within the context of colonization. The term 'colonial city,' however, is problematic, 'blurring as
many features of the reality as it illuminates.' What is a colonial city? Most
cities in history might in some sense be viewed as colonial in that they
have subordinated their agrarian hinterlands in a manner analogous with
a colonizing power. 'The local relationship of town-to-country,' Anthony
King has noted, 'becomes the metropolis–colony connection on a world
scale.'[1] At the same time, municipal authorities in the second half of the
nineteenth century mobilized many of the same instruments in order to
regulate the behavior of native city dwellers at home and abroad. To this
extent, at least, 'Bombay and Manchester were "colonized" in the same
way.'[2]

The aim in this chapter is to chart different epidemic histories through
the biographies of Asian cities from the late eighteenth to the early twentieth century in order to illuminate facets of the interrelationship between
epidemic disease and urbanization. As a process, urbanization may be
defined as the spatial concentration of a population that results from
the centralization of government and the clustering of economic activity. In the previous discussion, we considered the port cities of Manila,
Nagasaki, and Hong Kong as contact zones: sites of epidemics where different scales of mobility converged, generating friction and violence. In
this chapter, I develop these ideas to show how epidemics both propelled

---

[1] Anthony D. Smith, 'Colonial Cities: Global Pivots of Change.' In: Robert J. Ross and Gerard J. Telkamp, eds., *Colonial Cities: Essays on Urbanism in a Colonial Context* (Dordrecht:
Martinus Nijhoff Publishers, 1985), pp.7–32 (8).

[2] John Broich, 'Engineering the Empire: British Water Supply Systems and Colonial Societies, 1850–1900,' *Journal of British Studies*, vol.46, no.2 (2007): 346–365 (365).

and stymied urban growth, even as cities produced different kinds of epidemic threats. In a European context, the historian Richard Evans has explored the inner life of Hamburg in relation to cholera epidemics – and in particular the epidemic of 1892 – demonstrating how disease highlighted social inequalities, shaped the city's municipal politics, and above all created the conditions for political reform.[3] Similarly, each of the four case studies in this chapter considers specific aspects and moments in the history of a city to shed light on the management of urban space and infectious disease.

In the first section, we explore Batavia, capital of the Dutch East Indies, at the turn of the eighteenth and nineteenth centuries in order to reconsider the factors that contributed to the walled city's decline and eventual abandonment. Reflecting on the history of old Batavia through the lens of epidemic disease may help to answer broader critical questions, such as: What are cities for? How do they work? What happens when cities cease to function – that is, when they lose their capacity for agglomeration and instead become forces for declension? A key focus, here, is on Batavia's relationship with its hinterland and the city's location within local, interregional, and global networks of trade.

The second case focuses on the re-planning of Hanoi, which became the French colonial capital in 1902 after the creation of the Indochinese Union (1887). The city was chosen in part because – unlike Saigon, the commercial center in the south (today's Ho Chi Minh City) – it provided what the French perceived as a blank canvas for building anew. This section considers the extent to which epidemic anxieties provided a rationale for the city's reorganization under the direction of Paul Doumer (1857–1932), appointed governor general of French Indochina in 1897. The dangers of urban epidemics were understood in environmental and social terms: as the effects of a malign tropical climate and as the consequences of unhygienic native habits. We discuss the racial ideologies that were manifest in the equation of disease threats with an indigenous Vietnamese population, and the strategic zoning and segregation policies that aimed to create 'safe' spaces for French colonials. The purpose is to show how the medical science that underpinned modern hygiene 'was as much a discourse of settlement as it was a means of knowing and mastering disease.'[4]

The third section investigates epidemics of venereal disease (VD) in Singapore during the late nineteenth and early twentieth centuries, with

---

[3] Richard J. Evans, *Death in Hamburg: Society and Politics in the Cholera Years, 1830–1910* (Oxford: Clarendon Press, 1987).
[4] Warwick Anderson, *The Cultivation of Whiteness: Science, Health, and Racial Destiny in Australia* (Durham, NC: Duke University Press, 2006), p.4.

a focus on debates about female trafficking and prostitution, and particularly on the interconnections between sex work and the production of urban spaces. Historically, the term VD has included the bacterial infections syphilis, gonorrhea, and chancroid. Today, the terms sexually transmitted infections (STIs) and sexually transmitted diseases (STDs), which are used interchangeably, are more commonly employed. Cities such as Singapore and Hong Kong owed their growth and prosperity predominantly to migrant coolie labor, and as a result they were overwhelmingly male societies. The government of Singapore countenanced prostitution as a way of assuaging this gender asymmetry, even as it sought to regulate and contain the threat posed by infectious disease. In this sense, VD was a by-product of government policy, raising critical issues about the state, public health, and the sexual economy.

The fourth and final case study returns to the plague, this time exploring Bombay between 1896 and 1897. How did the city create the conditions for plague to spread? What kinds of socio-cultural and political tensions did the plague reveal and intensify? In this section, we shift the conventional focus to explore the role that modern communication systems – and notably the railway – played in the epidemic. As the British statesman Lord Salisbury avowed in 1871: 'The great organizations and greater means of locomotion of the present day mark out the future to be one of great empires.'[5] Locomotives were central to the expansion of capital and the extension of empire. They were also instrumental in the development of Indian cities, not least in Bombay's phenomenal growth during the nineteenth and twentieth centuries. Here, we demonstrate the strategic significance of the railway, showing how stations, trunk lines, and locomotives became critical sites for both the propagation and management of urban disease.

By way of a conclusion, the chapter draws out the larger themes and considers epidemics in relation to the rapid urbanization that has taken place in Asia following the Second World War, and particularly over the last few decades, a period of demographic transition that has witnessed a dramatic reconfiguration of the relationship between the urban and the rural, with attendant concerns about sustainability and the looming threat of pandemics to come.

Imagining the urban

Modern cities have been shaped by local, regional, national, and global processes. They represent an 'extraordinary agglomeration of flows' – of

---

[5] *Hansard's Parliamentary Debates, Third Series*, vols. 1–356 (London: T. C. Hansard, 1821–1891), CCIV [1871], pp.1366–1367.

people, commodities, and capital – and they have played a key role in the creation of industrial modernity.[6] Cities may be understood as both the agent and product of modernity. From the late nineteenth and early twentieth centuries, urban theorists have tended to conceive of the city in terms of 'new modes of movement and restlessness.'[7] 'Towns are like electric transformers,' Fernand Braudel wrote in a well-known formulation: 'They increase tension, accelerate the rhythm of exchange and constantly recharge human life.'[8]

In seaborne empires, port cities were particularly important sites for urban development, helping to constitute and support networks of empire. The metaphor of the 'web' has been used to suggest the 'interconnected networks of contact and exchange' that existed between colonial sites: 'Empires, like webs, were fragile and prone to crises where important threads were broken or structural nodes destroyed, yet also dynamic, being constantly remade and reconfigured through concerted thought and effort.'[9] Cities were also, on account of their concentrated populations, often dangerously unhealthy places. As Anne Hardy has observed, 'The history of the infectious diseases in modern times remains inextricably intertwined with the history of the cities that spawned them.'[10] Sedentism – the shift from nomadic to settled human existence that took place some 10,000 years ago – marked a transitional phase in the relationship between human beings and the environment, particularly in relation to changing patterns of epidemic disease distribution. The massing of human beings in cities provided pathogens with a sustainable chain of transmission. Pollution from the disposal of waste and the proximity of humans to domesticated animals also furnished conditions for diseases to evolve and cross species. The domestication of animals led to closer human–animal contact, with infections such as smallpox crossing between species in what has been called 'the lethal gift of livestock.'[11]

If cities are spaces where epidemics can take hold, they are also concentrated spaces that make population surveillance and regulation feasible. Historically, cities have not only been characterized by flow, but

---

[6] Ash Amin and Nigel Thrift, *Cities: Reimagining the Urban* (Cambridge: Polity, 2002), p.42.

[7] Urry, *Mobilities*, p.22.

[8] Fernand Braudel, *The Structures of Everyday Life: The Limits of the Possible*. Translated by Siân Reynolds (London: Collins, 1981), p.479.

[9] Tony Ballantyne and Antoinette Burton, 'Introduction: Bodies, Empires, and World Histories.' In: Tony Ballantyne and Antoinette Burton, eds., *Bodies in Contact: Rethinking Global Encounters in World History* (Durham, NC: Duke University Press, 2005), pp.1–18 (3).

[10] Anne Hardy, *The Epidemic Streets: Infectious Disease and the Rise of Preventive Medicine, 1856–1900* (Oxford: Clarendon Press, 1993), p.293.

[11] Diamond, *Guns, Germs and Steel*, p.195.

also by government attempts to regulate or stifle it. As we saw in the previous chapter, the experience of cholera in late nineteenth-century Japan gave rise to the incorporation of a public health agenda and state-sponsored endeavors to build institutions around the precepts of hygienic modernity. This 'distinctive constellation of space, society, and technology' has been termed 'the bacteriological city.'[12] Increasingly intrusive forms of technical and managerial expertise were applied to city populations. Municipal governance was shaped by disease epidemiology, which also influenced civil engineering, planning, and public health.

The development of colonial cities across Asia was often closely connected to urban expansion in Europe. While the metropole relied upon colonial materials and markets, the infusion of capital and expertise from the metropole was also instrumental in the relative prosperity of many colonial cities.[13] Nonetheless, historians have tended, perhaps, to over-simplify the distinctions between Western and Asian cities. Braudel characterized European cities in terms of their economic enterprise and autonomy, distinguishing the dynamism of early modern cities from their feudal hinterlands. In contrast, he depicted cities in Asia as 'enormous, parasitic, soft and luxurious.' Although they were vast in size, they were not vital commercial hubs, but rather fed passively off the surplus produced by a downtrodden peasant class. Moreover, they appeared to lack strong institutions of municipal government, which were salient features of Western cities.

This argument about the 'parasitic' Asian city echoes that of the German sociologist Max Weber (1864–1920), who had earlier contended that European cities evolved a distinctive civic identity and a level of autonomy in contradistinction to cities in the East. What explains this great divergence? The perceptions of a dichotomy between Western and Eastern cities may have originated in part from early European travelers to Asia. As the sociologist Ravi Arvind Palat has noted: 'Arriving in Asia, they were confronted with a variety of relational networks and cultural manifestations completely alien to their expectations and experiences.'[14] While Southeast Asian cities are often treated as alien impositions, they are, in fact, indigenous: 'Cities are ancient to the region and home to

---

[12] Matthew Gandy, 'The Bacteriological City and its Discontents,' *Historical Geography*, vol.34 (2006): 14–25 (14).

[13] Anthony D. King, *Urbanism, Colonialism, and the World-Economy: Cultural and Spatial Foundations of the World Urban System* (London: Routledge, 1990).

[14] Ravi Arvind Palat, 'Symbiotic Sisters: Bay of Bengal Ports in the Indian Ocean World-Economy.' In: Reşat Kasaba, ed., *Cities in the World-System: Studies in the Political Economy of the World-System* (Westport, CT: Greenwood Press, 1991), pp.17–40 (17–18).

almost a third of its people, but somehow scholars assume the "real" Southeast Asia is off in the countryside and back in the past.'[15]

Underlying these concerns is a broader question: How should we define a city? Is it a question of demography and density of population, of economic status, or of the social and political institutions cities house? Across Asia, urbanization has been driven by many factors and there is a good deal of diversity in the characteristics of urban environs between countries and regions. Before the nineteenth century, there were numerous thriving port-cities in Southeast Asia, including Batavia, Malacca, and Manila, with close trade links to China, India, Europe, and the Americas (Chapter 1). There were also important sacred cities, such as Pagan (today's Bagan in Burma), which were places of pilgrimage, drawing people from afar. However, in contrast to South and East Asia, the region's rural interior had a much lower population density.

Imperial expansion during the nineteenth and early twentieth centuries changed existing patterns of settlement, acting as a spur to rapid urban development. Burgeoning colonial cities were not only administrative hubs, but also commercial pivots: they connected rural hinterlands to wider trans-regional and global pathways of trade, functioning as strategic connectors between the colonial economy and the metropole. Beyond the larger cities – many of them coastal – were other kinds of settlement that grew up around infrastructural networks, particular those linking ports to extractive industries. Meanwhile, the vast majority of the population remained rural and engaged in subsistence farming, and across much of Southeast and East Asia this was focused on rice production. Examining cities in relation to epidemic disease may shed light on these continuities and discontinuities in patterns of urbanization, and in particular on the different forces that have driven urban development across Asia: markets, political power, agricultural interests, and so forth. It may also provide a new perspective on how infectious diseases have been understood and how urban systems have developed in response to them.

Batavia: Storehouse of disease

The city of Jayakarta, the principal port of the Kingdom of Sunda, and subsequently part of the Muslim Sultanate of Banten, was conquered by forces of the VOC in the early seventeenth century (1619) and renamed Batavia after the 'Batavi,' an ancient Germanic people who were the

---

[15]   Richard A. O'Connor, 'Indigenous Urbanism: Class, City and Society in Southeast Asia,' *Journal of Southeast Asian Studies*, vol.26, no.1 (1995): 30–45 (44).

purported forebears of the Dutch nation. The new city was strategically located near the Sunda Strait, between Java and Sumatra, connecting the Indian Ocean, the Java Sea, and the South China Sea. For some 200 years it served as the headquarters of VOC operations.

After their acquisition of Jayakarta, the Dutch tore down the existing town and began a process of re-planning and building. Influenced by the design ideas of the Flemish military engineer and mathematician Simon Stevin (1548–1620), a walled city was constructed reminiscent of a Dutch city, bisected with 16 canals that diverted the flow of the Ciliwung River and were lined with trees. The seafront was dominated by the white coral battlements of a castle. Further developments saw the addition of a moat along with the piecemeal extension of the stone wall to enclose the city. By 1650, Batavia was complete and in the subsequent decades acquired the epithet 'Queen of the East.' As the traveler and VOC employee Johan Nieuhof (1618–1672) noted during his three-year stay in Batavia in the late 1660s, the location of the city in a bay scattered with islands to break the wind made it 'one of the safest Harbours of the whole World.' The air and climate were 'as temperate and healthy as any place whatever in the *Indies*,' while 'the soil about *Batavia* [was] so rich, that the seeds brought hither out of *Holland*, *Persia*, and from *Suratte*, thrive extremely, and yield plentiful fruits.' The elegance of the city's design was a counterpart and extension of this fecund nature: 'All of the Buildings of this City are well contriv'd, most even of the private Houses having handsome gardens, well planted with Fruit-trees and Plants and Flowers.' Although Nieuhof observed that in the recent past 'a certain contagious distemper' had raged through the city, the menace of disease was countered by a municipal resolve to build 'a pest-house, where such as were seiz'd with this evil, might be provided with lodgings, diet, and suitable remedies.'[16]

The plans for Batavia largely ignored the shape of the pre-Dutch city. Indigenous urban settlements appeared haphazard to the colonizers with no clearly demarcated bounds. 'Batavia to the Dutch was a European creation,' observes Susan Abeyesekere, 'built by them out of nothing from entirely new materials.'[17] The new plans suggested a harmonious and rational space clearly inspired by the arrangements of an Italian Renaissance city. This was an idealized urban blueprint that was to influence the form of other Dutch colonial cities in Asia, such as Cochin (Kochi),

[16] John Nieuhoff [Johan Nieuhof], *Voyages and Travels into Brasil and the East-Indies*, 2. vols. (London: Printed for Awnsham and John Churchill, 1703), II, pp.302, 323, 304, 313.
[17] Susan Abeyesekere, *Jakarta: A History*. Revised edition (Singapore: Oxford University Press, 1989), p.3.

Colombo, and Malacca.[18] As the historian of the Dutch East Indies, Leonard Blussé, has commented, Batavia was a 'visible city,' frequently depicted in engravings. Artists and engravers produced idealized illustrations of Batavia's main buildings and street scenes, which displayed the city's pageantry and depicted boats gliding down the pristine waters of the city's grand canals (Figure 2.1).

By the early nineteenth century, however, the city had gained a reputation for unhealthiness and was in decline. Sir Thomas Stamford Raffles (1781–1826), the English colonial administrator who visited Batavia in 1811, famously called it a 'storehouse of disease.' In the appendices to his history of Java, Raffles reported on the city's unwholesomeness, attributing it to a number of environmental factors: an insalubrious climate, surrounding swamps, and the eruption of Mount Salak in 1699, which silted up the rivers; lime kilns and plantations in the environs, which impeded the free circulation of air; and stagnant, polluted canals. 'History,' he affirmed, 'attests that this city has been highly pernicious to the health both of Europeans and Natives, almost from its foundation, and recent experience concurs with the testimony of history.'[19]

Raffles was not alone in his condemnation of the city. 'The whole city of Batavia,' wrote another commentator contemptuously, 'is proverbially unhealthy, not so much from the heat of the climate, as from its injudicious situation and misplaced embellishments.' By the early nineteenth century, few Europeans ventured 'to sleep within the limits of [Batavia's] pestilential atmosphere.'[20] The rational elements of the city's original design, such as its canals, which were imported from Holland and designed to improve city life and commercial efficiency, were perceived to have countervailing effects. Furthermore, the city was tainted by toxic emissions from artisanal enterprises, such as breweries, tanneries, and slaughterhouses.[21] As the writer and statesman Sir John Barrow (1764–1848) noted in his *Voyage to Cochinchina* (1806):

[18] Robert C. M. Weebers and Yahaya Ahmad, 'Interpretation of Simon Stevin's Ideas on the Verenigde Oostindische Compagnie (United East Indies Company) Settlement of Malacca,' *Planning Perspectives*, vol.29, no.4 (2014): 543–555; Marsely L. Kehoe, 'Dutch Batavia: Exposing the Hierarchy of the Dutch Colonial City,' *Journal of Historians of Netherlandish Art*, vol.7, no.1 (2015): doi:10.5092/jhna.2015.7.1.3.

[19] Sir Thomas Stamford Raffles, *The History of Java*, 2 vols. (London: John Murray, 1830) I, Appendix A, pp.viii–xiii.

[20] Walter Hamilton, *The East India Gazetteer* (London: John Murray, 1815), pp.90–96 (91).

[21] Luc Nagtegaal, 'Urban Pollution in Java, 1600–1850.' In: Peter J. M. Nas, ed., *Issues in Urban Development: Case Studies from Indonesia* (Leiden: Research School CNWS, Leiden University, 1995), pp.9–30; Jean Gelman Taylor, *The Social World of Batavia: European and Eurasian in Dutch Asia* (Madison: University of Wisconsin Press, 1983), p.52.

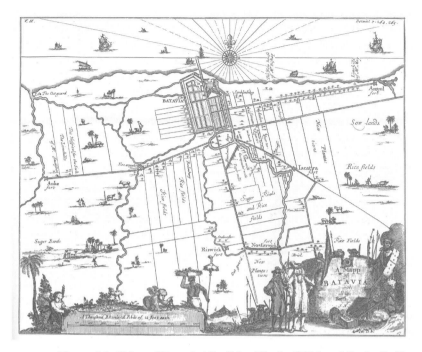

Figure 2.1. 'Map of Batavia.' In: John Nieuhoff [Johan Nieuhof], *Voyages and Travels into Brasil and the East-Indies*, 2 vols. (London: Printed for Awnsham and John Churchill, 1703), II, pp.302–303.

A seventeenth-century view of Batavia

The United East India Company, known as the VOC, was a chartered company established in 1602 and granted a monopoly on the lucrative spice trade in Asia by the States General of the Netherlands. The VOC was vested with the authority to conduct military campaigns, conclude treaties and agreements, issue coinage, and establish colonies. However, by the late eighteenth century the Company was insolvent. After its dissolution in 1799, its possessions were acquired by the Dutch government. Batavia remained the capital of the Dutch East Indies until the Japanese occupation in 1942, after which the city was renamed Jakarta. Figure 2.1 is an engraved map of old Batavia, signed by Johan Nieuhof and taken from his book *Voyages and Travels to the East*

Indies, which appeared posthumously in Dutch in 1682 and in an English edition in 1700. Accused of stealing from the Company during a period of employment in Tuticorin (Thoothukudi), a Dutch port in India on the Coromandel Coast, Nieuhof spent three years in Batavia, from 1667 to 1670, before returning to Europe to clear his name with the directors of the VOC. Lavishly illustrated, Nieuhof's book provides many insights into seventeenth-century VOC trading cities in Asia. In particular, Nieuhof's stay in Batavia gave him the opportunity 'to take a full view of the city, not only to make draughts of all its public structures, but also of such plants and trees as grow in and about that city.' Some of the illustrations in the book appear to have been drawn on the spot. Others are the work of commissioned artists. However, even Nieuhof's sketches were clearly worked up by Dutch engravers, who added numerous details and fanciful embellishments. The figures in many of the illustrations are depicted in classical poses reminiscent of European paintings. They tell us much about European preconceptions of Asia, even as they provide glimpses into life in Batavia in the seventeenth century. Although Nieuhof's map was produced before the sugar plantation boom from the 1680s, note the development of the city's hinterland with 'new' plantations encroaching upon the rice fields.

In making choice of the present site of the city of Batavia, the predilection of the Dutch for a low swampy situation evidently got the better of their prudence; and the fatal consequences that have invariably attended this choice, from its establishment to the present period, irrefragably demonstrated by the many thousands who have fallen sacrifice to it, have nevertheless been hitherto unavailing to induce the government either altogether to abandon the spot for another more healthy, or to remove the local and immediate causes of a more than ordinary mortality. Never were national prejudices and national taste so injudiciously misapplied, as in the attempt to assimilate those of Holland to the climate and the soil of Batavia.[22]

Of course, these were British views of Batavia and hardly impartial given intense Anglo-Dutch rivalry. In 1811, during the Napoleonic Wars, the British had launched an attack on Java and temporarily seized control of Batavia from a Franco-Dutch expeditionary force. Raffles was

---

[22] John Barrow, *A Voyage to Cochinchina, in the Years 1792 and 1793* (London: T. Caddell and W. Davies, 1806), p.171.

briefly lieutenant governor of British Java (1811–1815) and subsequently governor general of Bencoolen (1817–1822) on the west coast of Sumatra (today's Bengkulu). All the same, numerous travelers of other nationalities also reflected on Batavia's degeneration. They noted prevalent 'fevers,' which they invariably attributed to miasmic vapors emanating from the swampy terrain around the city. A particularly dramatic rise in mortality after 1733 underlined the danger posed by disease.[23] Above all, numerous visitors identified the contaminating role of the city's malodorous canals, which functioned as sewers and were in need of frequent and expensive dredging by convicts and Javanese laborers. The canal system became a breeding ground for water-borne diseases to the extent that those tasked with dredging them 'had been virtually handed a death sentence.'[24] Although the agent and transmission route of malaria were not discovered until the final decade of the nineteenth century (Chapter 3), the murky canal water was identified as a source of disease. As John Splinter Stavorinus, a captain in the service of the VOC, asserted in the second half of the eighteenth century:

The stagnant canals, in the dry season, exhale an intolerable stench, and the trees planted along them impede the course of the air, by which in some degree the putrid effluvia would be dissipated. In the wet season the inconvenience is equal; for then these reservoirs of corrupted water overflow their banks in the lower part of town, and fill the lower stories of the houses, where they leave behind them an inconceivable quantity of slime and filth.[25]

By the end of the eighteenth century, an exodus from the fetid city had commenced. Governor General Pieter Gerardus van Overstraten (in office 1796–1801) had begun to relocate his headquarters from Batavia further inland to Weltevreden by 1800. A few years later, Governor General Herman Willem Daendels (in office 1807–1811) transferred the city's administration and the military there. The buildings in the old city were demolished to be used in the construction of the new: the castle and walls of the city were pulled down, and the canals buried.

Why was Batavia overtaken, as contemporary accounts suggest, by epidemic disease? How did this transformation of the city come about – from the healthy port celebrated by Nieuhof to Raffles' 'storehouse of disease'?

---

[23] P. H. van der Brug, 'Malaria in Batavia in the 18th Century,' *Tropical Medicine and International Health*, vol.2, no.9 (1997): 892–902.

[24] Kerry Ward, *Networks of Empire: Forced Migration in the Dutch East India Company* (Cambridge: Cambridge University Press, 2008), p.101.

[25] John Joseph Stockdale, *Sketches, Civil and Military, of the Island of Java and Its Immediate Dependencies*. Second edition (London, 1812), pp.133–134.

The causes of old Batavia's decline have been the subject of much discussion and debate. Most historians, following Raffles, have cited a combination of contributory environmental factors. And yet a comparison with other cities, facing similar pressures and environmental problems, suggests that we look elsewhere to explain Batavia's decay. A case in point is the city of Calcutta (today's Kolkata), located on the east bank of the Hooghly River in West Bengal. Calcutta was developed by the British from the end of the seventeenth century, when the EIC was granted a trading license by the Nawab of Bengal. From a fortified mercantile base, the city grew to become the administrative capital of India under the EIC and later the capital of the British Raj until 1911. Like Batavia, however, Calcutta's location was far from ideal: it was situated in flood-prone marshlands in an area where cholera was endemic. 'The dissemination of cholera from Calcutta by soldiers and sailors, pilgrims and migrant labourers,' writes David Arnold, 'reflected the wider patterns of human and disease mobility in India and throughout the vaster region of which it in some senses served as capital.'[26] Nineteenth-century commentators fulminated against the city's pollution and squalor, noting how much of Calcutta's population lived in a condition of destitution. So why did Calcutta prosper – a city founded in an ecologically unsuitable locality as an administrative and military center and a hub for trade – while Batavia declined?

The answer must be sought in the nature of the city itself, as a social, political, and economic space – and above all in the relationship of the city to the hinterland, and its independence from the metropole. Batavia was a VOC city controlled by the Company for the prime purpose of trade. Despite its expansion, the VOC had little interest in administering a territorial state. Neither did it encourage the development of an independent civic society, which would have challenged its authority. In effect, Batavia served as 'a kind of super trade-factory,' with policy geared to maximizing the Company's profits. Private traders, or burghers, were deemed to be competition and regulations were put in place to impede entrepreneurial initiatives. Citizens were denied political autonomy and privilege, while the city suffered from a lack of independent institutions. The reliance on the VOC meant that the city's prosperity and future were inextricably linked to that of the Company. The VOC's bankruptcy at the end of the eighteenth century inevitably spelled the end of the city. Old Batavia, notes Blussé, 'survived the VOC [by] a mere decade.'[27]

[26] Arnold, 'The Indian Ocean as a Disease Zone,' pp.10–11.
[27] Leonard Blussé, 'The Story of an Ecological Disaster: The Dutch East India Company and Batavia (1619–1799).' In: *Strange Company: Chinese Settlers, Mestizo Women and the Dutch in VOC Batavia* (Dordrecht: Foris Publications, 1986), pp.15–34 (18).

The VOC's monopolistic stranglehold on the city's development was perhaps most conspicuous in the opening up and opportunistic exploitation of Batavia's hinterland – known in Dutch as the *Ommelanden* – for sugar cultivation after 1680. The development of sugarcane as a cash crop by the Chinese, but under the supervision of the VOC, constrained the possibilities of developing more sustainable forms of cultivation that would have benefitted the city. The dependence on exports exposed the city to market volatility when prices fell with demand. Above all, sugar production caused environmental degradation. In the late 1660s, Nieuhof had commented on the fertility of the city's hinterland, which supported plentiful flora and fauna, and consisted of 'impassible forests and wildernesses.' In the decades after 1680, the land was progressively transformed. Water was diverted for irrigation, affecting the land's natural ecology. Trees were felled to provide wood for the sugar refineries, leading to deforestation, as well as to the pollution of rivers. Soil erosion diminished crop yields. The river to the port silted up, stagnating the canals and clogging the bay. The castle was left stranded inland, now separated from the sea by obnoxious smelling mudflats.[28]

In short, then, Batavia's demise was not caused by the impact of some external force – an imported epidemic, for example. It was not the result of a natural disaster or simply the faulty planning of a Dutch city misplaced in the tropics. It was an 'ecological disaster,' as Blussé has termed it. Exploring the role of disease in the history of Batavia's eclipse thus helps to illuminate the dynamic interrelationship between environmental, biosocial, economic, and political processes in the making and unmaking of a city.

Colonial Hanoi and the blueprint of disease

Discussion so far has focused on the ecological circumstances that led to a city's decline. The emphasis has been less on how disease was understood than on tracing the different factors that contributed to Batavia's decay. In the next case, we explore how changing attitudes to disease in the late nineteenth century impacted upon city planning. Increasingly during the nineteenth century, earlier assumptions about the role of the environment in disease causation gave way to a biomedical emphasis on germs and disease vectors.[29] In colonial discourse, the focus shifted onto native

---

[28] Blussé, 'The Story of an Ecological Disaster.' In: *Stange Company*, pp.26–28.

[29] Hans Pols, 'Notes from Batavia, the Europeans' Graveyard: The Nineteenth-Century Debate on Acclimatization in the Dutch East Indies,' *Journal of the History of Medicine and Allied Sciences*, vol.67, no.1 (2012): 120–148.

populations as disease carriers.[30] How did these new ideas influence the way in which cities were constructed and regulated? Hanoi, the capital of French Indochina from 1902, provides a particularly striking example of how anxieties about epidemics influenced city planning and policies of urban zoning at a moment when scientific and medical knowledge was transforming the way disease was understood.

The French had consolidated their hold on Tonkin (northern Vietnam) with the Sino-French War of 1884–1885. The Indochinese Union was formally established in 1887 as a consolidation of Tonkin, Annam, and Cochinchina (corresponding to present-day Vietnam) with Cambodia. Laos was annexed in 1893 after the Franco-Siamese War. 'Indochina' was thus constructed by the French within 'a complex region of intermingling civilizations' marked by great diversity.[31] Situated in Tonkin, in the northeast-most portion of French territory, Hanoi occupied a strategic position on the western frontiers of the Qing Empire. While the port of Saigon in Cochinchina – captured by the French in 1859 – was the largest city and certainly the most important commercial hub, Hanoi was chosen as the capital of the Indochinese Union for a number of reasons. The city had been the royal center of political power in Vietnam until 1802, after which it was overshadowed by Huế, the capital under the Nguyễn dynasty. If Hanoi offered a royal pedigree, it also furnished the new colonial regime with more opportunities than Saigon for remodeling according to the blueprint of a colonial city – and, in the process, for demonstrating French power. As Paul Doumer, governor general of Indochina between 1897 and 1902, remarked in his memoirs, Saigon 'was a city that was already made, which one could simply complete and embellish, whereas Hanoi was a rough-hewn city, waiting to be made.'[32] Tonkin was also advantageously sited for the commercial exploitation of southern China. The scramble for China had intensified following the Qing Empire's defeat in the First Sino-Japanese War and Japan's annexation of Taiwan in 1895. French dominance over Tonkin held out the possibility of developing a trade route into Qing territory that sidelined the treaty ports of the Chinese coastal provinces, with the ultimate aim of

---

[30] Warwick Anderson, *Colonial Pathologies: American Tropical Medicine, Race, and Hygiene in the Philippines* (Durham, NC: Duke University Press, 2006).

[31] Pierre Brocheux and Daniel Hémery, *Indochina: An Ambiguous Colonization, 1858-1954*. Translated by Ly Lan Dill-Klein (Berkeley: California University Press, 2009), pp.1–14 (1–2).

[32] Paul Doumer, *L'Indo-Chine française (souvenirs)*. Second edition (Paris: Viubert et Nony Editeurs, 1905), p.124.

absorbing Yunnan into Indochina.[33] Doumer, supported by the imperialist minister of foreign affairs, Gabriel Hanotaux (1853–1944), was
intent on extending French influence and accessing the Chinese markets
of Yunnan, Guangxi, and Guangdong. In 1898, the Chinese territory of
Kwang Chow Wan (Guangzhouwan) on the east coast of the Leizhou
peninsula was ceded to the French on a 99-year lease. While linking
Hanoi with Yunnan, the Red River gave the city access to deep-water
anchorage at Haiphong on the Bay of Tonkin.

Hanoi's geographical position on the border of Yunnan, however, also
exposed it to epidemic disease. The drive to extend French influence
across the frontier was thus qualified by concerns about the risks that
counter-flows of infection posed to Indochina. It was, at least in part,
with a view to countering such threats that French medical dispensaries
were established close to the northern frontier of Indochina in the 1890s.
In a report from Yunnan to the governor general of Indochina in 1893,
the French colonial official Émile Rocher had noted the spread of plague
in China and concluded: 'Without being a pessimist, it seems to me that
there are good reasons for studying the development of the disease and to
take precautions in order to prevent its spread into our colony.'[34] It was
the prospect of a plague epidemic in Tonkin that had induced the authorities to dispatch the physician and bacteriologist Alexandre Yersin to Hong
Kong, where he discovered the plague bacillus in June 1894 (Chapter 1).
As Yersin noted in his paper 'The Bubonic Plague at Hong Kong':

> The disease had been raging for a very long time in an endemic state on the high
> plateaus of Yunnan and from time to time had appeared quite near the frontier
> of our Indo-Chinese possessions at Mengzi, Longzhou, and Pakhoi . . . The great
> commercial movement between Canton and Hong Kong, on the one hand, and
> between Hong Kong and Tonkin, on the other, and the difficulty in establish-
> ing on the littoral of these lands a really effective quarantine makes the French
> government fear that Indochina will be invaded by the epidemic.[35]

From the early years of conquest in the 1850s and 1860s, the French
had been preoccupied with health in the colony and with some reason: early mortality figures were high, and diseases including malaria,

---

[33] Robert Lee, *France and the Exploitation of China, 1885–1901: A Study in Economic Imperialism* (Hong Kong: Oxford University Press, 1989), pp.230–266.

[34] Florence Bretelle-Establet, 'From Extending French Colonial Control to Safeguard-
ing National Prestige: The French Medical Dispensaries in Southern China.' In: Iris
Borowy, ed., *Uneasy Encounters: The Politics of Medicine and Health in China, 1900–1937*
(Frankfurt: Peter Lang, 2009), pp.63–92 (63–64, 65).

[35] Alexandre Yersin, 'La peste bubonique à Hong-Kong,' *Annales de l'Institut Pasteur*, vol.8
(1894): 662–667 (662).

dysentery, and cholera sapped the military. Reports and guide books, employing a language of extreme and excess (too hot, too humid), invariably attributed ill-health to the deleterious effects of the torrid climate and landscape. As Eric Jennings has observed: 'Disease – and not just malaria – actively shaped French priorities in Southeast Asia from the outset.' In the early years of the colony, the sick were repatriated for convalescence or sent to recuperate at a sanatorium in the Japanese treaty port of Yokohama. At Doumer's insistence, however, efforts were made to locate the site for a convalescence center in Indochina, 'where functionaries and settlers alike will be able to rebuild their strength.' This led to the establishment in 1897 of the hill station of Dalat on the Lang Biang highland plateau 150 miles northeast of Saigon. 'Discovered' by Yersin, Dalat was envisaged as a haven from the tropical heat and developed into a European-style resort with villas, hotel, and boarding schools nestled in Alpine-like environs of pine trees and artificial lakes.[36]

Dalat was built from scratch as a sanitary safe zone. Remodeling a preexisting urban center – even when it provided more scope for change than Saigon – proved more difficult. Although French visitors to Hanoi from the 1880s frequently lauded the city's handsome buildings and well-laid out streets, epidemics exposed a glaring discrepancy between grandiose claims and the practical exigencies of governing a recently colonized city. The disparity between appearances and practices was periodically revealed. 'The vulnerability and very artificiality of French authority in Indochina,' the architectural historian Gwendolyn Wright has observed, 'encouraged a ruthless colonial policy – and strong resistance.'[37]

From the 1880s, Hanoi underwent major re-planning and reconstruction. This impetus for infrastructural development gained new momentum in 1897 after Doumer's appointment as governor general with a mandate to centralize government and expand the administrative machinery. It is within the context of this bureaucratic overhaul and efforts to further erode the authority of the Nguyễn and Cambodian monarchies, that we should view Doumer's city-building initiatives. The aim in Hanoi, particularly from the late 1890s, was to create a stately and ordered space, modernizing the ancient Vietnamese city. Between 1902 and 1903, Doumer organized an exhibition in the capital to showcase the transformative powers of French urban planning and technologies in creating a modern, hygienic city in an inauspicious tropical terrain (Figure 2.2).

[36] Eric T. Jennings, *Imperial Heights: Dalat and the Making and Undoing of French Indochina* (Berkeley: University of California Press, 2011), pp.7, 13.
[37] Gwendolyn Wright, *The Politics of Design in French Colonial Urbanism* (Chicago, IL: University of Chicago Press, 1991), pp.161–163.

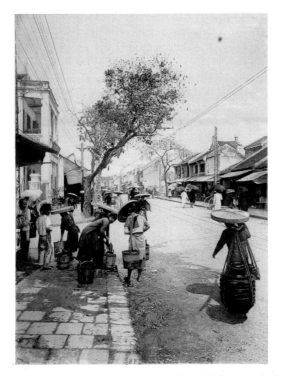

Figure 2.2. 'La rue du Coton, Hanoi.' In: Louis Salaun, *L'Indochine* (Paris: Imprimerie Nationale, 1903), pp.364–365.

A street view of Hanoi

The colonial official Louis Salaun published his book *L'Indochine* in 1903 in the immediate aftermath of the colonial exhibition in Hanoi. Figure 2.2 is reproduced from Salaun's book and shows the rue du Coton (Phố Hàng Bông), a street in the 'native' quarter of the city, where cotton was produced. In 1908, there was an outbreak of plague in the area. The text by Salaun accompanying the image emphasizes the importance of science, medicine, and hygiene for colonial governance. Public works, supported by medical institutions, such as the 'Indochina Medical College' established in Hanoi in 1902 – now the Hanoi Medical University – and directed by Yersin, were perceived as vital in the 'civilizing' of native populations.

There were discrete phases to Hanoi's modernization. The first, in the 1880s, was functional and carried out largely by military engineers.[38] The military played a critical role in pacifying the native population and quelling dissent. Grid roads were constructed, allowing access to troops and emergency services. The royal citadel was remodeled and the Kinh Thiên Palace demolished. As Doumer later observed in an attempt to vindicate the destruction of Vietnamese historical buildings, in tropical climates health considerations and the ever-present menace of infectious disease outbreaks justified most actions.[39] In the second phase, beginning in the late 1890s, smart villas and shaded walkways were erected, eclipsing the dirty and overcrowded native quarter known as the 'Thirty-Six Streets.' The European section of the city was equipped with a modern sewerage system and flushing water. Under Doumer, Hanoi's damp, swampy environs were to be transformed and its reputation as a place of fevers would be revised.[40]

Yet the construction of the new city produced other, unforeseen effects. The process of construction itself drew thousands of workers to the city, contributing further to Hanoi's expansion and to an increased threat of disease, which this influx posed – as well as to potential native unrest. As Doumer noted, the growth of the population of Hanoi in the five years after his accession as governor in 1897 had been 'extremely rapid, prodigious, as had the development of the city.'[41] Makeshift dwellings were put up along the banks of the Red River and in the surrounding villages, a blight that shattered the harmonious effect of the city's elegant streets and stone buildings. Shanty towns appeared near the Doumer Bridge (Long Biên Bridge), a centerpiece in the modernization of Hanoi, which was constructed by the French engineering firm Daydé et Pillé between 1899 and 1902 as a vital link to Saigon in the south and onwards to Yunnan and China. After 1900, Hanoi continued its growth as rural populations flooded into the city. Writing in the early 1930s, in the aftermath of the second investment boom of the 1920s, the novelist Vũ Trọng Phụng (1912–1939) captured the alienation of this drifting rural population in his exposé *Household Servants* (1936). There, uprooted villagers look for poorly paid work as servants or laborers in an unaccommodating 'modern' city. As the protagonist waits amongst a crowd of workers, he reflects on their predicament:

---

[38] William S. Logan, *Hanoi: Biography of a City* (Sydney: University of New South Wales Press, 2000), p.92.

[39] Doumer, *L'Indo-Chine*, p.123.   [40] Logan, *Hanoi*, pp.92, 76.

[41] Doumer, *L'Indo-Chine*, p.124.

The city lures people from the countryside who leave dry fields and dead grass, and who starve a second time after they have abandoned their homes. It reduces people to the level of animals; it often drives young men into prison and young women into prostitution.[42]

Authorities viewed this deracinated population – created, at least in part, by the city's development – as a menace. It contributed to the insalubrity of the city's overcrowded 'native quarter.' As one commentator observed:

Because of the [Vietnamese] population density, the closeness of the houses in the native quarter, the carelessness of the Annamites in regard to even the most basic rules of hygiene, the capital of Tonkin, as well as the other population centers of the colony, could quickly become a wonderful field test for the plague, if – as certain persons, whose competence in this matter is indisputable, predict – the illness reappears and invades the country.[43]

Policies were directed against native thatched houses or *paillotes* in the so-called 'indigenous city' (*ville indigène*), where the stink of accumulated waste was an affront to French authority. Disease and foul odors characterized the native city, associated both with the filthy native body and with the environment that these bodies inevitably produced. Natives were accused of dumping their rubbish in Hoàn Kiếm Lake, turning it into a noxious swamp where infectious disease fomented. As one traveler noted in 1883,

native huts crowded its shores; to go down to the water it was necessary to weave through narrow alleys leaving the city's passable roads ... to run into a thousand detours [formed by a jumble of] ... straw huts where a destitute population swarmed, to hop among stinking puddles and piles of garbage ... [44]

As a preventive measure, the stilted huts around the lake were removed and household waste diverted to cesspits. Water channels and pumping stations were constructed to deal with malaria and dysentery.

Epidemic disease remained a constant threat to the colonial regime and a reminder, when outbreaks did occur, of the interdependencies that existed in the city between colonial and native populations, as well as the futility of colonial efforts at segregation. The first officially recorded cases of plague in Indochina occurred in Nha Trang, southern Vietnam, in June 1898. This was not coincidental: Yersin had established his laboratory close to the port city, and in fact had just returned from a trip

[42] Vũ Trọng Phụng, 'Household Servants.' In: *The Light of the Capital: Three Modern Vietnamese Classics*. Translated by Greg Lockhart and Monique Lockhart (Kuala Lumpur: Oxford University Press, 1996), pp.121–156 (130).

[43] Michael G. Vann, 'Of Rats, Rice, and Race: The Great Hanoi Rat Massacre, an Episode in French Colonial History,' *French Colonial History*, vol.4 (2003): 191–203 (195).

[44] Logan, *Hanoi*, p.73.

to India, where plague was raging and where he had been experimenting with an anti-plague serum. The general supposition was that lax security had enabled the plague to leak out of Yersin's research facility. The irony that a plague epidemic had occurred 'at the very site created for its control and prevention' was not lost on Governor Doumer.[45]

As noted above, Doumer had staged an international exhibition in Hanoi to promote French achievements in the colony. However, overseas consignments delivered for the exhibition had in all likelihood contained rats, which infested the city's sewers and led to an outbreak of plague in 1903.[46] Such episodes were reminders that despite concerted efforts at modernization and disease control, infections were hard to keep at bay. In 1906, plague broke out in Saigon, with the source of infection allegedly being infected cargo from Canton coming through Hong Kong. There were also intermittent recurrences of the disease in Hanoi. Coercive public health interventions exacerbated tensions between colonial authorities and the local population with resentment flaring up 'into an open conflict along clear racial lines.'[47] Famine in Bắc Ninh province to the east of Hanoi in March 1906, which had been preceded by a series of natural disasters, led to a social crisis, driving desperate villagers onto the city's streets.[48] Meanwhile, Hanoi's City Council reported that inhabitants were fleeing the city in droves, resulting in an economic slump. Urban refugees spread the disease to the countryside, compounding the disruptions already created by famine.[49]

The 1903 plague outbreak underlined the vulnerabilities of the European district, with rats infesting the new sewers. Authorities sent out teams of native rat-catchers, thereby ironically re-introducing native bodies into the heart of the European district. Although health regulations and disease surveillance focused on the native quarter could reduce the severity of outbreaks, the plague – and other infectious diseases, notably cholera – remained a major concern throughout French rule. In the summer of 1910, an outbreak of cholera caused panic in the city.[50] This was

[45] Au, *Mixed Medicines*, pp.44–45.
[46] Michael G. Vann, '"All the World's a Stage," Especially in the Colonies: L'Exposition de Hanoi, 1902–3.' In: Martin Evans, ed., *Empire and Culture: The French Experience, 1830–1940* (Basingstoke: Palgrave Macmillan, 2004), pp.181–191.
[47] Michael G. Vann, 'Hanoi in the Time of Cholera: Epidemic Disease and Racial Power in the Colonial City.' In: Monnais and Cook, eds., *Global Movements, Local Concerns*, pp.150–170 (155).
[48] Van Nguyen-Marshall, *In Search of Moral Authority: The Discourse on Poverty, Poor Relief, and Charity in French Colonial Vietnam* (New York: Peter Lang, 2008), pp.34–41.
[49] Vann, 'Of Rats, Rice, and Race,' p.199.
[50] Vann, 'Hanoi in the Time of Cholera.' In: Monnais and Cook, eds., *Global Movements, Local Concerns*, pp.159–160.

by no means the first appearance of the disease there: cases of cholera had been reported through the 1880s and 1890s.

The history of Hanoi in the late nineteenth and early twentieth centuries suggests that for all the grand schemes of urban re-planning and building, colonial control of the urban environment remained tenuous. The 'racial ecology' of the city – legitimated through hygiene and medical science – served to undermine rather than bolster colonial authority.[51] Debates about epidemic disease in Hanoi were closely connected to broader concerns about power, race, and health. Epidemic disease brought to the fore tensions between different conceptualizations of the city, raising further questions about what cities were for, and how precisely they were to be governed. While natives were viewed through the lens of disease, the threat of disease provided a critical rationale for the city's planning. The subjection of place and of an indigenous people were inextricably bound up with the taming of disease.

As a case study, Hanoi thus foregrounds a number of contradictions that informed colonial urban planning, particularly the way that colonial authorities perceived and responded to the native Vietnamese. On the one hand, the indigenous population was viewed suspiciously as a destabilizing presence. On the other hand, it was seen as docile and oblivious to the progressive and dynamic qualities of Western civilization. Administrators sought to confine natives to designated areas of the city, or to reorganize and reinvigorate native 'village' life by imposing civic models from the West. Although there was a long history of city-dwelling in Vietnam, the village was understood to be the essential unit of native life. It was inevitably viewed as representing the homogeneous, inward-looking, and static dimensions of indigenous culture. As John Kleinen reminds us, however, there is no such thing as 'the' Vietnamese village, 'simply because such a village does not exist. Variations in landscape, physical attributes, socio-cultural circumstances and historical background do not warrant a comprehensive description of "the" Vietnamese village.'[52]

Sex in the city: Venereal disease in Singapore

As I suggested in the previous chapter, today intensified and accelerated human mobility is presenting major challenges for global health, with Asia at the forefront of this mass migration. Most accounts of the history of migration in the nineteenth and twentieth centuries tend to emphasize

---

[51] Vann, 'Hanoi in the Time of Cholera.' In: Monnais and Cook, eds., *Global Movements, Local Concerns*, p.151.

[52] John Kleinen, *Facing the Future, Reviving the Past: A Study of Social Change in a Northern Vietnamese Village* (Singapore: Institute of Southeast Asian Studies, 1999), p.2.

the movement of male indentured laborers, with relatively little discussion of women. This is not surprising, given that men formed the overwhelming majority of those who migrated and were key to the development of port cities. Labor in industry and shipping relied on a male workforce, while many Indian and Chinese migrants were sojourners – that is, migrants who arrived without their families, intending to return home to their native villages. The 1891 census in Hong Kong counted 40,492 Chinese women and 127,690 men, a ratio of close to 1:3. This was a pronounced shift from the 1860s, when some four-fifths of the coolie population had been men; a difference that prompted Hong Kong's registrar general, James Stewart Lockhart (1858–1937), to remark approvingly in 1891 on the increase in 'Chinese families,' noting how anti-Chinese agitators in the United States and Australia used the argument about the lack of Chinese women accompanying male migrants to oppose Chinese immigration.[53] In the Chinese community of Singapore, however, the gender ratio was 6:1 in 1871, and in the Straits Settlements the coolie population remained over 90 percent male until the twentieth century.[54] What were the effects of these skewed ratios on infectious disease? Colonial commentators were in no doubt: it propagated crime. 'Female immigration,' wrote the lawyer Jonas Daniel Vaughan of the Straits Settlements in 1879, 'should be encouraged by our Government to prevent, if for no other reason, the fearful crimes that prevail amongst the Chinese in consequence of the paucity of females.'[55]

In this section, I focus primarily on Singapore to explore how this demographic asymmetry led to a booming commercial sex sector, which in turn resulted in an explosion of venereal disease (VD) and concomitant anxieties about the state's ability to manage the risks of infection. While colonial authorities sought to crack down on disease, they were also conscious of the importance of prostitution in a city that was disproportionately male. The drive to regulate brothels reflected a tacit recognition that in overwhelmingly male societies, prostitutes were a necessary evil. In the words of Sir Frank Swettenham (1850–1946) – a colonial official in British Malaya and later governor of the Straits Settlements – given the demographic imbalance, prostitutes were a means of channeling male sexual impulses and thereby preventing men from engaging in even more

---

[53] 'Census Report 1891,' *Hongkong Sessional Papers 1891*, no.30, pp.373–395 (374).

[54] Lenore Manderson, 'Migration, Prostitution and Medical Surveillance in Early Twentieth-Century Malaya.' In: Lara Marks and Michael Worboys, eds., *Migrants, Minorities and Health: Historical and Contemporary Studies* (London and New York: Routledge, 1997), pp.49–69 (51); Philippa Levine, *Prostitution, Race, and Politics: Policing Venereal Disease in the British Empire* (New York: Routledge, 2003), pp.25, 28.

[55] J. D. Vaughan, *The Manners and Customs of the Chinese of the Straits Settlements* (Singapore: The Mission Press, 1879), p.9.

'unnatural and abominable vices.'[56] Moreover, the willingness of authorities in Singapore to tolerate brothel prostitution, despite growing opposition within Britain, might be viewed as a critical factor in the city's
economic success. As the historian James Francis Warren has suggested:
'Without a labor policy of unrestricted male immigration, prostitution
would not have retained its considerable importance.' Accordingly, the
toleration of brothels was integral to the policy goals of colonial officials
and urban planners.[57]

Prostitution may be understood as a by-product of 'coolie capitalism' –
an industrial system in the colonies that was dependent on plentiful supply of cheap, indentured or contracted labor (see Chapter 1 for discussion
of 'coolies'). Urban space, gender, and migration may also be viewed in
relation to a complex interplay of socio-political and economic factors.
Government attempts to contain sexually transmitted infections in 'red-
light' districts of the city led to a spatial ordering that underscored the role
of race and class, as well as gender, in the sexual economy. While prostitution shaped the colonial urban landscape, the forces driving it were
located, not only in the city, but elsewhere: in Qing China, where profound economic and socio-political transformations were taking place,
and in the modernization and industrialization of Japan after the Meiji
Restoration in 1868. In other words, economic growth and urbanization in Southeast Asia were part of a broader interregional dynamic that
extended to East Asia. Histories of Chinese and Japanese female migrants
are therefore not so much 'background' material to the story of Singapore's development as integral parts of that story.

In 1893, the Qing government formally revoked a law prohibiting overseas emigration. However, for decades before this, millions of Chinese
had left the coastal provinces of Fujian and Guangdong in southern
China, many of them traveling through Hong Kong and the treaty ports,
bound for Southeast Asia and other regions of the world where there
were Chinese communities. Migrants were driven abroad by internal conflicts within the increasingly fractured Qing dominions (Chapter 1), by
harvest failures and famines, and by pressures of over-population. Many
were propelled by the economic boom in Southeast Asia and the Pacific,
and by the discovery of gold in California and Australia. The expansion
of Singapore, like Hong Kong, was the result of this vast emigration of
Chinese coolies, particularly from the 1880s. The establishment of the
Straits Settlements as a British crown colony in 1867 (hitherto they had

---

[56] Manderson, 'Migration, Prostitution and Medical Surveillance.' In: Marks and Worboys,
eds., *Migrants, Minorities and Health*, p.52.
[57] James Francis Warren, *Ah Ku and Karayuki-san: Prostitution in Singapore, 1870–1940*
(Singapore: Oxford University Press, 1993), p.153.

been administered from India), along with the consolidation of British control over Malaya in the 1870s, acted as stimuli to economic development, and spurred demand for labor. The opening of the Suez Canal in 1869 further enhanced Singapore's trade, augmenting the traffic of steamships, and transforming the city into a military and commercial node. The ensuing inflow of migrants inevitably shaped the character of Singapore and other cities in the region. The Chinese worked on plantations and in mines; they labored in construction, on the docks, and in the factories of the booming port city.

The mass scale of this human migration heightened fears of potential epidemics and, particularly with the third plague pandemic from the 1890s (further discussed below), resulted in increasingly heated debates about the need for a more coordinated trans-colonial and international system of quarantining, as well as regulation to control the surge of migrants (Chapter 1). Concerns about plague slotted into earlier anxieties about cholera. These concerns also drew additional force from another infectious threat: VD. From the mid-century, high levels of VD amongst the British armed forces had led to calls for regulating prostitution, resulting in the passing of the first Contagious Diseases Act in Britain in 1864. Syphilis, an STI caused by the bacterium *Treponema pallidum*, was untreatable before the development of the drug Salvarsan by the German physician Paul Ehrlich (1854–1915) in 1908. The availability of the antibiotic penicillin from the early 1940s was a further breakthrough in the treatment of the disease.

Across the British Empire, attempts were made to regulate prostitution with a view to curbing the threat of VD, chiefly syphilis and gonorrhea (an infection caused by the bacterium *Neisseria gonorrhoeae*). As the historian Philippa Levine has noted: 'The rhetoric of venereal disease control as a war within a war developed quickly in Britain and its colonies.'[58] However, disease control differed significantly between colonial sites, and legislation passed in the colonies was often more sweeping than that applied at home. In Hong Kong, Governor Sir John Bowring (1792–1872) introduced an Ordinance for Checking the Spread of Venereal Disease in 1857, five years before the first Act in Britain. A Contagious Diseases Ordinance was passed in the Straits Settlements in 1870 and came into effect in 1872. Amongst the Ordinance's 44 provisions, brothel keepers were required to register their premises and provide a list of the 'inmates' working there; if infected women were found in brothels, keepers were liable to a fine; and women were subject to medical inspection with their detention for treatment in a hospital

---

[58] Levine, *Prostitution, Race, and Politics*, p.146.

when they were found to be infected.[59] The overriding motivation for the new legislation was a worry about the high numbers of naval and military personnel at risk, although this practical concern often merged with a paternalistic emphasis on moral restitution. The avowed mission of the colonial state, as proclaimed by many of its agents, was to save women from 'lives of slavery and debauchery.'[60] Although the inspector general was originally in charge of the Ordinance's enforcement, in 1881 this was transferred to the Chinese Protectorate – an administrative agency set up to oversee the welfare of Chinese residents.

If VD was a gendered disease, in the Asian colonies it also became a distinctly racially inflected infection, predominantly associated with Asians, and in particular with the Chinese, who made up the majority of working women. A racial bias informed the inspection process: whereas prostitutes who served a Chinese clientele were inspected once a month in the 1870s, those who catered to all nationalities were inspected every week, suggesting that the health of non-Chinese communities was a greater priority. Prostitution was also an urban problem. Overcrowded cities and their distorted sex ratios were understood to be drivers of commercial sex, along with other forms of criminal activity, including membership of 'secret societies.' The city was a locale where 'underground' spaces overlapped with the public sphere. The publicly registered brothel was precisely such a locus: an ambiguous place, at once hidden but highly visible, where the private and the public converged. It was this conjunction that made prostitution and disease particularly difficult to manage. As they endeavored to reorganize urban space in order to neutralize the infective threat of prostitution and the scourge of VD, colonial authorities delineated other kinds of economic, social, and cultural relations.

This spatial ordering of the city and its rationale in policies of epidemic prevention will be considered in more detail below. Before doing so, however, we should briefly consider the history of these female migrants. Who were they? Why and how did they come to work in Singapore? In many regions of Asia, women played an important role in the expansion of industry, moving from rural areas to cities, where they labored in factories. In early twentieth-century China, women and child labor fueled the booming textile mills. Prior to 1949, women accounted for two-thirds of the workforce in Shanghai's cotton, silk, and tobacco factories.[61] The

---

[59] John Augustus Harwood, ed., 'Ordinance No. XXIII of 1870.' In: *The Acts and Ordinances of the Legislative Council of the Straits Settlements, from the 1st April 1867 to the 1st June 1886*, 2 vols. (London: Eyre and Spottiswoode, 1886), I, pp.310–317.

[60] Vaughan, *The Manners and Customs of the Chinese*, p.10.

[61] Emily Honig, *Sisters and Strangers: Women in the Shanghai Cotton Mills, 1919–1949* (Stanford, CA: Stanford University Press, 1986), p.1.

rise of female wage labor was evident in Japan, too, where women were central to the textile industry, one of Japan's major industrial sectors in the years prior to the Second World War. Young women were brought from the countryside by recruiters on short-term contracts, and this growing female workforce generated attendant anxieties. What were the social and physical corollaries of this feminization of labor and the urbanization of rural Japan? Critics pointed to the nation's deteriorating health and the specter of infectious disease, which undercut the push for modernization. Young migrant women employed in silk or cotton mills were targeted as one of the main causes of the spike in TB, a disease which became epidemic from the 1880s as the country began to industrialize. From 1900 to 1919, a period during which Japan's textile industry matured, TB posed a major challenge. Female workers who resided in mill dormitories became the object of invasive public health initiatives aimed at halting the spread of the disease.[62]

Industrialization and urbanization were also closely connected to prostitution. In a number of cosmopolitan Chinese cities, such as treaty-port Shanghai, a rapidly increasing and diversifying population in the late nineteenth century, along with an expansion in foreign trade, contributed to the growth of prostitution.[63] To deal with this expansion in commercial sex – from courtesans in brothels to streetwalkers – municipal authorities, influenced by developments in Japan and Europe, implemented a range of administrative measures, including registration, taxation, and various forms of monitoring. These processes were important in extending the hitherto circumscribed functions of local government during the late Qing period. Prostitution provided a significant impetus to local state-building, not only in terms of the revenue it generated through taxation, but in terms of the expanding range of regulatory and supervisory functions it called forth. Thus, while the state shaped the institution of prostitution, prostitution also played a transformative role in the state's administrative apparatuses to the extent that 'gender needs to be written into the story of statebuilding in China, even though women, generally barred from political life at that time in China, were not visible political actors.'[64]

---

[62] Janet Hunter, 'Textile Factories, Tuberculosis and the Quality of Life in Industrializing Japan.' In: Janet Hunter, ed., *Japanese Women Working* (London and New York: Routledge, 1993), pp.69–97.

[63] Christian Henriot, *Prostitution and Sexuality in Shanghai. A Social History, 1849–1949.* Translated by Nöel Castelino (Cambridge: Cambridge University Press, 2001).

[64] Elizabeth J. Remick, *Regulating Prostitution in China: Gender and Local Statebuilding, 1900–1937* (Stanford, CA: Stanford University Press, 2014), p.2.

The development of global trading hubs such as Hong Kong and Singapore provided new opportunities for profit to be gained from illicit networks of exchange, including human trafficking and sex work. There was an extensive trade in young women between Hong Kong and Chinese port cities up the coast, including Amoy, Swatow (Shantou), Shanghai, and Canton. Hong Kong served as a 'redistributive depot' in this circulation of prostitutes, predominantly those from rural southern China migrating east to Singapore and to other cities in Southeast Asia, or across the Pacific to the United States.[65] Singapore was also a regional center for traffickers moving women to Malaya, Siam, Borneo, and the Dutch East Indies. Economic necessity and family obligation appear to have driven Chinese women into prostitution. One estimate suggests that only five percent of prostitutes in Shanghai had entered into sex work as 'free persons.' Most had been kidnapped, pawned, or sold to brothel owners by their families or traffickers.[66] In Malaya and the Straits, Chinese prostitutes seldom worked independently but were forced to pay protection money to Chinese gangs or 'secret societies,' surrendering a portion of their earnings to brothel keepers (Figure 2.3).[67]

There was also a migration of prostitutes to Southeast Asia from Japan. The so-called *karayuki-san* – the ideograms translate literally as 'a person who goes to China' – were women from impoverished families in northeastern Kyushu who worked abroad as prostitutes after the restoration of the Meiji dynasty, when restrictions on foreign travel were lifted (Chapter 1). The *karayuki-san* have conventionally been viewed as representatives of the underside of Japan: the consequences of a rural–city dislocation, and emblems of the adverse effects of Japan's rapid modernization on traditional rural society.[68] This is the view most often presented in histories and reinforced in popular works, such as the bestselling book *Sandakan No. 8 Brothel* by Yamazaki Tomoko, first published in 1972 and adapted for film by Kei Kumai. Yamazaki's tale draws extensively on oral testimony and follows the life of a woman who was sold into prostitution by her family. The story is told in flashbacks from the perspective of an elderly and impoverished former *karayuki-san* called Osaki, who recalls her life from the 1920s. We learn how she was taken from Kyushu to Sandakan in British North Borneo (today's Malaysian state of Sabah)

---

[65] Warren, *Ah Ku and Karayuki-san*, p.74.

[66] Gail Hershatter, 'The Hierarchy of Shanghai Prostitution, 1870–1949,' *Modern China*, vol.15, no.4 (1989): 463–498 (476).

[67] Ah Eng Lai, *Peasants, Proletarians, and Prostitutes: A Preliminary Investigation into the Work of Chinese Women in Colonial Malaya* (Singapore: Institute of Southeast Asian Studies, 1986), p.28.

[68] Mikiso Hane, *Peasants, Rebels, and Outcastes: The Underside of Japan*. Second edition (Lanham, MD: Rowman & Littlefield, 2003), pp.209–225.

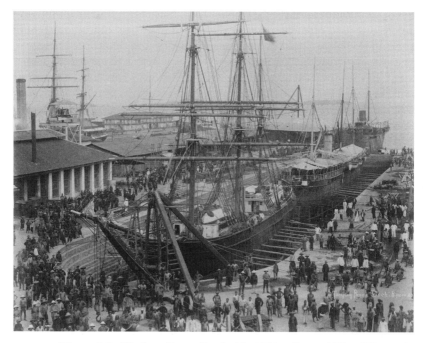

Figure 2.3. 'Tanjong Pagar Dock. 20, 1890s: General View.' From the Lee Kip Lin Collection. All rights reserved. Lee Kip Lin and National Library Board, Singapore 2009.

Booming trade in Singapore

The German photographer G. R. Lambert established a photographic studio in Singapore in the late 1860s. Figure 2.3 shows the docks owned by the Tanjong Pagar Dock Company, which was later expropriated by the government and eventually transmuted into the Singapore Harbour Board. After its establishment in 1819, Singapore became the center of the Chinese junk trade, as well as a strategic port for British trade in Asia, including opium. The city functioned as a coaling station for steamship traffic and became a hub servicing the Malay peninsula. Transport networks were developed to bring tin, oil, and rubber from the hinterland to Singapore where they were processed and shipped globally.

believing that she was going to work as a maid, only to discover that Sandakan No.8 is a brothel and she must work as a prostitute. The fear of contracting disease there is constant: 'Syphilis – if you got that, you know, your body would rot. Your whole body would be covered with pustules and you would die a terrible death, or you would go mad.'[69]

From another perspective, however, we might consider the *karayuki-san* as exemplifying a new form of global wage labor; as 'urban pioneers' at the forefront of capital expansion across the region.[70] Certainly, overseas Japanese prostitution was a repercussion of the country's 'opening up' from the late 1850s and a by-product of Meiji–Taisho modernization. As Bill Mihalopoulos has argued, the *karayuki-san* were in effect part of a new global workforce, even though their 'work' jarred with official ideals of hygienic modernity and womanhood.[71] Exploring these conflicting views of the *karayuki-san* rehearses many ongoing historiographical debates about the status of prostitutes and prostitution: first, about whether prostitution should be regarded as a form of labor – 'sex work' – or whether such a designation implies volition and underplays the institution's manifestly coercive and stigmatizing character. Second, about the possibility of restoring historical agency to women who have been rendered passive victims of male abuse (Figure 2.4).

The influx of prostitutes to colonial cities such as Hong Kong and Singapore produced new stress points, since prostitutes were considered the principal vectors of disease. In the blunt words of Thomas C. Mugliston, who became Singapore's colonial surgeon in 1888, women were the 'chief disseminators of disease.'[72] From the 1860s to the 1880s, many colonial states sought to construct systems of registration, brothel inspection, and mandatory medical examination to regulate the commercial sex market in response to a perceived 'epidemic' of VD. In Hong Kong, the licensing of brothels from the 1860s created what was tantamount to a segregated city: foreign-frequented brothels clustered in the Central District, while Chinese brothels were, for the most part, located in the Western District. This spatial ordering reflected a sexual economy

---

[69] Tomoko Yamazaki, *Sandakan Brothel No.8: Journey into the History of Lower-Class Japanese Women.* Translated by Karen Colligan-Taylor (Abingdon: Routledge, [1999] 2015), pp.69–70.

[70] Luise White, *The Comforts of Home: Prostitution in Colonial Nairobi* (Chicago, IL: University of Chicago Press, 1990), p.34.

[71] Bill Mihalopoulos, *Sex in Japan's Globalization, 1870–1930: Prostitutes, Emigration and Nation-Building* (London: Pickering & Chatto, 2011); Hiroshi Shimizu and Hitoshi Hirakawa, *Japan and Singapore in the World Economy: Japan's Economic Advance into Singapore, 1870–1965* (Abingdon: Routledge, 1999), pp.19–50.

[72] Lenore Manderson, *Sickness and the State: Health and Illness in Colonial Malaya, 1870–1940* (Cambridge: Cambridge University Press, 1996), p.177.

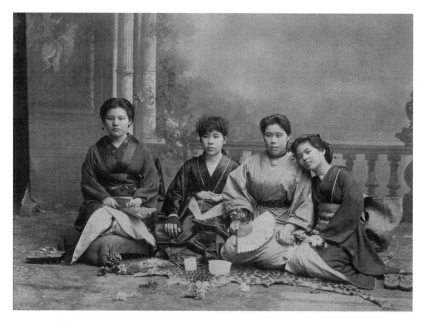

Figure 2.4. 'Japanese women in traditional dress, Singapore (1890s).'
Courtesy: National Archives of Singapore.

Coolie women

While male coolies exemplified unencumbered labor, female coolies
were viewed more ambiguously. Given that a woman's place was
taken to be at home with the family, the female coolie – like the
prostitute – was often perceived as posing a moral threat, undermining the social order. At the same time, a lack of women was
identified as a cause of high rates of suicide among migrant laborers.
Whereas British colonial authorities sought to deal with this problem of discrepant gender ratios, private interests resisted pressures
to encourage more female coolies, viewing women and children as
burdens that reduced profitability. It was only in the twentieth century that employers encouraged family life as a way of consolidating
the workforce, although single women were recruited as indentured
labor: for example, taking ship from southern India to work on the
sugar plantations of British Guiana.

Jan Breman, *Taming the Coolie Beast: Plantation Society and the
Colonial Order in Southeast Asia* (Delhi: Oxford University Press,
1989), pp.94–96, 159–160, 191–193.

Gaiutra Bahadur, *Coolie Woman: The Odyssey of Indenture*
(Chicago, IL: University of Chicago Press, 2014).

that was constructed through 'cultural ascription and socio-political negotiation,' which revealed 'the limits as well as the reach of the colonial biopolitical state.'[73]

By the final decades of the nineteenth century, Singapore had assumed a distinctive form with its central business district, administrative quarters, a European residential district, and a Chinatown. In contrast to these clearly delineated spaces, the Asian areas of the city 'were complicated mosaics of specialized trade areas, bazaars, densely packed tenement housing, and concentration of eating houses, theatres, and brothels.'[74] According to a visitor from Shanghai in 1885, 'Along Kereta Ayer [a road in Chinatown], brothels are as many and as close together as the teeth of a comb.'[75] Prostitution clustered primarily in two 'red-light' districts to the west and east of the Singapore River, which bisected the city. Brothels servicing the Chinese were located in the so-called 'big town' or 'greater town,' a predominantly coolie area to the west; brothels catering to the non-Chinese were mainly to be found in the 'lesser town' to the east, in the area around Malay Street. The toleration of these sex enclaves was, in part, a practical solution for managing the public health threat that prostitution was understood to pose. Zoning sex work in this way facilitated the regulation of brothels and the medical inspection of prostitutes. Beyond that, it functioned as a means of relegating problem areas to 'safe' districts in the city; de-compression areas, where the pent-up pressures of sex, disease, and the working-classes could, at least in theory, be safely managed.

In 1886, the Contagious Diseases Acts were repealed in Britain, with colonies such as Hong Kong and Singapore soon forced to follow. By 1894, despite petitioning from the colonial government, the registration of brothels in Singapore was abolished with mandatory medical inspection replaced by a voluntary system. There was widespread opposition to this move, which was viewed as opening the floodgates to infection. Particularly vocal in their opposition to the repeal of the Ordinance were members of the Chinese elite who argued that legislation was required to avert disease and prevent the ill-treatment of Chinese prostitutes. Colonial officials also argued that social conditions in Singapore were exceptional and incomparable to those in Britain. In Singapore, the asymmetric sex ratio had particularly 'evil consequences': fears about the

---

[73] Philip Howell, *Geographies of Regulation: Policing Prostitution in Nineteenth-Century Britain and the Empire* (Cambridge: Cambridge University Press, 2009), pp.212–218 (217).

[74] Brenda S. A. Yeoh, *Contesting Space in Colonial Singapore: Power Relations and the Urban Built Environment* (Singapore: NUS Press, 2003), p.48.

[75] Warren, *Ah Ku and Karayuki-san*, p.43.

spread of disease were intertwined with arguments about the need to protect women from abuse.[76]

The Women and Girls' Protection Ordinance was introduced in 1887 (and in revised form in 1888) as an attempt to safeguard women from unscrupulous traffickers and the activities of the 'secret societies.' It also functioned as a means of plugging the surveillance gap left by the repeal of the Contagious Diseases Ordinance. Under this new legislation, the Chinese Protectorate was vested with the authority to control brothels. While it was permitted to conduct raids on brothels, its powers were circumscribed and a proposal in the Legislative Council in 1896 to grant the Protector 'extraordinary powers to carry out his duty' was defeated. Simultaneously, there was a drive to establish more medical clubs where prostitutes could pay to be medically inspected. Few women – aside from Japanese prostitutes – voluntarily submitted to inspection at the free lock hospitals, since they were reluctant to stand in queues and undergo a humiliating examination by a European doctor. The medical clubs also proved unpopular and in the aftermath of the repeal of the Contagious Diseases Ordinance there was mounting concern about an epidemic of VD. This apprehension was well founded as incidences of infection rose. While women suffered from a wide range of diseases, including syphilis, gonorrhea, genital ulcers, and urinary tract infections, colonial anxieties focused predominantly on the city's male population. The most visible victims were the military, and cases of VD in the forces surged: in the Tanglin Barracks the ratio of infection stood at 618 per thousand in 1895. Similarly, the number of VD cases admitted to the Tan Tock Seng Pauper Hospital after 1888 considerably outstripped previous years, while prison reports reveal a similar rise, suggesting the spread of STIs into poorer sections of the coolie population at large.[77]

In this section, we have explored the interconnections between prostitution, VD, and the development of Singapore as a coolie city and imperial nexus in Southeast Asia. We have examined the growth of the port city in relation to transformations in China and Japan, showing how migration fueled urban expansion, and underlining the role that women played in this process. A major theme has been the ambiguity of the administration's attitude to prostitution and its efforts to manage infection. On the one hand, prostitutes and brothel keepers were censured as the spreaders of disease. On the other hand, by seeking to regulate commercial sex, colonial authorities conceded their importance. Like

[76] Tan Beng Hui, '"Protecting" Women: Legislation and Regulation of Women's Sexuality in Colonial Malaya,' *Gender, Technology and Development*, vol.7, no.1 (2003): 1–30 (5).
[77] Warren, *Ah Ku and Karayuki-san*, pp.129–133.

the so-called 'secret societies,' brothels were in fact far from secret: they were highly visible institutions that occupied 'safe' zones embedded in the heart of the city.

In the final case, we consider another booming Asian city: Bombay. Here, too, epidemic disease is explored in relation to the intertwined social and political forces driving urban expansion, focusing on Bombay's modernity; on those distinctively modern features, and notably the railway, which made the city susceptible to an old disease: plague.

Bombay: Disease in a 'world of wonder'

At the close of the nineteenth century, a tripartite model of disease history, structured around a disease's 'ancient,' 'medieval,' and 'modern' manifestations, was widely promoted. While it drew on earlier humanist thinking, this tripartite model reflected late nineteenth-century assumptions about the progressive nature of history. A similar periodization was applied to a wide array of cultural artifacts, ranging from language to architecture. Accounts of the bubonic plague in the 1890s thus invariably traced the disease back to the fourteenth-century Black Death and to the Justinian plague in the sixth century, which had devastated the Byzantine Empire. Part of the panic provoked by the third plague pandemic, however, was plague's residual status as an 'old' disease. For many Western commentators, the plague represented the re-emergence of an obdurate old world into the new.

A persistent association of the plague with the past, and the emphasis in late nineteenth-century reports on the backward urban environments where plague germs fomented, have tended to eclipse discussion of the newness of the Asian cities where outbreaks occurred. Accounts of the epidemic in Hong Kong, for example, are prone to ignore the colony's technological edge. While the plague was raging in the Chinese districts, an elevator was ascending in the Hongkong Hotel, installed by Otis in 1888. Street lights illuminated Queen's Road Central, Battery Path, and Upper Albert Road. Hong Kong was networked through the telegraph and the telephone.

In the 1890s, Bombay, too, was in many respects a pre-eminently modern city characterized by novel technologies and monumental landmarks. As the journalist James Furneaux noted in his photographic history of India in 1895, Bombay was 'essentially a modern city, a city of the present and the future, but not of the past.'[78] The Parsee politician and lawyer Sir

[78] J. H. Furneaux, *Glimpses of India A Grand Photographic History of India, the Greatest Empire of the East* (Bombay and London: C. B. Burrows & Co., 1896), p.196.

Dinshaw Wacha (1844–1936) celebrated this sense of novelty in his recollections of the city's transformation in the 1860s and early 1870s into
'a great emporium of trades and manufactures, of vast enterprise and
of a cosmopolitan character.' For Wacha, Bombay's emergent modernity
contrasted with the grime and stink of the old city, where the streets were
heaped with rubbish, and noxious gases 'saturated the atmosphere with
foul exhalations.'[79] Under the governorship of Sir Bartle Frere (1815–
1884), the seventeenth-century ramparts of the old fort were demolished and the city was re-planned to accommodate an industrial future.
Land was reclaimed and swamps drained so that by the 1890s Bombay's islands had been joined and the metropolis had assumed its modern
form. Above all, new public buildings were erected along the Esplanade to
house the city's burgeoning civic institutions: the Town Hall, the Rajabai
Clock Tower, the High Court, the University Library and Convocation
Hall, the Government Secretariat, the Central Telegraph Office, and the
Bombay Municipal Corporation Building. Ironically, the spirit of technological modernity was expressed through Neoclassical, Italianate, and
Gothic architectural forms, exemplified by Bombay's spectacular Victoria Terminus Station (today known as the Chhatrapati Shivaji Terminus and classified in 2004 as a UNESCO World Heritage site), which
served as the central terminal for the Great Indian Peninsula Railway.
Begun in 1879, and designed by the architectural engineer Frederick
William Stevens (1847–1900), the station was thrown open for traffic in
1882 but officially inaugurated for the Queen's Golden Jubilee in 1887
(Figure 2.5). With a height of 100 meters and a length of 366 meters, the
station was reminiscent of a cathedral, with stained glass windows, tessel-
lated floor, and ornate iron work. 'The hall is as large as that so familiar
at Euston,' observed Furneaux, 'but infinitely grander.' The building's
exterior was fittingly adorned with figures personifying Commerce, Agriculture, and Engineering, while Progress held a flaming torch aloft, with
a winged wheel in the other hand:

As to the station proper it may be mentioned that the total length of roof is 600
feet, and it covers eight lines of rails and four large platforms, two for arrivals and
two for departures, the main roof of corrugated iron with air spaces under the
apex, having two spans each of 120 feet clear... From an architectural point of
view, however, the crowning point of Mr. Stevens' triumph is undoubtedly the
large massive dome which surmounts the main building.[80]

---

[79] Sir Dinshaw Wacha, *Shells from the Sands of Bombay – Being My Recollections and Rem-
iniscences, 1860–1875* (Bombay: T. K. Anklesaria, The Indian Newspaper Co., 1920),
p.478.
[80] Furneaux, *Glimpses of India*, p.203.

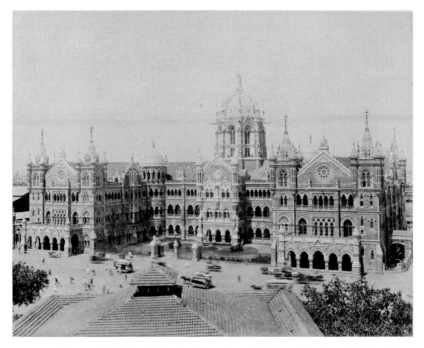

Figure 2.5. 'The Victoria Terminus Railway Station GIPR [Great Indian Peninsula Railway] Bombay (1880s).' © The British Library Board.

The Victoria Terminus epitomized imperial modernity and was expressive of the power of capitalist commerce and industry. Indeed, railways were instrumental in the extension of empire and the expansion of capital, linking cities to hinterlands, and connecting local economies to global markets.[81] As Karl Marx prophesied in 1853 – the year that saw the inauguration of India's railway system – locomotives would be the chief driver of industrialization on the subcontinent:

You cannot maintain a net of railways over an immense country without introducing all those industrial processes necessary to meet the immediate and current wants of railway locomotion, and out of which there must grow the application

---

[81] Clarence B. Davis and Kenneth E. Wilburn Jr., with Ronald E. Robinson, eds., *Railway Imperialism* (Westport, CT: Greenwood Press, 1991).

of machinery to those branches of industry not immediately connected with railways. The railway-system will therefore become, in India, truly the forerunner of modern industry.[82]

By 1890, 15,842 miles of track had been laid and by 1910 the Indian railway had become the fourth-largest in the world.[83] Bombay's Victoria Terminus also underscored the importance of the locomotive in the city's transformation. In its early colonial history, Bombay had been primarily a port for trans-shipments with few linkages to the hinterland. However, during the American Civil War (1861–1865) the Southern Confederate ports were blockaded by the North, preventing the export of cotton and leading to rising prices. English cloth manufacturers turned to India for substitute supplies of raw cotton. Commercial institutions 'sprang up like mushrooms' around Bombay's thriving cotton trade, observed the politician Sir Richard Temple: banks, financial associations, shipping, insurance, and joint-stock companies.[84] In part to manage the slump that followed the cessation of conflict and the United States' re-entry into the cotton market – as well as to counter the dominance of European firms in trade – Parsee, Jewish, and Bhatia industrialists sought to develop the city as a manufacturing hub by establishing new steam-powered mills.[85] By 1890, there were 70 mills in Bombay, employing nearly 76,000 workers. The railway underpinned Bombay's expansion and functioned, as Ian Kerr has put it, as 'an engine of change.' While it contributed to the expansion of port cities such as Bombay, Calcutta, Madras (Chennai), and Karachi, it did so at the expense of inland centers where high transport costs disadvantaged industry.[86] Tunneling through the Western Ghat mountain range, the railway connected Bombay to the cotton growing areas of the Deccan Plateau in west-central India and to Gujarat further north, spurring the growth of industry, and opening up Bombay to supplies of cheap labor. Thousands of migrants flocked to find work in the docks and mills. By 1891, Bombay's population was estimated to be over 820,000. According to the 1901 census of India, Bombay was

---

[82] Karl Marx, 'The Future Results of British Rule in India.' In: Ian J. Kerr, ed., *Railways in Modern India* (New Delhi: Oxford University Press, 2001) pp.62–67 (65).

[83] John M. Hurd, 'Railways.' In: Dharma Kumar, ed., *The Cambridge Economic History of India, vol.2: c.1757–1970* (Cambridge: Cambridge University Press, 1983), pp.737–761 (739, 737).

[84] Sir Richard Temple, *Men and Events of My Time in India* (London: John Murray, 1882), pp.269–270.

[85] Rajnarayan Chandavarkar, *The Origins of Industrial Capitalism in India: Business Strategies and the Working Classes in Bombay, 1900–1940* (Cambridge: Cambridge University Press, 1994), pp.21–71.

[86] Ian J. Kerr, *Engines of Change: The Railroads That Made India* (Westport, CT: Praeger, 2007); Hurd, 'Railways.' In: Kumar, ed., *The Cambridge Economic History of India*, pp.757–758.

'admitted to be the most crowded city in the world.'[87] As Sir George W. Forrest declared in *Cities of India* (1903), Bombay was 'a world of wonder.'[88]

The city's newness, then, served as a backdrop to the plague when it arrived in the late summer of 1896. On 18 September, the Goan-born physician Dr. Accacio G. Viegas (1856–1933) had identified the first case in the area of Mandvi close to the docks, a diagnosis that was confirmed after bacteriological analysis. Officials conjectured that the disease had been imported from Arabia, the Persian Gulf, or Hong Kong, which seemed most likely. As in Hong Kong, some attributed the epidemic to abnormal climatic conditions: to an unusual monsoon season, which had seen heavy rains and floods followed by protracted dry spells, leading to an acute water shortage.

Historians of the plague have generally emphasized the sanitarian crisis sparked by the epidemic and the increasing focus by agents of the colonial state on the overcrowded Indian tenements, or *chawls*, which became particular targets of draconian public health interventions. The emphasis, in other words, has been on the dark, foul-smelling city where disease was understood to fester. In this section, however, the aim is to refocus on those modern institutions and civic landmarks that exemplified the state's increasingly technocratic management of urban space. While the epidemic exposed the fragility of Bombay's institutions, it also revealed what could happen when their function was inverted and they worked in reverse, undermining the order they were established to uphold. In other words, perceptions of the plague as an old affliction – the 'Black Death' – had obscured its identity as a modern disease, spread through the pathways enabled by expanding technology.

Even before the plague outbreak, there had been concerns about the possibility that railways might function as vehicles for disease transmission. For the British writer Rudyard Kipling (1865–1936), overcrowded Indian trains, in particular, were lethal vectors of infection:

The people crowded the trains, hanging on to the footboards and squatting on the roofs of the carriages, and the cholera followed them, for at each station they dragged out the dead and the dying.[89]

This specter of locomotive communication as a force of infectious declension undermined visions of the railway as a modern instrument of

[87] 'Notes from India (The Plague in India),' *Lancet*, vol.1, no.3891 (March 26, 1898): 898–899 (899).

[88] G. W. Forrest, *Cities of India* (London: Archibald Constable, 1903), pp.33–34.

[89] Rudyard Kipling, *Without Benefit of Clergy* (New York: Doubleday and McClure Co., [1890] 1899), pp.64–65.

civilization that would mesh the country, promoting – in the words of the governor general of India, Lord Dalhousie (1812–1860) – 'similar progress in social improvement that has marked the introduction of improved communications in various Kingdoms of the Western World.' The railway would propagate education, help to dismantle the caste system, and prevent famine by facilitating the distribution of food.[90] In contrast to this vision of productive integration, Marx had noted what he called 'the double mission' of British colonialism, exemplified by the transposition of the railway system to India: the creation of a modern, industrial society entailed the systematic 'annihilation' of the old.[91]

As the report of the Plague Committee noted, to escape the epidemic, 'a large number of upper-class Hindus' moved out to temporary accommodation by the railway in Salsette, commuting into the city by train.[92] Increasingly, however, as disease spread, the railway system became a focus of government intervention and a flashpoint of conflict. Originally, private companies had been contracted to build the lines, but from 1869 the government had begun to assume responsibility for their construction. After 1879, when it took over the East Indian Railway, the government acquired ownership of the large railway companies, but with management remaining predominantly in private hands. 'In the appearance of the plague,' writes Laura Bear, 'the dream of circulating commerce and passengers became the nightmare of indiscriminate passage of disease in the bodies and parcels of the Indian public.'[93] As another historian has expressed it, 'plague rode the rails.'[94] Trains were used in a mass exodus of the city and special trains (known as 'specials') departed from Bombay carrying those fleeing the epidemic:

When the plague was at its height, and the exodus in full flow, the scenes at the railway stations were striking, a motley crowd of natives of every caste and creed, pressing, and shouting for tickets, and then, as the train steamed in a hurrying anxious throng, old and young alike, tottering under enormous bundles of household goods.[95]

[90] W. H. Macpherson, 'Investment in Indian Railways, 1845–1875,' *Economic History Review*, vol.8, no.2 (1955): 177–186 (177).

[91] Marx, 'The Future Results of British Rule in India.' In: Kerr, ed., *Railways in Modern India*, p.63.

[92] Sir James MacNabb Campbell, *Report of the Bombay Plague Committee* (Bombay: Printed at the 'Times of India' Steam Press, 1898), pp.17–18.

[93] Laura Bear, *Lines of the Nation: Indian Railway Workers, Bureaucracy, and the Intimate Historical Self* (New York: Columbia University Press, 2007), p.43.

[94] Ira Klein, 'Plague, Policy and Popular Unrest in British India,' *Modern Asian Studies*, vol.22, no.4 (1988): 723–755 (743, 737).

[95] M. E. Couchman, *Account of Plague Administration in the Bombay Presidency from September 1896 till May 1897* (Bombay: Printed at the Government Central Press, 1897), p.21.

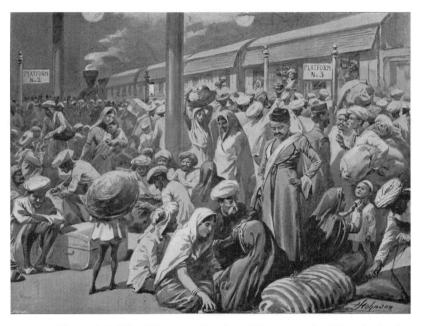

Figure 2.6. 'The Plague at Bombay: Natives at the Victoria Station Leaving the Town by Special Train.' Lithograph after a drawing by Herbert Johnson, *Graphic* (January 30, 1897), p.121. Courtesy: Bridgeman Images.

An illustration in the January 30, 1897 edition of the *Graphic* depicted panicked crowds on the platform of the Victoria Terminus during the plague (Figure 2.6). Similar sketches of crowds at stations appeared in other metropolitan publications, including a full-page lithograph by Amédée Forestier in the *Illustrated London News*.[96] Writing from Bombay, the *Graphic*'s correspondent noted: 'The trains and small steamers daily take thousands of fugitives from the city. Victoria terminus every evening is a sight not to be forgotten. Over a thousand natives swarm together tightly packed at the barriers of the platforms, and on the gates being opened they struggle and fight to get seats in the trains, which become so overcrowded that special trains have to be added.'[97] The municipal commissioner described the scene as residents sought to leave Bombay by rail at the end of 1896:

[96] 'The Plague in India: The Exodus from Bombay,' *Illustrated London News* (February 6, 1897).
[97] *Graphic* (January 30, 1897), p.121.

As special after special left the stations, the relics of the disappointed crowds, sooner than miss the next opportunity, would quietly settle down to sleep on the platforms. The busy scenes at the station stood out in marked contrast to the quietness of Bombay; whole streets of shops were closed, business was paralysed, and the desolate emptiness of thoroughfares ordinarily teeming with life was most remarkable, and continued throughout the months of December and January, when the population had been reduced to its lowest figure.[98]

Early on in the epidemic, concerns were articulated about the likelihood of the railway system spreading disease. In October 1896, the railway companies were consulted about measures 'for the prevention of the conveyance of plague infection by Railway passengers.' Under provisions in the Railway Act, 1890 (Sections 71 and 117), a railway company had the 'power to refuse to carry persons suffering from infectious or contagious disorder,' and offending passengers could be removed from the railway carriage. As Bear observes of the clampdown on travel during the plague: 'It was a short step from the existing power of railway staff to the tight imposition of control over passengers during this period.'[99] Passengers were examined leaving Bombay through the city's two main stations, the Victoria Terminus and the Grant Road station – the terminus of the Central India Railway, which connected Bombay to Surat.[100] The scale of the flight from Bombay, however, soon put pressure on these preliminary efforts. In February 1897, it was decided to shift the focus with inspecting medical officers dispatched to examine all passengers passing through the stations of Kalyan and Palghar (Figure 2.7). Government officials were alarmed at the prospect of the disease spreading from Bombay to other cities on the subcontinent via the railway. In October 1896, the colonial administrator Herbert Risley (1851–1911), speaking before the Corporation of Calcutta and responding to news of the plague in Bombay, had declared: 'with the communications which existed between the two cities a microbe which was so infinitesimal and so long-lived might come from Bombay at any moment and propagate infinitely.' To avert such an outcome, it was imperative for railway companies to take the 'utmost precaution,' and Risley called for the medical inspection of passengers on platforms.[101]

The Epidemic Disease Act, brought in by the Government of India in February 1897, reinforced the authority of the local government. Officials

[98] Couchman, *Account of Plague Administration in the Bombay Presidency*, pp.21–22.
[99] Bear, *Lines of the Nation*, pp.43–44.
[100] James Knighton Condon, *The Bombay Plague: Being a History of the Progress of Plague in the Bombay Presidency from September 1896 to June 1899* (Bombay: Printed at the Education Society's Steam Press, 1900), p.141.
[101] Bear, *Lines of the Nation*, pp.43–44.

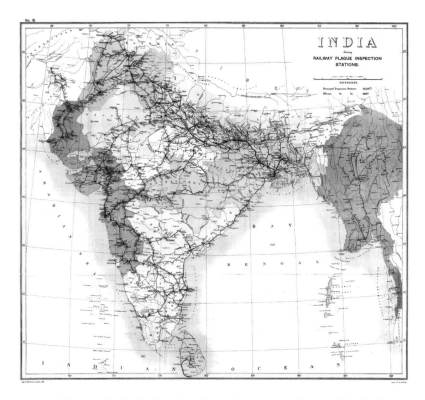

Figure 2.7. 'India Showing Plague Inspection Stations.' In: R. Nathan, *The Plague in India, 1896, 1897. Maps and Plates* (Calcutta: Office of the Superintendent, Government Printing, India, 1898), IV, plate 16.

were vested with the right to detain those suspected of being infected, as well as disinfecting – and in the last resort demolishing – contaminated dwellings. It also allowed for the inspection of stations and the establishment of 'segregation camps' at suitable places on railways. The railway system was deemed more important to quarantine than shipping, given that 'the length of time spent on a railway journey is generally less than on a sea voyage, and therefore in the case of arrival by sea the chance of Plague showing itself before or on arrival was greater than in the case of passengers by rail.' Season ticket holders and first-class passengers, 'except in the case of delicate or sickly persons, were not generally considered necessary.' Second-class passengers were inspected for disease in the carriages, while third-class passengers were examined on the platforms: 'Local passengers were examined before the arrival of trains and kept in a barricaded portion of the station until after the inspection of passengers arriving by trains.' From October, with the increase in the number of people arriving in Bombay from infected districts, surveillance at train stations was strengthened. At the Victoria Terminus, the Great Indian Peninsula Railway 'set apart and fenced in a portion of the station known as the Arcade for the sorting and examination of passengers.' From November 1897 through April 1898, a camp was established adjacent to the Victoria Terminus, 'surrounded by a bamboo mat fence' with a holding capacity of 2,500 persons.[102] In some instances, trains were stopped at random, and plague 'suspects' were pulled off. The Bombay press railed at the opprobrious treatment of Indian lawyers and '[n]ative gentlemen of position,' who were treated like third-class passengers at the Victoria Terminus.[103] Aside from those fleeing the plague, the movement of grain aid to the famine-affected rural areas in turn ferried rats and fleas from city to village. Railway companies were anxious about the likelihood of disturbances at stations, as well as the disruption of train services.[104]

The plague was driven, in part, by the railway – an institution that had come to represent Bombay's ascendancy as the 'urbs prima in Indis.' Like the telegraph, which had been conceived as a way of meshing the subcontinent but came to be subverted as a tool for Indian nationalism, so, too, did the railway work in reverse. The institutions that marked Bombay out as modern: hospitals, the Crawford Market – the first building to have electric light in Bombay – and the city's stations, were also sites of conflict. While the clock tower at the Crawford Market was shot at during riots, the Arthur Road Hospital was also attacked in 1897. Both were emblems of colonial rule, exemplifying an imperial vision of civic modernity.

To be sure, 'overcrowding' became a key concern for urban authorities at the turn of the century. Epidemics revealed the problems of city living: dirt and defective infrastructure. Diseases such as smallpox, syphilis, typhoid, and TB thrived in densely populated port cities, which were reliant on migrant labor (Chapter 1) and serviced by often inadequate water and waste systems. Indeed, the plague underlined the close connection between migration, urbanization, and disease in port cities.

---

[102] Campbell, *Report of the Bombay Plague Committee*, pp.8, 34, 37, 40, 76.
[103] David Arnold, 'Touching the Body: Perspectives on the Indian Plague.' In: Ranajit Guha and Gayatri Chakravorty Spivak, eds., *Selected Subaltern Studies* (Oxford: Oxford University Press, 1988), pp.391–426 (424).
[104] Mark Harrison, *Public Health in British India: Anglo-Indian Preventive Medicine, 1859–1914* (Cambridge: Cambridge University Press, 1994), pp.140–141.

In this way, it shaped novel approaches to urban planning.[105] Bacteriological breakthroughs and a new understanding of the etiology of disease converged with environmental thinking to influence the construction and policing of cities. After the plague, there was a fresh impetus to construct urban infrastructure, including sewage systems and waterworks – evidence of the 'sanitarian syndrome.'[106] In Bombay, and other cities, plague improvement trusts were established to clear slums, construct roads, and build new dwellings.

The Bombay City Improvement Trust: Plague and urban planning

When plague broke out in Bombay in 1896, the disease was attributed in part to overcrowding in the poor, working-class districts of the city. The congested living conditions there were understood to be drivers of infection – a connection reinforced by the statistics: death rates in these neighborhoods exceeded 12 percent. The Bombay City Improvement Trust was established in November 1898 to address the housing question and improve sanitary conditions in the slum areas, which the Bombay Municipal Corporation had proven incapable of dealing with (similar improvement trusts were subsequently established in other cities, such as Calcutta in 1911). There was an economic imperative to the Trust's mission since the plague had paralyzed the economic life of the city. Over half of Bombay's population are estimated to have fled, including some 30 percent of the city's mill workers and many workers involved in essential services, such as street cleaning and night-soil removal. Commerce and industrial production were inevitably severely disrupted. The Trust was charged with clearing unsanitary housing, widening roads, and draining low-lying ground. It was also vested with the authority to redevelop sections of the city to increase the housing supply and construct residential suburban estates, making use of undeveloped sites belonging to the government and the Municipal Corporation, as well as acquiring private land for which it paid compensation to owners. However,

---

[105] William Beinart and Lotte Hughes, *Environment and Empire* (Oxford: Oxford University Press, 2007), pp.167–183.

[106] Maynard W. Swanson, 'The Sanitation Syndrome: Bubonic Plague and Urban Native Policy in the Cape Colony, 1900–1909,' *Journal of African History*, vol.18, no.3 (1977): 387–410.

the Trust exacerbated old problems, while creating new ones. Critics argued that it fueled property speculation and led to a hike in rents, reducing rather than increasing the availability of housing. Overcrowded, insanitary tenements continued to pose health risks, while the interests of property developers and industrialists, notably the mill owners, undermined the Trust's mission. If the plague epidemic highlighted the need for a more integrated urban design and provided the impetus for reform, it also exposed competing interests and entrenched views, which obstructed change.

Prashant Kidambi, 'Housing the Poor in a Colonial City: The Bombay Improvement Trust, 1898–1918,' *Studies in History*, vol.17, no.1 (2001): 57–79.

Accounts of these post-plague urban development initiatives are prone to pit the modern against the old, progress against backwardness, health against disease. However, as I have sought to suggest above, understanding the role of the modern city and its technologies in producing epidemics suggests a more complex interplay between modernity and disease. It was precisely this interplay which Mahatma Gandhi (1869–1948) underlined in his critique of Western society's faith in science and technology. Gandhi singled out 'locomotive ambition' and the railway for particular censure, arguing that the re-engineering of social life that the railway effected had brought about a psychological and moral disequilibrium. In his book *Hind Swaraj* (*Indian Home Rule*), published in 1908, Gandhi considered the material consequences of rail travel:

It must be manifest to you that, but for the railways, the English could not have a hold on India as they have. The railways, too, have spread the bubonic plague. Without them, masses could not move from place to place. They are the carriers of plague germs. Formerly we had natural segregation. Railways have also increased the frequency of famines, because, owing to facility of means of locomotion, people sell out their grain, and it is sent to the dearest markets.[107]

The railways are condemned for imposing an imperial order on India, even as they subject the population to an exploitative capitalist system that creates the conditions for famine. The railways are also imagined as vectors of disease: for Gandhi, colonial cities were the 'real plague-spots of Modern India.'[108]

[107] Rohit Chopra, *Technology and Nationalism in India: Cultural Negotiations from Colonialism to Cyberspace* (Amherst, NY: Cambria Press, 2008), p.98.
[108] David Smith, *Hinduism and Modernity* (Malden, MA and Oxford: Blackwell, 2003), p.30.

Conclusion: Disease entrepôts

During the nineteenth and twentieth centuries, cities such as Calcutta, Bombay, Singapore, and Hong Kong functioned as critical nodes in a global pattern of disease transmission. As Arnold has observed, they 'performed much the same function in epidemiological terms as they did in commercial ones. They were disease entrepôts: the principal points of entry for arriving pathogens.'[109] The geographical location of port cities, as well as their social constitutions, created an environment for infectious disease to spread.

This chapter has explored a number of epidemics – of malaria, cholera, VD, and plague – in relation to four colonial cities: Batavia, Hanoi, Singapore, and Bombay. Each of these epidemics throws light on an aspect of the city's life (and death): on urban hinterlands and the city's economic base, segregationist politics, gender and sexual economies, and technology. Within these broad contexts, several themes have been considered. First, how specific disease identities – plague as an 'old' disease or VD as a coolie-prostitute's disease – produced specific urban spaces, just as these urban spaces shaped how epidemics were understood; second, the stresses that epidemics placed on urban institutions; third, the governmental technologies that epidemic crises called forth; fourth, the interactions between different communities, institutions, and professionals in these moments of crisis; and fifth, the local fabric of colonial cities, as well as their transnational connections and multi-city networks. Studying cities in this way, I have suggested, helps us to think about the socially produced and negotiated aspects of epidemic events.

Part of the story has also been the tension between how cities are imagined and how they are actualized or experienced; between the blueprint of the city as a site of hygienic modernity – a map, as it were, where an embedded order prohibits disease – and the city as an unsettling material presence that pushes back in messy ways against this ideal. Of course, discourses of 'health' and 'disease' do shape cities, as Rogaski has shown in her history of Tianjin, a treaty port in northern China, where the concept of *weisheng* (hygiene), variously interpreted by Meiji, Qing, and Kuomintang (KMT) rulers, was instrumental in determining public health policy and practice in the city.[110]

The cities explored in this chapter were not only sites of epidemics, however; they were also places where scientific knowledge was produced

---

[109] Arnold, 'The Indian Ocean as a Disease Zone,' p.10.
[110] Rogaski, *Hygienic Modernity*.

and professional expertise developed. Hospitals, medical schools, and scientific research facilities defined the urban landscape. Institutions such as the Indochina Medical College in Hanoi stood out as prominent landmarks in the colonial city: bastions of scientific rationality that embodied the munificent authority of colonial power, they were also reflections of civic pride. The exclusive character of these colonial establishments, however, began to change as they opened to 'native' Asian doctors and nurses. Meanwhile, wealthy Parsees and Chinese funded hospitals in Bombay and Singapore.[111] Indeed, while we have emphasized government attempts to rationalize, regulate, and segregate urban space, it is important to emphasize that cities were also places of contestation and fundamental dis-order – places where social boundaries were redrawn and hierarchies could dissolve.

What about the explosive growth of the contemporary Asian city? Following the bombing of Pearl Harbor in December 1941 and Japan's entry into the Second World War, much of Southeast Asia – including parts of China, Hong Kong, Manila, Singapore, Penang, and Rangoon – came under Japanese occupation. Disruption caused by military conflict in many rural areas led to an inflow of refugees to urban centers, including Hanoi and Jakarta, in search of food. In other areas there were reverse flows, as people fled the targeted bombing of cities. Overwhelmingly, however, the Second World War and its after-effects of revolution fundamentally reconfigured urban–rural relations. After 1945, in the wake of independence from colonial powers, urban development accelerated across Asia, fueled by economic expansion. This pace of change transformed social structures, institutions of government, and lifestyles, bringing fresh challenges and leading to the growth of squatter settlements or shanty towns in many parts of South and Southeast Asia.

Today, cities such as Beijing, Delhi, Jakarta, Karachi, Manila, Mumbai, Seoul, and Shanghai each have populations exceeding 20 million, with greater Tokyo set to hit 40 million. Urbanization on this scale is a phenomenon across Asia, where cities swell collectively by over 40 million people every year. The growth of Asia's megacities has been predominantly dependent on mass internal migration as rural populations relocate in search of opportunities. The PRC has become the center of this rapidly urbanizing world. According to the 2010 census, those living in cities accounted for 50 percent of the population, an increase of 210 million people since 2000. Meanwhile, the rural population had depleted during the same period by 133 million. It is anticipated that the megacities around the Pearl River Delta, including Guangzhou, Shenzhen,

---

[111] Arnold, 'The Indian Ocean as a Disease Zone,' pp.18–19.

Dongguan, and Foshan, will soon merge to create a vast urban agglomeration. In China, the growth of urban centers, such as Guangzhou, has been driven by the devolution of economic decision-making to municipal governments, who are incentivized to boost economic competitiveness by implementing strategic development plans (Chapter 5).[112] It is estimated that by 2030, 65 percent of China's population will be living in cities, meaning an expansion of 300 million people. As in most countries in Asia, this urbanization will be driven by migration, which is likely to create further segregation within cities, while urban sprawl will be difficult to contain, posing environmental challenges (Chapter 3).[113]

Many cities in Asia are expanding with minimal planning and dangerously high levels of air pollution, traffic congestion, and poverty. According to a 2014 WHO report, Delhi has the worst air pollution of any urban center. India and China consistently top the list of countries with the most polluted cities. A World Bank report in 2007 attributed an estimated 750,000 deaths to pollution in China and noted the high level of chronic respiratory disease and infection amongst children. A 2015 study, drawing on official data across eastern China, has claimed that air pollution contributes to 1.6 million deaths per year.[114] The increasingly global interconnectedness of Asian megacities through material circulations of people and commodities also poses new challenges for preventing the spread of infectious disease, as we shall explore in Chapter 5 in a discussion of SARS, influenza, and 'globalization.'[115] Information flows may trigger panic, producing markets perturbations and affecting inward investment adversely. By the same token, however, the networks that link these global cities may serve as counter-measures to the spread of disease, enabling the transfer of critical information, knowledge, and policy. Yet the projected continuation and intensification of this urban development is likely to strain the sustainability of governance, management, and infrastructure, with consequences for the emergence and re-emergence of infectious disease in the future.

---

[112] Fulong Wu and Jingxing Zhang, 'Planning the Competitive City-Region: The Emergence of Strategic Development Plan in China,' *Urban Affairs Review*, vol.42, no.5 (2007): 714–740.

[113] Wu and Gaubatz, *The Chinese City*, pp.275–280.

[114] Angel Hsu, 'Seeing Through the Smog: China's Air Pollution Challenge for East Asia.' In: Paul G. Harris and Graeme Lang, eds., *Routledge Handbook of Environment and Society in Asia* (Abingdon and New York: Routledge, 2015), pp.160–175 (160–161); Robert A. Rohde and Richard A. Muller, 'Air Pollution in China: Mapping of Concentrations and Sources,' *PLoS ONE*, vol.8, no.8 (2015): e0135749.

[115] S. Harris Ali and Roger Keil, 'Introduction: Networked Disease.' In: S. Harris Ali and Roger Keil, eds., *Networked Disease: Emerging Infections in the Global City* (Malden, MA and Oxford: Wiley-Blackwell, 2008), pp.1–7 (5).

3   Environment

Natural disasters, such as hurricanes and tsunamis, have long been viewed as the result of external biophysical forces acting upon human societies. They have been understood, in other words, as implacable natural processes beyond human control. More recently, particularly as a result of concerns about global climate change, there has been a shift of emphasis onto the anthropogenic causes of such adverse events. By destroying features of the environment, such as mangroves and wetlands, that provide protection from storm surges, humans are amplifying the effects of these extreme occurrences. While earlier histories tended to minimize the role of the social in natural disasters, more recent approaches have stressed the part played by human agency.[1] Human history is increasingly viewed within an ecological framework. Expressed somewhat differently, we might say that the emphasis on human-made determinants of natural disasters reflects a deeper notion that people are 'inescapably part of a larger ecosystem.'[2]

Epidemics share many characteristics with natural disasters. They are the result of identifiable natural processes that lead to loss of human life and damage to property, infrastructure, and business; their impact may be mitigated by a population's preparedness; and above all, of course, they require susceptible populations. Disease outbreaks – or fear of them – are often a by-product of other species of disaster. The 2004 Indian Ocean earthquake and tsunami, which killed an estimated 280,000 people across South and Southeast Asia, with a million displaced into temporary camps, gave rise to concerns about epidemics of water-borne and food-borne infectious diseases, such as salmonellosis, typhoid fever, cholera, hepatitis, and shigellosis. By and large, these fears were not realized, but the specter of epidemics nonetheless shaped emergency responses to the tsunami. In this chapter, I probe the role of human

---

[1] Jonathan Bergman, 'Disaster: A Useful Category of Historical Analysis,' *History Compass*, vol.6, no.3 (May 2008): 934–946.
[2] Nash, *Inescapable Ecologies*, p.1.

agency in disease emergence and consider epidemics as episodes that foreground the convergence of human and natural ecologies. To what extent should epidemics be understood as the outcome of environmental crises? What countervailing effects have been produced by attempts to intervene with the environment to mitigate disease threats? How have evolving conceptions of disease shaped environmental change? And, finally, what role does politics play in determining human–environment relations?

As we saw in the previous chapter, cities have been important catalysts in Asia's environmental transformation, drawing in migrants to work in expanding industry. As urban populations grew, so did their requirements for basic resources: water, staple crops, livestock, as well as wood for construction and fuel. To meet these needs, land was cleared in the hinterlands, embankments and irrigation systems built, along with other essential infrastructure, including trunk lines, roads, and canals. The introduction of the plantation complex in the nineteenth century, where a few commodity crops were grown for export on large estates, changed the nature of agriculture, linking it to global markets. The case of the Dutch city of Batavia is particularly illustrative, suggesting the inadvertent health consequences that human interactions with the environment can have: there, the over-development of sugar plantations in the eighteenth century under the rule of the VOC was responsible for silting up of the city's principal river. This, in turn, led to the stagnation of the canal system, which became a breeding ground for mosquitoes, the vector of malaria – a mosquito-borne infectious disease caused by parasitic protozoa, first identified in 1880 by the French physician Charles A. Laveran (1845–1922).

In Dutch-controlled Java, the development of a cash crop agriculture meant that production in the hinterland was increasingly influenced by market fluctuations. Following their victory in the Java War (1825–1830), the Dutch consolidated their control of the island. From the 1830s, the so-called 'Cultivation System' (*Cultuurstelsel*) was instituted to raise state revenue by profiting from export markets. In order to pay the government a tax in cash, farmers were required to reserve part of their land for the cultivation of government-specified crops for export, such as sugarcane and coffee, which they were obliged to sell to the Netherlands Trading Company – an institution that monopolized trading – at a fixed price.[3] In other words, the transformation of the environment in Java was linked to economic developments, to an increasingly market-oriented society,

[3] R. E. Elson, *Village Java under the Cultivation System, 1830–1870* (Sydney: Asian Studies Association of Australia/Allen & Unwin, 1994), pp.42–98.

and to a centralized colonial polity, which profited from the revenue that this reorganized agriculture generated.

This chapter reflects on epidemics as environmental events produced by the stresses of these natural, economic, social, and political convergences. It also explores the racial politics that informed and shaped colonial and modernizing environmental practices. In the first of four case studies, epidemics are considered in relation to the development of industrial-scale rubber plantations in Southeast Asia, with a particular focus on the Federated Malay States (today's Peninsular Malaysia) – a federation of four protected states established by the British in 1895. Technological developments in the late nineteenth century, including the popularity of the bicycle and the rise of the automobile industry after 1900, led to the rapid expansion of the tire industry and to a consequential boom in rubber production in South and Southeast Asia, with Malaya becoming the leading producer.

In 1926, Leo Amery (1873–1955), British secretary of state for the colonies, identified 'the marriage of tropical production to the industrial production of the temperate zone' as being a defining feature of 'modern industrial development.'[4] What were the environmental impacts of this hybrid model of tropical–industrial production? How did the region's integration into a global economy, and the material processes that this involved, affect ecosystems, producing conditions ripe for the spread of malaria? In engaging with these questions, we track the interconnections between disease, environmental change, and a profit-driven plantation system reliant on migrant labor. Investigating plantation culture in this way enables us to rethink colonization in Asia not solely in terms of the refashioning of the environment, but also in terms of the social transformations it necessitated. Modernization extended from the landscape to the regulation of those who worked and lived there; it involved an everted process of 'medicalized nativism,' wherein non-native colonial agents routinely associated 'native' and contracted labor with disease.[5] The aim is thus to break down divisions between environmental, social, and economic histories – locating epidemic history at the intersection of all three.

In the second case, I explore Japanese anti-malarial campaigns in Taiwan in the early twentieth century. Taiwan was Japan's first colonial possession, acquired after its victory over China in the First Sino-Japanese War of 1894–1895. As noted in Chapter 1, the restoration of the Meiji

---

[4] Michael Havinden and David Meredith, *Colonialism and Development: Britain and Its Tropical Colonies, 1850–1960* (London and New York: Routledge, 1993), p.169.

[5] Alan M. Kraut, *Silent Travelers: Germs, Genes, and the 'Immigrant Menace'* (Baltimore, MD: Johns Hopkins University Press, 1995), p.3.

Emperor in 1868 inaugurated a program of concerted modernization in Japan, in which science, technology, and medicine played key roles. This modernization drive was also evident in Japanese overseas possessions. As in its other colonies – such as the Kwantung (Guandong) Leased Territory on the Liaodong peninsula, a territorial concession acquired in 1898 following China's defeat in the Sino-Japanese War, as well as Korea, which was annexed by Japan in 1910 – there was an emphasis on constructing a modern infrastructure and promoting public health technologies to safeguard colonial commercial interests and the health of the colonial population. Censured by the Japanese for its insalubrious environment, Taiwan became a particular object of public health intervention as the colonial state sought to prevent and control malaria epidemics. These measures were initially targeted at the population, but after 1919 increasingly focused in parallel on vector control through strategic environmental management. The aim in this section, then, building on the first case, is to examine the inconsistencies and tensions that arose from a policy that shifted between an emphasis on eradicating malarial parasites in native bodies to one that viewed the environment as the prime locus of disease emergence.

The third section investigates Mao Zedong's campaign against schistosomiasis in the PRC during the Great Leap Forward (1958–1962). It argues that the fight to 'annihilate' infectious disease in China – and specifically schistosomiasis, an infection caused by parasitic worms carried by fresh water snails – should be viewed in relation to broader policies geared to maximizing agricultural production and spurring development through collectivization. Ironically, this very process of rationalization, which involved radically reconfiguring the environment with irrigation works and dams, produced stresses on the natural ecology, creating potential conditions for the spread of vector-borne diseases. At the same time, the schistosomiasis campaign was prefigured by the 1952 Patriotic Health Campaign during the Korean War (1950–1953), when rural communities were mobilized to help counter the threat of alleged US biogerm warfare. To what extent did this mobilization against a foreign aggressor overlap with and pre-empt Mao's 'war' against nature viewed in the context of the push for disease 'annihilation'? How was an endemic disease reframed as an epidemic?

Finally, the fourth section traces the history of the Nipah virus (NiV), a species of henipavirus that is naturally hosted by the fruit bat. NiV, which may cause acute respiratory syndrome and fatal febrile encephalitis in those infected, was first identified in Malaysia in 1999 and named after the town where the initial outbreak occurred (Kampung Sungai Nipah). Since its emergence in Malaysia, there have been cases in India, and particularly in Bangladesh. An outbreak there in 2013, which was linked to the drinking of raw and contaminated date-palm sap, resulted in 21 deaths. This section explores the multiple factors that contributed to the Malaysian epidemic, including anthropogenic impact on the environment. It also investigates how the epidemic became entangled in Malaysia's complex ethnic politics, aggravating tensions between the majority Muslim Malays and the Chinese community. The epidemic began on a pig farm, with pigs the intermediate hosts for the virus. Given that pork and pork-related products are forbidden in Islam, pig farms and abattoirs in Malaysia are largely managed by the Chinese. The NiV outbreak was viewed by many Malays as a Chinese problem, triggering ethnic tensions that influenced the official handling of the epidemic. Meanwhile, NiV led to the closing of farms and to the culling of livestock, which severely affected the Chinese economically, particularly coming as it did after the 1997 Asian financial crisis.

Each of the four cases is thus concerned with charting disease emergence in relation to changes in human–environment interactions. The creation of vast rubber plantations entailed the felling of indigenous rainforests, which profoundly altered the ecological dynamics across South and Southeast Asia, with ramifications for human health. How was this transformation – and the 'insatiable appetite' that drove it – perceived and understood at the time?[6] In addressing this question, we consider how changing conceptions of disease were instrumental in the transformation of Asia's varied environment. The aim is not only to show how diseases were connected to specific places, but to demonstrate how particular communities associated with those pathogenic places were targeted for surveillance and became the object of often coercive regulation.

Managing nature in Asia

Environmental change has varied widely across Asia. In contrast to South and East Asia – notably India and China – many areas of island and continental Southeast Asia had comparatively low population densities until the nineteenth and twentieth centuries. 'Most of the region was still covered by jungle as late as 1800,' writes Anthony Reid, 'so that attacks by tigers were not uncommon even on the outskirts of substantial population centers.' Of course, there were exceptions even in Southeast Asia, where fertile and low-lying alluvial regions, such as the plain of the Chao Phraya River in Thailand, the Irrawaddy Delta in Burma, or the Mekong

---

[6] Richard P. Tucker, *Insatiable Appetite: The United States and the Ecological Degradation of the Tropical World* (Berkeley: University of California Press, 2000).

and Red River Deltas in southwestern and northern Vietnam, sustained much larger populations.[7] Today, there continues to be wide diversity across the region, with more remote areas inhabited by ethnic minorities who retain their distinct identities. Nonetheless, by the turn of the nineteenth and twentieth centuries, development had brought profound changes. An aerial view of the Malaysian state of Sarawak on the island of Borneo reveals extensive tropical rainforests that provide a habitat for abundant plant and animal species, including Asia's only large ape, the orangutan, which has become emblematic of Borneo's rich biodiversity. It also reveals the extent to which this primary forest is fast disappearing under the pressure of mining, logging, and agricultural expansion. The effects of timber harvesting by licensed logging companies and illegal tree-felling activities have been amplified by land clearance for palm-oil, pulp, and paper operations (Figure 3.1). The grid-like symmetry of Sarawak's palm-oil concessions, cut out of the rainforest, reflects the imposition of a new socio-economic order on the land. It reminds us, too, of the extent to which contemporary culture and society are 'built on, and absolutely dependent on, a sharply alienating, intensely managerial relationship with nature.'[8]

In many parts of Asia, this transformative process was begun when European empires established new models of statehood that territorialized Asian landscapes, imposing formal frontiers and instituting foreign forms of proprietorial rights that overrode indigenous patterns of land tenure. Rural hinterlands were opened up and new crops introduced: tobacco and rubber from South America; tea in Southeast Asia from India; oil palm from West Africa. Mines were dug and tracts of swampland converted to agricultural land. Today, extensive rice fields dominate the irrigated lowlands; areas such as the Central Thai Plain and the Mekong Delta have been developed to meet an expanding rice market, resulting in far-reaching social change. The convoluted feedback loops between ecosystem and societal transformations have been studied by the anthropologists Lauriston Sharp and Lucien Hanks who chart the vicissitudes of a Thai rice farming community in Bang Chan as it responds to new rice-growing technologies and shifting markets. More recent work has demonstrated the extent to which the history of rice, as a food and commodity, is interconnected with histories of colonialism, industrial capitalism,

---

[7] Anthony Reid, 'Economic and Social Change, c.1400–1800.' In: Tarling, ed., *The Cambridge History of Southeast Asia*, pp.460–507 (460–461).

[8] Donald Worster, *Rivers of Empire: Water, Aridity, and the Growth of the American West* (New York: Pantheon, 1985), p.5.

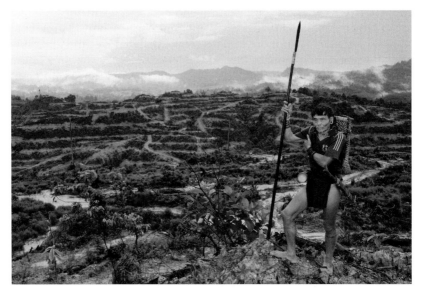

Figure 3.1. 'An indigenous blowpipe hunter in Sarawak, Malaysia, stands in front of land cleared of rainforest. Logging operations and palm-oil plantations are rapidly engulfing the land.' Photograph by Mattias Klum.

Biodiversity and the plantation complex

Plantations are mass agro-industrial enterprises, usually in tropical or subtropical environments. They are generally monocultures: that is, they involve the cultivation of a single commodity crop grown on a large estate. Examples of crops include trees for timber production, cocoa, cotton, coffee, tobacco, sugarcane, sisal, and rubber. Historically, slavery and indentured labor have underpinned the plantation economy. In the twentieth century, the meaning of 'plantation' converged with that of 'estate.' Land clearance required for plantations reduces biodiversity and results in loss of habitat (Figure 3.1). The consequential depletion of topsoil and vegetation affects rainwater absorption, producing fertile ground for *Anopheles* mosquitoes to breed and spread malaria. Campaigns to protect biodiversity, which are invariably linked to claims about conservation and health, often run up against opposition not only from private companies with interests in exploiting the land, but from local communities whose livelihoods may also be threatened by state injunctions to protect the environment. Indigenous populations, state officials, journalists, epidemiologists, environmental activists, and conservation biologists all have very different notions of what the 'environment' is, and how it should be defined, used, and preserved.

> Subhrendu K. Pattanayak and Junko Yasuoka, 'Deforestation and Malaria: Revisiting the Human Ecology Perspective.' In: Carol J. Pierce Colfer, ed., *Human Health and Forests: A Global Overview of Issues, Practice and Policy* (London and Sterling, VA: Earthscan, 2008), pp.197–217.

and the integration of rice growing regions into global markets.[9] If the intensification of rice production wrought momentous environmental and social changes across Asia, so too did the emergence of the plantation complex in the late nineteenth century. For one, plantations were dependent on a massive importation of labor, predominantly from India and China. Secondly, they required substantial inflows of capital, essential infrastructure, and state protection. The regimental plantations across much of South and Southeast Asia embody a landscape that has been engineered for profit: capitalist exploitation and environmental conquest have been inextricably linked.

European colonial commentators often conjured up an image of Western engineers enforcing an order on an unruly tropical landscape. In the mid nineteenth century, the British imported over a million indentured and contracted laborers from central India to transform the 'jungle' of Assam in the northeast of the subcontinent into an imperial 'garden' of tea plantations.[10] The term 'jungle' to refer to tropical nature was itself loaded: the word is of Hindi and Sanskrit origins and came to designate land with untamed vegetation that calls for ordering.[11] Many French colonial commentators, for example, viewed the reclamation of large areas of the Mekong Delta in Vietnam and the construction of a

---

[9] Lauriston Sharp and Lucien M. Hanks, *Bang Chan: Social History of a Rural Community in Thailand* (Ithaca, NY: Cornell University Press, 1978); Francesca Bray, et al., eds., *Rice: Global Networks and New Histories* (Cambridge: Cambridge University Press, 2015).

[10] Jayeeta Sharma, *Empire's Garden: Assam and the Making of India* (Durham, NC: Duke University Press, 2011), p.5.

[11] Michael R. Dove, 'Forest Discourses in South and Southeast Asia: A Comparison with Global Discourses.' In: Paul R. Greenough and Anna Lowenhaupt Tsing, eds., *Nature in the Global South: Environmental Projects in South and Southeast Asia* (Durham, NC: Duke University Press, 2003), pp.103–123 (107–108).

canal and levee system there from the 1860s as a way of bringing to heel an essentially wild and unwholesome environment of swamp and marsh.

Environmental change, however, was not only the result of colonization. Recent research on China has pointed to the ecological ramifications of water exploitation, deforestation, and mineral extraction over the last four millennia – suggesting, among other effects, the emergence of vector-borne diseases. Road building under the Qin and Han dynasties from the third century BCE, attempts to recourse the Yellow River in the twelfth century, and human interventions to build up the sediment in the Pearl River Delta in order to reclaim fertile farmland: all of these led to the progressive 'simplification of natural ecosystems.' Although 'traditional' forms of agriculture may appear sustainable, they have in fact induced profound environmental alterations.[12]

All the same, colonization and the development of modern engineering and farming technologies enabled an intensification of this process. In the Mekong Delta, the French did effect dramatic change, even if they inherited a landscape that had been worked on before them and was by no means a 'wilderness.' The area of land under cultivation expanded from 200,000 hectares in 1879, to over two million hectares by the late 1920s.[13] In the Mekong Delta, deforestation, channelized rivers, an intricate canal system – as well as subsequent hydropower development – interacted with equally complex transformations in the geopolitics of the region. Reclamation projects were closely connected to French pacification efforts, which ultimately had countervailing effects, sparking local revolts and longer-term anti-colonial resistance.[14] The example of the Delta and its reconstruction into a 'modern hydraulic landscape' reminds us that environmental transformations were not only driven by economic requirements, but by political imperatives. It also underlines how the promotion of health and efficiency through a reordering of the land could have unforeseen effects: inciting resistance and amplifying disease.

Another good example of such counterproductive colonial attempts to 'improve' the environment is provided by the British in West Bengal, an area inundated by the annual monsoon floodwaters of the river Ganges. In order to increase efficiency and prevent flooding, the British

---

[12] Robert B. Marks, *China: Its Environment and History* (Lanham, MD: Rowman & Little-field, 2012), p.334.

[13] David Biggs, 'Problematic Progress: Reading Environmental and Social Change in the Mekong Delta,' *Journal of Southeast Asian Studies*, vol.34, no.1 (2003): 77–96 (79).

[14] David Biggs, *Quagmire: Nation-Building and Nature in the Mekong Delta* (Seattle: University of Washington Press, 2010), p.11.

dammed rivers and streams, creating a new irrigation system. Embankments were also constructed to open up the region for exploitation, allowing better access with new roads and railways. These developments in the second half of the nineteenth century spurred an expansion in rice production and an intensification in agriculture. As a consequence, the region's ecology was modified: rivers silted up, the ground became waterlogged, providing an ideal breeding ground for a species of *Anopheles* mosquito that had hitherto been confined to limited areas of Bengal. Furthermore, farmland was deprived of the benefits of the flooding, which fertilized the soil. As a result of these multiple and interlinked factors, there was a marked reduction in productivity as farmers abandoned their land, precipitating further ecological decline. 'British policies inadvertently brought "death by development" to colonial India,' Ira Klein has observed. Particularly from the 1860s, epidemics of malaria ravaged Bengal. According to one estimate, three-quarters of some village populations succumbed to malaria, with a mortality rate of 25 percent.[15]

Many contemporary observers were aware of the unanticipated consequences of these interventions. They wrote about the degradation of the land, expressing 'environmental anxieties' about the economic and health repercussions of development.[16] 'When the jungle is rudely swept away, man seems to conquer,' noted Malcolm Watson (1873–1955), a pioneer of malaria control in Malaya. 'In reality,' he concluded, 'a condition of "unstable equilibrium" has been produced; or rather it can be described more correctly as the beginning of a war that can only end in man's defeat, however long it may be prolonged: man with knife and axe and fire; the jungle with its myriads of aerial troops.'[17]

By the early twentieth century, new knowledge about the role of insect vectors in the diffusion of disease had led to a fresh focus on entomological research. Although some diseases, such as smallpox, could be controlled through vaccination, other diseases, such as malaria, posed more intractable challenges and there was growing appreciation of the ecological complexities within which these diseases were produced.[18] While the

[15] Randall M. Packard, *The Making of a Tropical Disease: A Short History of Malaria* (Baltimore, MD: Johns Hopkins University Press, 2007), pp.3–5; Ira Klein, 'Development and Death: Reinterpreting Malaria, Economics and Ecology in British India,' *Indian Economic and Social History Review*, vol.38, no.2 (2001): 147–179 (147, 162–163).

[16] James Beattie, *Empire and Environmental Anxiety: Health, Science, Art and Conservation in South Asia and Australasia, 1899–1920* (Basingstoke: Palgrave Macmillan, 2011).

[17] Malcolm Watson, *The Prevention of Malaria in the Federated Malay States: A Record of Twenty Years' Progress* (New York: E. P. Dutton and Co., [1911] 1921), p.291.

[18] Helen Tilley, 'Ecologies of Complexity: Tropical Environments, African Trypanosomiasis, and the Science of Disease Control in British Colonial Africa, 1900–1940,' *Osiris*, vol.19 (2004): 21–38.

immediate cause of an epidemic might be exposure to a pathogen, the forces that converged to produce and sustain outbreaks were multifaceted and interconnected, making solutions problematic. As the environmental historian Richard Grove has observed, European colonial expansion promoted an awareness of the environment's vulnerabilities and underlined the extent to which human societies could precipitate ecological change. An incipient environmental 'movement' in tandem with state policies of conservation, which were driven by science, sought to mitigate environmental threats by 'protecting' nature.[19]

The causes and drivers of many infectious diseases are now understood to be multifactorial and may include ecological changes, shifts in human demographics and behavior, and microbial adaptation.[20] It is likely, for example, that malaria spread as a result of climate change at the end of the last glacial period 10,000 years ago, together with the development of agriculture. Slash-and-burn farming methods transformed the environment, increasing the population of *Anopheles* mosquitoes. Crop choices, housing patterns, and cultural practices have also influenced the spread of malaria.[21] As we have already noted, many new and emerging infections are zoonoses: that is, infections that have crossed the species barrier from animals to humans. The emergence of new zoonotic diseases has been attributed to a number of factors, including human encroachment on wild habitats where pathogens exist in natural reservoir hosts. The high concentrations of animal populations in industrial livestock rearing processes are also likely to spread infection, while large-scale monocultures – the practice of breeding genetically similar or identical livestock to ensure greater yields – are producing new vulnerabilities to disease (Chapter 5).

Plantation fever: Malaria and the rubber boom

The first plantations were developed in the European colonies of the Americas in the sixteenth and seventeenth centuries. It was not until the mid nineteenth century that an industrial-scale cash crop cultivation system was introduced to Asia. As the historian Philip Curtin has argued, plantation economies exhibit certain definable characteristics,

[19] Richard H. Grove, *Green Imperialism: Colonial Expansion, Tropical Island Edens and the Origins of Environmentalism, 1600–1860* (Cambridge: Cambridge University Press, 1995).

[20] Stephen S. Morse, 'Factors in the Emergence of Infectious Diseases,' *Emerging Infectious Diseases*, vol.1, no.1 (January/March 1995): 7–15.

[21] Peter J. Brown, 'Culture and the Global Resurgence of Malaria.' In: Marcia C. Inhorn and Peter J. Brown, eds., *The Anthropology of Infectious Disease: International Health Perspectives* (Amsterdam: Overseas Publishers Association, 1997), pp.119–141.

including: the production of one (or at least very few) crops for export; a dependence on coerced – often migrant – labor; a system of management that assumes state-like oversight and disciplinary functions; reliance on mass-transportation networks; and metropolitan political and economic control.[22]

Rubber was one of the most important crops in the plantation economies of South and Southeast Asia. The industry was based on the extraction of latex, the sap from the *Hevea brasiliensis*, a tree native to Amazonia. In 1839, the American manufacturing engineer, Charles Goodyear (1800–1860), had developed the chemical process of vulcanization, which converted natural rubber into a more durable material. John Boyd Dunlop's (1840–1921) development of the pneumatic tire in the late 1880s contributed to a rubber boom. The growth of the automobile industry after 1900, and the need for car and truck tires that this stimulated, further expanded the global demand for rubber.

In the 1870s, 70,000 rubber tree seeds were allegedly smuggled out of Brazil to Britain by the explorer Henry Wickham, where they were cultivated at the Royal Gardens in Kew, outside London.[23] Seedlings were then sent out from Britain to the colonies: to Ceylon, India, Singapore, and British Malaya. The rubber production initiative at this stage came largely from the Colonial Office, which was keen to ensure a stable supply for the burgeoning manufacturing industry in Britain. The aim was also to reduce Malaya's reliance on tin and to mitigate losses from mining. A basic stock of trees was grown in the Singapore Botanic Gardens, where the director, H. N. Ridley, developed a technique of herring-bone 'tapping' in the 1890s; this involved slicing the bark to collect the sticky milk-like sap, known as latex, which was then refined into rubber before processing (Figure 3.2).

The pace of production gathered momentum in Malaya from the late 1890s, as the price of rubber surged due to demand for car and truck tires. This followed the peninsula's political reorganization, as the British extended their control to create a federation of Malay states under the putative leadership of Malay sultans (prior to 1867 Malaya had been governed as part of India). As a result of the increasing demand for rubber, estate owners progressively abandoned the production of other export crops such as sugar and coffee, which experienced a price slump. By 1906, some 39,000 hectares had been planted with rubber. By 1921,

---

[22] Philip D. Curtin, *The Rise and Fall of the Plantation Complex: Essays in Atlantic History*. Second edition (Cambridge: Cambridge University Press, 1998), pp.11–13.

[23] Joe Jackson, *The Thief at the End of the World: Rubber, Power, and the Seeds of Empire* (New York: Viking, 2008), p.176.

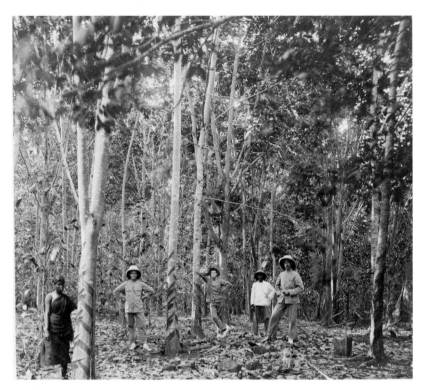

Figure 3.2. 'Rubber plantation in Singapore (ca.1890).' Courtesy: US
Library of Congress.

Cultivating rubber in the Straits Settlements

The botanist Henry Nicholas Ridley (1855–1956) was director of
the Singapore Botanic Gardens from 1888 until his retirement in
1911, responsible for forestry and gardens in the Straits Settlements. Aside from pioneering a new method of 'tapping,' which
entailed removing only sections of a Para tree's bark in order to
preserve the tree, Ridley also pursued research into the best planting and processing methods, as well as the most efficient means of
packing and shipping rubber. Particularly from the 1890s, Ridley
was instrumental in persuading coffee planters to switch to rubber.
The transition was facilitated by the boom in rubber demand from
the automobile industry, as well as the devastating consequences of

Hemileia vastatrix, a fungus that caused coffee leaf rust on coffee plantations in Malaya.

D. J. M. Tate, *The RGA History of the Plantation Industry in the Malay Peninsula* (Kuala Lumpur: Oxford University Press, 1996), pp.193–204.

there were some 907,000 hectares under cultivation and the Federated Malay States had emerged as a major producer of plantation rubber.[24]

The intensive capital outlay required to set up a large plantation encouraged the formation of joint-stock companies, which could tap overseas capital markets. Between 1903 and 1912, approximately 260 rubber companies were registered in Britain with operations in Malaya, as well as Ceylon, India, Burma, and the Dutch East Indies. The London-based Rubber Growers' Association was established in 1907 to represent their interests to government.[25] The emergence of powerful rubber companies, in part as a consequence of the capital-intensive nature of industrial-scale cultivation, was to generate friction between private interests and the state over their respective responsibilities. In particular, there were disagreements about health and disease prevention policies.[26]

The introduction and development of rubber plantations across Malaya had profound impacts on the natural and social ecologies of the peninsula. For one, the rubber boom created an unprecedented demand for labor, resulting in the influx of thousands of Tamils from southern India recruited to work on the plantations. In order to ensure the steady supply of Indian laborers, the government passed the Tamil Immigration Fund Ordinance in 1907, subsequently called the Indian Immigration Fund Ordinance. The associated costs of recruiting labor were henceforth to be met by employers with a quarterly tax paid into a designated government fund. Second, transportation systems were constructed to link expanding areas under cultivation to coastal ports, precipitating a further 'opening up' of the country. The advent of industrial-scale plantations led to the amalgamation and expansion of

---

[24] Colin Barlow, *The Natural Rubber Industry: Its Development, Technology, and Economy in Asia* (Kuala Lumpur: Oxford University Press, 1978), p.26; John H. Drabble, *Rubber in Malaya, 1876–1922: The Genesis of the Industry* (Kuala Lumpur: Oxford University Press, 1973), Appendix 3, p.215.

[25] Drabble, *Rubber in Malaya*, p.53.

[26] Liew Kai Khiun, 'Planters, Estate Health & Malaria in British Malaya (1900–1940),' *Journal of the Malayasian Branch of the Royal Asiatic Society*, vol.83, no.298 (2010): 91–115.

earlier transport networks that had grown up to meet the needs of the tin mining industry in western Malaya – including the construction of the trunk line linking Singapore in the south to Butterworth, opposite Penang on the northwest coast.[27]

Third, and above all, was land clearance. The mining industry, along with plantations of crops such as sugarcane and coffee, had resulted in some clearance from the mid-century. Tin mining was a particularly wood-intensive industry, requiring firewood for the pumping engines. But deforestation intensified dramatically with the rubber boom. To reduce costs, plantations tended to be sited where land was less expensive in 'isolated frontier areas, far from towns and mining settlements.'[28] 'The land chosen for rubber estates in the Federated Malay States is, with very few exceptions, virgin jungle,' remarked John Bennett Carruthers, director of agriculture and government botanist in 1908. 'Upon receiving the grant of the land, which is a permanent title giving all the rights of freehold,' Carruthers noted in an overview of the rubber industry in Malaya, 'if the conditions of rent, &c., are duly carried, the planter proceeds to get rid of the jungle.'[29] Land clearance led to changes in patterns of water absorption, increasing the incidence of malaria: 'A signal indicator of human intrusion into the moist tropical environment was the scourge of malaria.'[30]

As in Malaya, the transformation of the East Coast of Sumatra as a result of the introduction of plantations was also spectacular: within decades, the landscape changed 'from a jungle into a vast commercial garden.'[31] There, multinational corporate capital, with the support of the Dutch colonial state and the collusion of the local Malay aristocracy, acquired large tracts of prime agricultural land, creating a land shortage for the indigenous population of Malays and Bataks. While tobacco plantations had taken off from the 1870s in Sumatra, after 1907 there was a rubber boom. Tens of thousands of Chinese and Javanese indentured laborers were imported into Sumatra each year. As a result of this

[27] Amarjit Kaur, 'The Impact of Railroads on the Malayan Economy, 1874–1941,' *Journal of Asian Studies*, vol.19, no.4 (1980): 693–710.

[28] Amarjit Kaur, 'Indian Labour, Labour Standards, and Workers' Health in Burma and Malaya, 1900–1940,' *Modern Asian Studies*, vol.40, no.2 (2006): 425–475 (450).

[29] J. B. Carruthers, 'Rubber.' In: Arnold Wright and H. A. Cartwright, eds., *Twentieth Century Impressions of British Malaya: Its History, People, Commerce, Industries, and Resources* (London: Lloyd's Greater Britain Publishing Co., 1908), pp.345–351 (348).

[30] Jeyamalar Kathirithamby-Wells, *Nature and Nation: Forests and Development in Peninsular Malaysia* (Honolulu: University of Hawaii Press, 2005), p.165.

[31] Clark E. Cunningham, *The Postwar Migration of the Toba-Bataks to East Sumatra* (New Haven, CT: Southeast Asia Studies, Yale University, 1958), p.15.

immigration, the population of East Sumatra had almost doubled by 1940.[32] Under the terms of the infamous Coolie Ordinance of 1880, known as the 'penal sanction,' migrant workers were repatriated after a maximum of three years: 'laborers who ran away, refused to work, or otherwise transgressed the rigorous rules inscribed in their contracts were subject to imprisonment, fine, and/or forced labor above and beyond the duration of the initial agreement.' Resentment often boiled over into violence directed at European planters. 'By the 1920s,' writes Ann Laura Stoler, 'assaults on white plantation personnel had escalated to such a level that Sumatra's East Coast had become infamous throughout the Indies.'[33]

A graphic description of the environmental and social transformations wrought in Sumatra by the development of plantations is provided by the Hungarian writer and entrepreneur László Székely (1892–1946) in his semi-autobiographical novel *Tropic Fever* (originally entitled *From Primeval Forest to Plantation*), which was first published in English in 1937. The book is set in 'Deli,' as the area around Medan in Sumatra was known, during the rubber takeoff at the beginning of the twentieth century, when Székely had himself lived and worked there as a planter. A sense of loss, alienation, and regret informs the narrative. As the protagonist concludes:

No trace could now be seen of the virgin forest, in place of the jungle stood rubber trees in endless rows. With loud hooting automobiles passed over straight, smooth asphalt roads. The steaming railroads rattled over the high embankment. Smoking steamers plied between Bagan Lampur and Bukit Djempol, and from the plantation little lorries clattered along narrow-tracked rails to the harbour, carrying rubber pressed into wooden boxes.

This description of the environment's transformation is offered in part as evidence of progress, since the virgin forest is consistently evoked in terms of danger and disease. Thus, we are told: 'The forest was marshy, in every little depression stood unpalatable, putrid water that swarmed with mosquito larvae, frog-lime [sic] and small water animals. No matter how many times such unsanitary water was boiled and filtered, a European would get ill from it.' As the English title of the book suggests – *Tropic Fever* – the pioneer period of the boom years was one of feverish

---

[32] Karl J. Pelzer, *Planter and Peasant: Colonial Policy and the Agrarian Struggle in East Sumatra, 1863–1947* (The Hague: Martinus Nijhoff, 1978), p.116.

[33] Ann Laura Stoler, *Capitalism and Confrontation in Sumatra's Plantation Belt, 1870–1979* (New Haven, CT: Yale University Press, 1985), pp.28, 47.

speculation, when Europeans went out to Southeast Asia to make their fortunes. It was also a world of disease, where workers and particularly colonials invariably succumbed to fever. Upon arrival in Sumatra to run a tobacco estate, for example, the protagonist immediately contracts malaria. 'Men died like flies in autumn,' he observes, before proceeding to conjure up a hallucinatory landscape of infection: 'The forest exhaled germs of disease. It breathed upon the intruders and, poisoned by its breath, the coolies died in shoals.'[34]

In Székely's book, we are given an account of the intertwined effects of colonization: environmental exploitation and the abuse of an indentured workforce comprised chiefly of Chinese, Tamil-speaking Indians, and Javanese who live in what is tantamount to a vast labor camp. Disease, which is pervasive, exists within the context of the repeated beatings inflicted on the coolies, the buying and discarding of concubines (*nyai*), and the brutal racial exchanges that characterize plantation life. At the same time, a tale of remorseless environmental exploitation is overlaid with another narrative that extols the human subjection of the wild, dark, snake-infested, and mosquito-riddled jungle. In the penultimate chapter of the book, the protagonist is described entering the 'gigantic virgin forest' to mark out the land for a new estate. As he walks through the 'nerve-killing' solitude of the forest with American 'geologists and pathologists' who have been sent out to verify the feasibility of the territory's exploitation, the protagonist conveys a sense that finally order is being brought to the recalcitrant wilderness. In other words, 'plantation' exists in relation to 'jungle,' while the jungle is viewed in different ways: 'as a resource in itself for export; as an impediment to capitalist agriculture, to be replaced with plantations; and as a source of fear and ambivalence.' Plantation texts, such as those by Székely, reflect a tension between the forest and the estate. In effect, the plantation functions as 'the diffracted image of the forest.'[35] Yet the notion of the forest, as the plantation's untamed antithesis, is complicated by an anxiety about the environmental destruction that this industrial-scale agriculture entails. Such anxieties reflect an ambiguity within the discourse of modernity between an impetus for exploitation and a counter-impetus for conservation.

[34] Ladislao Székely, *Tropic Fever: The Adventures of a Planter in Sumatra*. Translated by Marion Saunders with an introduction by Anthony Reid (Kuala Lumpur: Oxford University Press, 1979), pp.342, 335, 62.
[35] Maureen Sioh, 'Authorizing the Malaysian Rainforest: Configuring Space, Contesting Claims and Conquering Imaginaries,' *Ecumene*, vol.5, no.2 (1998): 144–166 (145, 147).

Disease and dissent: Life on a rubber plantation

Rubber plantations were also developed on an industrial scale in French Indochina. While Chinese and Javanese laborers were initially employed, the French later adopted a policy of moving peasants from Tonkin or Annam, in northern and central Vietnam, to work on plantations in the south. In his account of life on a French colonial rubber plantation in Cochinchina, Trần Tử Bình (1907–1967) emphasizes the exploitation of the impoverished workers from Tonkin and Annam who live and work on the plantation in the constant presence of disease. Under such harsh conditions, it was not surprising that many young men were radicalized and rose against the colonial regime. Trần Tử Bình himself led a strike on the plantation in 1930, which he describes in his memoirs. Subsequently, he became a general of the Democratic Republic of Vietnam (1948) and Vietnam's ambassador to the PRC (1959–1967).

The Phu-rieng plantation was part of the property of the Michelin rubber company. We were the first group of workers to arrive to clear the land ... We had to clear each section of forest to prepare it for planting the rubber trees. The early days of the clearing effort were especially hard and dangerous ... The forest was filled with mosquitoes, every one of them enormous and bright orange with glistening wings. They came buzzing through the air, then lighted and bit right through our clothes. These were malarial mosquitoes, and when they landed on us they arched their backs into the air. Even so, drinking water was not boiled. Whoever was thirsty just searched for some crevice or hole in the ground to drink from. So malaria spread among us extremely quickly. Within a month after we arrived at Phu-rieng there was not one among us who had not been stricken with the fever.

Margaret Slocomb, *Colons and Coolies: The Development of Cambodia's Rubber Plantations* (Bangkok: White Lotus Press, 2007).
    Trần Tử Bình, *The Red Earth: A Vietnamese Memoir of Life on a Colonial Rubber Plantation*. Translated by John Spragens (Athens: Centre for International Studies, Ohio University, 1985), pp.23–31.

Conditions on many early rubber estates in Malaya were similarly appalling. While hookworm was common, respiratory infections and diarrheal disease were aggravated by bad housing. Diseases of nutritional deficiency, such as beriberi, were also rife. There were periodic outbreaks of cholera, including one in the summer of 1906, which led to labor shortages across Malaya. As in many other plantation settings, however, the major scourge was malaria. There were epidemics in Malaya in 1907, 1911, 1920, 1928, and 1938. In 1908, it has been estimated that the death rate from malaria was over 20 percent across 21 estates. On the Midlands Estate between 1910 and 1912, 'nearly half the average population died.' As one report noted, 'no child was born and lived for more than seven years on the Midlands Estate.' According to an account in 1924, more than 90 percent of deaths among Indian workers were attributable to a cluster of diseases that included malaria, dysentery, pneumonia, pulmonary TB, and anemia.[36]

Given the importance of the rubber industry, colonial newspapers were replete with stories about the threat of malaria, and the press played an important role in promoting scientific ideas about disease and its management.[37] Many colonials were doubtless convinced 'that the risk of disease, like the impact of tropical forest deforestation and erosion, formed part and parcel of the march towards economic progress.'[38] Viewed from the perspective of an investor, estates assumed a rosy tincture. A former shareholder of the Highlands and Lowlands Para Rubber Company who toured a large estate in Batu Unjor in 1911 extolled its magnificence. Not only was it 'absolutely clean and free from weeds,' but compared to newer estates it was relatively free from malaria, too. As the rapturous tourist exclaimed, the estate 'might with advantage be tried as a health resort!'[39]

The difficulty in ensuring a constant supply of laborers led to an increasing focus on preserving workers' health. Economic success and operational efficiency, after all, depended on the strength of the workforce. 'A dead or broken-down coolie,' noted the Malayan health officer P. N. Gerrard in his 1913 essay *On the Hygienic Management of Labour in the Tropics*, 'is of no practical use on any estate.'[40] Or, as Carruthers put it, planting 'like other commercial enterprises, has to be managed from a practical view of pounds, shillings, and pence.'[41] However, company interests could run up against government attempts to regulate, as demonstrated by the clashes between planters and malaria control

---

[36] Kaur, 'Indian Labour,' pp.466–467.

[37] Liew Kai Khiun, 'Making Health Public: English Language Newspapers and the Medical Sciences in Colonial Malaya,' *East Asian Science, Technology and Society*, vol.3, nos.2/3 (2009): 209–229 (218).

[38] Kathirithamby-Wells, *Nature and Nation*, p.165.

[39] 'Highlands and Lowlands: The Estates Undoubtedly a Magnificent Property,' *The Straits Times* (February 8, 1911), p.12.

[40] Press review from *The Ceylon Observer*. In: P. N. Gerrard, *On the Hygienic Management of Labour in the Tropics* (Singapore: Printed at the Methodist Publishing House, 1913).

[41] Carruthers, 'Rubber.' In: Wright and Cartwright, eds., *Twentieth Century Impressions of British Malaya*, p.350.

boards and town councils.[42] From the perspective of officials, malaria was an issue of security. 'The time is one of change and advancement in our ideas of colonial development,' Sir Ronald Ross (1857–1932) – the Indian-born British physician who received the Nobel Prize in 1902 for establishing that the malarial parasite was transmitted by the mosquito – asserted in the foreword to Malcolm Watson's *The Prevention of Malaria in the Federated Malay States*, first published by the Liverpool School of Tropical Medicine in 1911.[43] Watson, the author of such works as *Rural Sanitation in the Tropics* (1915), had joined the Malaya Medical Service in 1900 and became a pioneer of malaria control. Writing in the *Singapore Free Press* in the late 1930s in an appeal for donations to support Ross in his retirement, Watson declared: 'If we had dropped all methods of preventing malaria devised as a result of Sir Ronald Ross's discovery, it would shut down the naval base, it would [have led] to appalling death rates in Singapore, Kuala Lumpur and other towns and it would paralyze half the rubber estates in the colony.'[44] In 1911, the year in which the Malaria Advisory Board was established to advise the government of the Federated Malay States, Watson had identified *Anopheles maculatus* as a malaria vector. The frontispiece to the second edition of his book *The Prevention of Malaria* is a photograph, captioned with text that reads:

THE SILENT WAR

Somewhere in Malaya – the ruins of a coffee store on an estate abandoned on account of Malaria. The jungle is beginning to take possession.

Colonial society is engaged in a ceaseless civilizational struggle to push back the encroaching jungle. As Ross observed, in this new era of 'scientific administration,' the greatest threat posed to prosperity was 'widespread disease.' The issue was one of national import, 'and perhaps the very first effort which must be made in new countries is to render them reasonably safe, not only from human enemies, but from those small or invisible ones which in the end are so much more injurious.'[45]

The high rate of mortality on the plantations prompted the government to pass legislation that required plantation estates to construct hospitals for their laborers. Initially, the government had proposed that each estate should provide enough hospital space to cater for five percent of the labor employed at any given time.[46] Planters resented the expense that

[42] Manderson, *Sickness and the State*, pp.127–165.
[43] Watson, *The Prevention of Malaria*, p.ix.   [44] Liew, 'Making Health Public,' p.218.
[45] Watson, *The Prevention of Malaria*, pp.ix–x.
[46] Drabble, *Rubber in Malaya*, p.56.

this would entail and pointed out the impracticability of the directive, lobbying against it through the Planters' Association of Malaya (1907). Colonial newspapers were filled with correspondence and commentaries criticizing the government for meddling with private business and shirking its responsibilities. As the *Penang Gazette* declared in a 1911 editorial:

It is preposterous absurdity for the government, which is harassing estate owners with all sorts of fancy rules and regulations for the preservation of health, to be killing off the laborers in scores by its own parsimony and lack of organization... There are some things over which a government may blunder without much harm resulting, but labour supply is not one of them, and labour supply will fail if Malaya gets a death trap reputation.[47]

As a compromise, it was agreed that two or more neighboring estates could combine in associations served by shared hospitals. By 1909, a chain of estate hospitals covered the main areas of rubber cultivation. The Estate Labourers (Protection of Health) Ordinance was enacted in 1911 as a result of the recommendations of a committee convened specifically to report on estate sanitation. And, in 1916, an official standard of housing was legally prescribed for the first time, setting out, among other things, the minimum dimensions required for workers' sleeping quarters on estates. The journalist Charles Edmond Akers noted in 1914 that malaria posed a particular problem throughout Malaya. 'Sanitary regulations are now enforced by Government ordinance on all estates,' he remarked. 'Adequate hospital accommodation,' he added, 'must be provided, with properly qualified medical attendance and supervision, and these hospitals are [sic] constantly visited by official medical officers.' Although planters complained about the expenditure and the intervention by the authorities who conducted regular medical inspections, 'it is obviously necessary to enforce all possible measures for the health of the labourers, both on account of the loss of work occasioned by sickness, and also in order to maintain a good reputation for the Malay plantations in the districts of Southern India where the coolies are recruited.'[48] As one planter commented in 1921, given that 'the supply of labour is very much below the demand, the first object of a manager is to make his labourers contented, and the rule is to do more rather than less than the required law.'[49]

---

[47] Liew, 'Making Health Public,' p.216.

[48] C. E. Akers, *The Rubber Industry in Brazil and the Orient* (London: Methuen & Co., 1914), p.210.

[49] J. Beckingham, 'The Malay States and Their Industries.' In: C. E. Ferguson-Davie, ed., *In Rubber Lands: An Account of the Work of the Church in Malaya* (London: The Society for the Propagation of the Gospel in Foreign Parts, 1921), pp.51–58 (56).

Scientific research on malaria was undertaken at strategic sites and locales of economic significance, such as cantonments and port cities. Rubber estates also became places of medical research and intervention.[50] In addition to the larger-scale anti-malaria work carried out by the Public Works Department under the supervision of the Malaria Advisory Board, district Mosquito Destruction Boards were established to coordinate local mosquito reduction efforts. Concurrently, plantation companies developed their own health programs and hospitals. In 1919, a separate system was established from the government-run Malacca Agriculture Medical Board.[51] Although there was certainly resistance from planters and company directors to government regulation, planters were also active in supporting malaria research. The Liverpool School of Tropical Medicine, established as a research and teaching institution in 1898, was backed by imperial commercial interests, including planters in Southeast Asia.

Human health became central to plantation management: from the quarantine centers at the ports where migrants disembarked and were processed before continuing on to the plantations, to the organization of the plantations themselves. According to Gerrard, it was essential that coolies were inculcated in disease awareness. In his manual detailing 'the commonest pitfalls on the road to Hygienic Estate Management,' which was directed at the planter community, Gerrard addressed what he saw as the principal sanitary and health issues. While the necessity of sleeping in mosquito nets had to be drummed into coolies, Gerrard was in favor of 'compelling them to wear shoes and gaiters or putties when at work, or in smearing their legs with some sticky substance.' Swampy ground was to be drained, oil poured onto stagnant water, buildings mosquito-proofed. The emphasis was also on inherent biological and cultural traits that made particular groups susceptible to infection. Thus, Tamils were deemed to be 'a delicate nationality, deeply infected with intestinal parasites.' Also apparent in such manuals was the tension between plantation priorities and government directives, specifically in relation to healthcare provisions on estates. According to the Indian Immigration Report for 1911, it was all too common for sick coolies not to be sent to hospital, while many of the estate facilities were considered 'very unsatisfactory, particularly in some parts of Selangor and it was difficult to get improvement effected.'

---

[50] Manderson, *Sickness and the State*, pp.127–165.

[51] J. Norman Parmer, 'Estate Workers' Health in the Federated Malay States in the 1920s.' In: Peter J. Rimmer and Lisa M. Allen, eds., *The Underside of Malaysian History: Pullers, Prostitutes, Plantation Workers* (Singapore: Singapore University Press, 1990), pp.179–192.

To mitigate the threat from infectious diseases there was an emphasis, too, on sanitary housing. As Gerrard pronounced, 'any labour badly housed on insanitary sites with questionable water and food supplies and insufficient medical attendance, must break down.' Medical and hygienic programs became explicitly political; preserving health might avert a physical 'break down,' while deterring 'labour troubles.'[52] Healthy housing assumed added significance, particularly when it came to 'new arrivals.' Some colonial experts argued that maintaining a clearing between buildings and vegetated areas would ensure the healthy circulation of air and plentiful access to light, which were held to be crucial for health. Speaking at an agricultural conference in Kuala Lumpur in 1917, one senior health officer noted a striking affinity between coolies and *Anopheles* mosquitoes: both preferred 'darkness and gloom' to light. Given that 'light will not hurt your coolies but anophelines will,' he recommended plentiful light, in addition to painting the walls, since 'anophelines are difficult to find in white-washed rooms whilst in adjoining rooms that have not been white-washed they may be found in numbers.'[53] Watson observed that 'destruction of the surrounding jungle, combined with drainage of the marshy ground,' could eradicate the breeding environs of the *Anopheles umbrosus* mosquitoes in many parts of Malaya. However, in other inland areas, where a different species of mosquito existed, the same procedures resulted in the opposite effect: opening up the jungle created new breeding places, while 'the better drained the area and the cleaner the hill stream, the more suitable does it become for this mosquito.' In such situations, the jungle clustered around hilly streams was left untouched. Breeding locations were doused with mixtures of mineral oil and kerosene, and dwellings were resited in places where continuous control was feasible.

The discussion so far has been concerned with situating infectious disease in relation to land, labor, capital, and the state. The development of large-scale plantations in the late nineteenth and early twentieth centuries transformed the natural and social ecologies of Southeast Asia. Farmers who had traditionally survived on subsistence farming became wage laborers, the farms of many smallholders were absorbed into bigger estates, and thousands of migrant workers swelled the population. Agrarian change led to the disruption of ecological systems, which affected the epidemiology of vector-borne diseases, such as malaria. Colonial concerns about infection were not only focused on the environment,

---

[52] Gerrard, *On the Hygienic Management of Labour*, p.xi.

[53] S. H. R. Lucy, 'Health and Sanitation on Estates.' In: L. Lewton-Brain and B. Bunting, eds., *Proceedings of the First Agricultural Conference, Malaya* (Kuala Lumpur: Printed at the Federated Malay States Government Printing Office, 1917), pp.123–134 (124).

however; they were also centered on the unhealthy bodies and practices of labor. If disease prevention measures were often a response to political and economic concerns, the interests of private capital and the state frequently diverged. At the same time, the shift of focus from environmental circumstances to the susceptible bodies of laborers was not only a manifestation of colonial racial assumptions; it also reflected tensions between different currents of biomedical thinking and practice. By the twentieth century, while there was a consensus on the etiology and diagnosis of many diseases, there were significant differences in approaches to their management. These differences, and the political contexts that determined them, are explored more fully in the next section.

Putting parasites in their place: Malaria in Japanese Taiwan

Taiwan is an island of approximately 14,000 square miles off the southern coast of China, opposite the province of Fujian. Although mountainous in the East, it is characterized by fertile plains in the West. Prior to the arrival of the Dutch and Spanish in the seventeenth century, when Han Chinese began immigrating, the island had been inhabited primarily by aborigine populations. In 1662, the Dutch were expelled and the first Han Chinese polity was established on the island, the Kingdom of Tungning. This was later subjugated by the Qing who annexed Taiwan in 1683. Following Japan's victory in the First Sino-Japanese War in 1895, the island was ceded to Japan by the terms of the Treaty of Shimonoseki and remained a Japanese colony until 1945.

Malaria appears to have been endemic in Taiwan. From the seventeenth century, there had been significant deforestation with irrigation systems constructed that served as breeding grounds for malarial mosquitoes. As the historian George Barclay noted: 'The moist heat, and the practice of admitting water into fields for irrigation in pools that were left to stagnate, helped to nurture the mosquitoes that spread the disease. Occasionally malaria broke out in epidemic form. It was likewise impossible to control, but was simply allowed to run its course. Even in the more fortunate years it served to undermine the strength of Taiwanese during much of the year, and probably their resistance to other sickness.'[54]

Such views, however, also echoed late nineteenth-century perceptions of Taiwan's environment and subtropical climate as particularly intemperate and unhealthy. Japanese commentators tended to emphasize the

---

[54] George W. Barclay, *Colonial Development and Population in Taiwan* (Princeton, NJ: Princeton University Press, 1954), p.135.

insalubrious nature of the land, which was compared unfavorably with Japan and described as particularly disease-ridden: overly hot, humid, with inhospitable forests and mosquito-infested marshes. To be sure, seventeenth-century Dutch sources had alluded to malaria-like fevers, as had Qing records, where fevers retrospectively identified as malaria were attributed to a variety of environmental factors and referred to as 'miasmas' (zhang). The term nueji, which had an ancient provenance, was subsequently used to describe modern malaria.[55] Yet the notion that Taiwan was an exceptionally unhealthy place was largely a construct of the late nineteenth century. Japanese convictions in the island's malignant properties were extended to views of the population as inherently sickly. Disease was construed as an impediment to industry and malaria became a developmental issue to be overcome through improvements. Such ideas were reinforced by – and filtered into – Western perceptions of the island. 'The dread malaria,' wrote the doctor and Presbyterian missionary George Leslie Mackay (1844–1901) in the 1890s, 'works havoc in every home.' It was not uncommon, he noted, 'to find half of the inhabitants of a town prostrated by malarial fever at once':

Because of it disease and death work terrible havoc among the inhabitants. Almost every form of disease is directly traced to this one source. Seldom do three months elapse without one or more members of every household being laid low. In the hot season the natives are suddenly attacked, and in many cases succumb in a few hours.

Mackay attributed the disease to 'malarial poison generated by the decomposing of organic matter,' observing that 'its intensity depends on the constitution, climate, and surroundings of the sufferer.'[56]

For the Japanese, Taiwan's unwholesomeness posed security challenges. First and foremost, malaria was a military predicament. During the Japanese invasion of 1874 – in retaliation for the murder by Taiwanese aborigines of 54 sailors shipwrecked off the coast of Taiwan – there had been several hundred Japanese casualties from malaria. According to the US journalist Edward H. House, 'the sudden outbreak of fever . . . rapidly prostrated a large proportion of the soldiers, and . . . hardly an individual connected with the expedition escaped . . . Of the thousands assembled there, no others were without attacks of more or less violent character. Some hundreds of the troops died – so many that it was necessary to fill

[55] Ts'ui-jung Liu and Shi-yung Liu, 'Disease and Mortality in the History of Taiwan.' In: Ts'ui-jung Liu, et al., eds., *Asian Population History* (Oxford: Oxford University Press, 2001), pp.248–269 (248–249).

[56] George Leslie Mackay, *From Far Formosa: The Island, Its People and Missions*. Fourth edition (New York: Fleming H. Revell Co., 1896), pp.206, 314, 43, 313.

the vacancies by successive reinforcements from Japan.'[57] In 1879, Japan had officially incorporated the Kingdom of Ryukyu, a chain of islands stretching between Kyushu and Taiwan, into the Okinawa prefecture. There, they had encountered the malignant form of malaria caused by the *Plasmodium falciparum*, which existed in Taiwan. In 1895, during the Japanese annexation of Taiwan, the mortality figures from the disease were far higher than they had been in the 1870s. Although there was little armed resistance and only 154 combat fatalities, there were over 4,000 deaths from malaria with many thousands of soldiers hospitalized.[58]

Western science and medicine were viewed as vital technologies in promoting modernization after the Meiji Restoration (Chapter 1). In Japan's first colony, disease control also became a key aspect of colonial governance, complementing more overt strategies of military subjugation and political assimilation. Medicine was espoused 'as a key to political welfare and doctors the agents of modern civilization.'[59] Japanese commentators noted that little attention had been paid by the Qing government to building a health infrastructure on the island. As Seiji Hishida asserted in 1907: 'Even Taihoku [Taipei], the capital of the island, was in a chronic state of filth, and swarmed with flies and mosquitoes. Malaria, black fevers and smallpox were common diseases among the natives.' Hishida contended that sanitation was a priority in the 'tropical zone.' 'Economic and social progress in a tropical colony,' he wrote, 'can be expected only where proper sanitary precautions are taken.'[60] This was a common theme in the early twentieth century. Writing at the same time about Japanese rule in Taiwan, the historian and politician Yosaburō Takekoshi (1865–1950) declared that in tropical colonies 'epidemic disease and malaria are the most formidable enemies man has to contend with.'[61]

Malaria was viewed as posing the most serious challenge, reflecting broader colonial anxieties about Japan's ability to govern. To an extent, the efficacy of anti-malaria measures became an index of Japanese authority. Soon after their occupation of the island, Japanese colonial officials sought to devise ways of preventing the disease. A medical school was established in Taipei in 1897 and two years later the governor general of Formosa ('Formosa' was the Portuguese name given to Taiwan)

---

[57] Edward H. House, *The Japanese Expedition to Formosa* (Tokyo, 1875), p.215.

[58] Barclay, *Colonial Development*, p.136.

[59] Ming-cheng M. Lo, *Doctors within Borders: Profession, Ethnicity, and Modernity in Colonial Taiwan* (Berkeley: University of California Press, 2002), p.39.

[60] Seiji Hishida, 'Formosa: Japan's First Colony,' *Political Science Quarterly*, vol.22, no.2 (1907): 267–281(274).

[61] Yosaburō Takekoshi, *Japanese Rule in Formosa*. Translated by George Braithwaite (London: Longmans, Green, and Co., 1907), p.283.

established the 'Committee on Taiwanese Endemic Diseases and Epidemics,' with a focus on malaria research. At the second Congress of the Formosan Medical Association, which convened in 1904, approaches to malaria prevention and control were discussed. While Japanese scientists were aware of Ross's discovery of the mosquito as the malaria vector and had conducted epidemiological studies of the disease, it was decided to focus on targeting the parasite in the human population.[62] This was the approach advocated by the German bacteriologist Robert Koch. In 1900, on a trip to the Dutch East Indies and northern New Guinea, a German protectorate between 1884 and 1914, Koch had studied the epidemiology of malaria. He had also developed a method for malaria prevention in the tropics that involved the systematic application of quinine therapeutically and prophylactically. Koch's focus was thus on antiparasite methods of control, since 'it is beyond human power to destroy or even considerably to reduce a species of insect like the anopheles in large districts.'[63] In contrast, Ross's emphasis was on eradication – or as he put it, on waging 'a war against our winged enemies' by destroying their natural breeding places. This approach was epitomized by Ross's call for the institution of quasi-military 'Mosquito Brigades,' headed by a 'superintendent or commandant-general,' as a core element of tropical hygiene.[64]

An economic rationale influenced public health policy. At least, this is suggested by the research of Kinoshita Kashichiro, a German-educated malariologist and member of the Committee on Taiwanese Endemic Diseases and Epidemics. Following an outbreak of malaria in 1906, which disrupted the camphor timber industry – of particular importance for the Japanese economy – Kinoshita was charged with producing a report on the most effective means of dealing with the disease. Based on a cost–benefit analysis, he advocated a parasite-focused approach involving blood testing and the taking of quinine, arguing that since mosquitoes bred in rice fields, which were ubiquitous, an eradication campaign was unfeasible.

---

[62] Lin Yi-ping and Liu Shiyung, 'A Forgotten War: Malaria Eradication in Taiwan, 1905–65.' In: Angela Ki Che Leung and Charlotte Furth, eds., *Health and Hygiene in Chinese East Asia: Policies and Publics in the Long Twentieth Century* (Durham, NC: Duke University Press, 2010), pp.183–203 (186).

[63] Hughes Evans, 'European Malaria Policy in the 1920s and 1930s: The Epidemiology of Minutiae,' *Isis*, vol.80, no.1(1989): 40–59 (51); Ku Ya-Wen, 'Anti-malaria Policy and Its Consequences in Colonial Japan.' In: Ka-che Yip, ed., *Disease, Colonialism, and the State: Malaria in Modern East Asian History* (Hong Kong: Hong Kong University Press, 2009), pp.31–48 (34–35).

[64] Ronald Ross, *Mosquito Brigades and How to Organise Them* (New York: Longmans, Green, and Co., 1902), pp.44, 13.

This policy was made official following a meeting convened in 1911 by the governor general to formulate a policy on malaria control. Legislation was passed designating districts that would be targeted in anti-malaria campaigns. Malaria control measures were to begin in 12 localities, expanding in due course to other highly malaria-affected areas. The authorities relied on detection and compulsory treatment of infected persons discovered within the specified districts.[65] The system co-opted the Taiwanese indigenous household and neighborhood surveillance network known as the *hōkō* or *baojia* in Chinese.[66] Headmen and local police were to help round up targeted populations for blood inspection, backed by corps of Japanese sanitary police.[67]

While the mobilization of the *hōkō* for state purposes might be viewed as a colonial tactic for suppressing local administrative institutions through assimilation, from another perspective it might be understood as an attempt to reinvigorate and reorganize such institutions by infusing them with a new purpose and connecting them to state directives. In other words, the colonial regime would work through local community structures, rather than superimpose a top-down order. Indeed, the German-educated physician and statesman Gotō Shinpei (1857–1929), appointed chief civil administrator of Taiwan in 1898, argued compellingly against policies of state-directed assimilation. Attempts to forcibly integrate colonial societies through the deployment of state institutions, he asserted, were as pointless as attempting to graft the eyes of a bream onto a flatfish.[68] Instead, in Gotō Shinpei's version of scientific colonialism, local customs were to be 'the groundwork for colonial governance.'[69] Reflecting on the achievements of Japanese colonialism in Taiwan, he observed:

Our first colony, Taiwan, had developed so rapidly that it took every country by surprise . . . In fact, these achievements were due to my suggestion of developing 'biological colonial policies.' In other words, we adhered to natural, instead of artificial, policies, which were developed and modified flexibly according to the abilities and characters of the colonized population.[70]

---

[65] Akihisa Setoguchi, 'Control of Insect Vectors in the Japanese Empire: Transformation of the Colonial/Metropolitan Environment, 1920–1945,' *East Asian Science, Technology and Society*, vol.1, no.2 (2007): 167–181 (171).

[66] Chin Hsien-Yu, 'Colonial Medical Police and Postcolonial Medical Surveillance Systems in Taiwan, 1895–1950s,' *Osiris*, vol.13 (1998): 326–338 (329–330).

[67] Ku, 'Anti-malaria Policy and Its Consequences in Colonial Japan.' In: Yip, ed., *Disease, Colonialism, and the State*, p.35.

[68] Christos Lynteris, 'From Prussia to China: Japanese Colonial Medicine and Gotō Shinpei's Combination of Medical Police and Local Self-Administration,' *Medical History*, vol.55, no.3 (2011): 343–347.

[69] Ku, 'Anti-malaria Policy and Its Consequences in Colonial Japan.' In: Yip, ed., *Disease, Colonialism, and the State*, p.42.

[70] Lo, *Doctors within Borders*, p.39.

In part, this was also an educational drive. A constant colonial refrain was the insouciance of the local population, who appeared oblivious to the dangers of malaria and uninformed about its etiology and mode of transmission. This nonchalance, stemming from ignorance, was understood to be one of the crucial drivers of disease. However, the overriding object of the Japanese anti-malaria program was to safeguard colonial interests – with key resource sites targeted in the anti-malaria push: waterworks, farmland, and plantations. In parallel to the focus on parasite identification, vector control was increasingly emphasized after 1919, when the government modified the 'Rules for Operation of the Law on Malaria Control Practice.' As Akihisa Setoguchi notes, '*Anopheles* mosquitoes were to be exterminated by destroying their habitats through civil engineering practices. Drainage canals, water pools, and other breeding places of mosquitoes were ordered to be cleaned or even filled.'[71] This was a more ambitious attempt to sanitize the Taiwanese environment and, through the environment, to reform its inhabitants. The context for this new policy was a rise in malaria deaths, as well as a political shift towards greater assimilation. After the First World War, the policy of 'Japanese Homeland Extensionism' – meaning the extension of Japanese cultural values outward to assimilate colonial cultures – was in the ascendant. Taiwan was now conceived as an extension of the Home Islands, and the Taiwanese were to be taught to assume their responsibilities as Japanese subjects. Japanese and Taiwanese co-education was promoted, local customs were derided as superstitions, Japanese norms were pushed, and health was championed as a crucial part of this emancipatory mission.

The emphasis was also on inculating new hygienic behavior in the local population. Those living in targeted malarial districts were obliged to drain pools and swamps, remove weeds from ditches, and cut back bamboo thickets. Land usage was monitored to enforce compliance, and Ross's idea of the 'Mosquito Brigades' was enthusiastically adopted. The transformation was also aesthetic: through these sanitary interventions the land would be reordered. While Yosaburō Takekoshi celebrated the development of a colonial medical service and advances in epidemic prevention, he puzzled over the statistical evidence that failed to reflect a drop in mortality. Takekoshi ascribed this anomaly to the fact that native Taiwanese were now less reluctant to come forth and seek treatment than they had been: 'A certain military doctor, who is thoroughly conversant with the conditions which prevailed some years ago in Taihoku and Taichu [Taichung], said to me one day: "When these two cities were surrounded as they used to be on all sides with flourishing forests, the

---

[71] Setoguchi, 'Control of Insect Vectors in the Japanese Empire,' p.172.

infectious bacteria accumulated to an amazing extent. But now that the forests are gone and the mosquitoes have no hiding-places, the sanitary conditions are vastly improved. It is strange, however, that the statistics do not show better results".[72]

Although the Taiwanese were marshaled to exterminate mosquitoes, there was resistance to Japanese hygienic interventions. Bamboo groves, for example, were invested with cultural significance and the Taiwanese were loath to destroy them. While some resented the intrusion into their daily lives, others were indifferent but begrudged the additional unpaid work that it entailed. Even within the Japanese scientific community there was opposition to the policy. Some argued that official statistics overstated the success of anti-malaria efforts. Others warned that mosquito eradication was doomed to failure, given Taiwan's harsh environment. However, many commentators wrote of Japanese anti-malaria efforts with approval. The British travel writer Owen Rutter, for example, declared in 1923: 'The Japanese have undoubtedly influenced the increase of the population, which has risen from 2,500,000 in 1896 to 3,250,000 at the present time. A considerable proportion of this increase is, of course, due to immigration; at the same time the death-rate has been materially reduced, and although malaria is still a prevalent disease, it is probable that as swamps in the neighbourhood of towns are drained, conditions will be further improved.'[73]

In November 1965, Taiwan was officially declared free of malaria by the WHO. For some, this represented a vindication of a century-long anti-malaria campaign and a constructive legacy of Japanese colonial rule, which had witnessed the introduction to Taiwan of modern biomedical and public health technologies. For others, however, biomedicine and public health had been utilized by the Japanese as coercive techniques for expanding state control.[74] There was, after all, a close connection between imperial medicine and the military. The island of Taiwan furnished a laboratory for Japanese military physicians to test out hypotheses, novel diagnostics, clinical practices, and treatments – just as Korea did after 1910. In particular, malaria occupied an important place in the history of this experimentation.[75]

---

[72] Takekoshi, *The Japanese Rule in Formosa*, p.289.
[73] Owen Rutter, *Through Formosa: An Account of Japan's Island Colony* (London: T. Fisher Unwin, 1923), p.156.
[74] Ku, 'Anti-malaria Policy and Its Consequences in Colonial Japan.' In: Yip, ed., *Disease, Colonialism, and the State*, p.31.
[75] Michael Shiyung Liu, *Prescribing Colonization: The Role of Medical Practices and Policies in Japan-Ruled Taiwan, 1895–1945* (Ann Arbor, MI: Association for Asian Studies, 2009), pp.114–125.

As it is told, however – either in terms of triumphant science or high-handed colonialism – the story of malaria's eradication in Taiwan washes over the uneven application of colonial policy, the contradictory emphases on place and person, the inconsistency with which policies were implemented, and the kinds of resistance it elicited. Changing policies reflected often irreconcilable views adopted by scientists whose opinions were determined by political and economic considerations. Although the focus had shifted from an anti-parasite to an anti-mosquito approach after 1919, by the 1930s optimism in malaria eradication had all but disappeared and an anti-parasite strategy was once again adopted, evidenced in the establishment of the Malarial Treatment Laboratory in 1929. Finally, anti-malaria measures did provoke resentment and opposition, underlining cultural differences in how disease was understood.

The case of malaria in Taiwan therefore underscores a number of critical issues. It suggests the shifting focus on place and person as objects of public health, and it points to the broader political contexts in which epidemic prevention policy is worked out and executed. On the one hand, efforts were made to co-opt local institutions in order to manage epidemics. On the other hand, assimilationist policies sought to reform the land and its people by inculcating Japanese norms. The next section explores another instance in which local institutions were mustered in state-sponsored efforts to 'annihilate' disease.

Mao's war against nature: Schistosomiasis

In January 1912, Sun Yat-sen (1866–1925) declared the establishment of the Republic of China, and the following month the child Emperor Xuantong (Puyi) abdicated. This brought a formal end to the Qing dynasty and to over two millennia of imperial rule. There followed an extended period of instability, with in-fighting between regional warlords. In 1931, Japan invaded Manchuria in northeast China and founded the puppet state of Manchukuo, with Puyi as the nominal head. After an offensive by the Soviet Union in 1945, Manchukuo collapsed. Civil War between the Chinese Communist Party (CCP) and the Nationalist Party, or KMT, raged from 1927 until the CCP's eventual victory in 1949, which saw the establishment of the PRC and Chiang Kai-shek's (1887–1975) retreat to Taiwan.

On October 1, 1949, standing by the Gate of Heavenly Peace in Beijing, Mao pronounced his vision for a modern China, a soon-to-be powerhouse on the world stage. Building the new China would involve a massive modernization drive, culminating in the Great Leap Forward (1958–1962), which sought to transform the nation through the rapid industrialization of rural areas, and the Cultural Revolution (1966–1976), which aimed to root out anti-revolutionary capitalist vestiges within Chinese society. At the same time, in the absence of any coherent healthcare system, and given the dislocations of war and widespread malnourishment, infectious diseases posed a threat to stability and to the prospects of social and economic development.

Infectious diseases became the object of concerted state campaigns. An article in the *Chinese Medical Journal* in 1949 declared that schistosomiasis – 'a devastating disease' – undermined 'the very existence of our nation which depends chiefly on agriculture for her national resources.'[76] In 1950, the First National Health Conference was convened and in the same year the Institute of Parasitic Diseases was established in Shanghai by the Chinese Academy of Medical Sciences, with research focusing on filariasis, hookworm, kala-azar, malaria, and schistosomiasis.[77] This last disease, which is also known as bilharzia after the physician Theodor Bilharz (1825–1862) who first discovered it in Egypt in 1851, is caused by water-borne parasitic trematode worms, or flukes, transmitted by freshwater snails. Of the five main species of blood fluke, *Schistosoma japonicum* occurs in China, Indonesia, and the Philippines. Livestock and rural populations working in rice fields are particularly susceptible to schistosomiasis through contact with water in ditches, dykes, and canals, which are home to the parasite's intermediary host. From the snail, the worm passes through the skin of its victims into the intestines, where it produces eggs that may be ejected in urine or feces. Once deposited in water, the eggs hatch into worms that breed in snails – thus completing the parasite's life-cycle.[78] Symptoms of infection include high fever, abdominal pain, diarrhea, with mortality in some instances. Fluid retention in the stomach, which results in severe bloating, explains the disease's colloquial designation in China as 'potbelly disease' or 'big belly' (*da duzi bing*).

While schistosomiasis's endemic status was recognized during the Republican era – with two US researchers, Ernest Faust and Henry Meleney, publishing their lengthy *Studies of Schistosomiasis japonica* in

---

[76] C. Ling, W. Cheng, and H. Chung, 'Clinical and Diagnostic Features of Schistosomiasis Japonica: A Review of 200 Cases,' *Chinese Medical Journal*, vol.67, no.7 (1949): 347–366 (347).

[77] Kenneth S. Warren, '"Farewell to the Plague Spirit": Chairman Mao's Crusade Against Schistosomiasis.' In: John Z. Bowers, J. William Hess, and Nathan Sivin, eds., *Science and Medicine in Twentieth-Century China: Research and Education* (Ann Arbor: Center for Chinese Studies, University of Michigan, 1988), pp.123–140 (128).

[78] F. R. Sandbach, 'The History of Schistosomiasis Research and Policy for its Control,' *Medical History*, vol.20, no.3 (1976): 259–275 (260–261); Miriam Gross and Kawai Fan, 'Schistosomiasis.' In: Bridie Andrews and Mary Brown Bullock, eds., *Medical Transitions in Twentieth-Century China* (Bloomington and Indianapolis: Indiana University Press, 2014), pp.106–125.

1924 under the imprimatur of the *American Journal of Hygiene* – a determined national treatment and prevention drive proved impossible at that time, given the political turbulence and inadequate resources.[79] In the 1950s, epidemiological surveys suggested that schistosomiasis was extensive along the Yangtze River and across large swathes of southern China. Out of a population of approximately 600 million, over 10 million people were infected, with another 100 million deemed to be at risk.

'Farewell to the Plague Spirit'

Mao Zedong (1893–1976) wrote poetry throughout his career and during the Cultural Revolution his poems and 'sayings' were widely memorized and displayed. The poem 'Farewell to the Plague Spirit' was written in 1958 during the anti-schistosomiasis campaign. According to Mao's own testimony, the verse was penned after learning from the *People's Daily* on June 30, 1958 that schistosomiasis had been eliminated from Yujiang County in the southeastern province of Jiangxi. Mao had been based in Yujiang in the 1920s and 1930s fighting the Nationalists. In the poem, composed like all of Mao's poetry in classical Chinese, the campaign against disease becomes symbolic of a bigger task: to purge China of the blights of the past.

> The waters and hills displayed their green in vain
> When the ablest physicians were baffled by these pests.
> A thousand villages were overrun by brambles and men were feeble;
> Ghosts sang their ballads in myriad desolate houses.
> Now, in a day, we have leapt round the earth
> And inspected a thousand Milky Ways.
> If the Cowherd [a constellation] asks about the God of Plagues,
> Tell him that with joy and sorrow he has been washed away by the tide.
>
> Thousands of willow branches sway in the spring wind;
> The six thousand million on this great land are all saintly.
> As they wished, the peach blossom have turned into waves
> And the green mountain ranges into bridges.
> On lofty Wuling rise and fall silver hoes.
> Iron arms shake the earth and tame the broad rivers.
> 'Where are you bound, God of Plagues?
> For your farewell we'll burn candles and paper boats.'

---

[79] John Farley, *Bilharzia: A History of Imperial Tropical Medicine* (Cambridge: Cambridge University Press, 1991), pp.94–96.

Warren, '"Farewell to the Plague Spirit": Chairman Mao's Crusade Against Schistosomiasis.' In: John Z. Bowers, J. William Hess, and Nathan Sivin, eds., *Science and Medicine in Twentieth-Century China: Research and Education* (Ann Arbor: Center for Chinese Studies, University of Michigan, 1988), pp.123–140 (124).

Jerome Ch'ên, *Mao and the Chinese Revolution with Thirty-Seven Poems by Mao Tse-tung*. Translated by Michael Bullock and Jerome Ch'ên (Oxford: Oxford University Press, 1965), p.349.

An article entitled 'Reds Fail to Halt Epidemic in China,' which was published in the *New York Times* in 1952, quoted extensively from an interview with a CCP health official in a Shanghai newspaper. 'Schistosomiasis,' the official conceded, was a 'fierce and stubborn enemy that threatens the broad masses of the people in East China.' The Party, he announced, was determined 'to prevent and combat the disease and eliminate it with resolution.'[80] In 1955, the so-called 'Nine-Man Subcommittee on Schistosomiasis' was set up with precisely this aim. The focus on schistosomiasis was reaffirmed as a political priority when Mao visited Zhejiang province in November 1955 and observed the effects of infection for himself. In his 'Seventeen Articles on Agricultural Work,' which outlined his program for reorganizing China's agricultural system through collectivization, the disease was singled out as a major pest. The following year, when the Party formally published its plans for agricultural development, an ambitious program was launched to eliminate the most debilitating diseases – schistosomiasis among them – within 12 years. Mao pushed for an intensification of the campaign with the blunt slogan 'schistosomiasis has to be eliminated.' The economic argument for the campaign was consistently made: the disease hampered development and productivity.[81] In this sense, the campaign was closely connected to Mao's agricultural policies. The natural environment required subjugating in order to maximize yields with large-scale water conservancy and reclamation projects. Grasslands were to be broken up, wetlands drained, and forests felled to feed furnaces. By the same token, pests had to be 'wiped out.' This was an essentially 'oppositional relationship to nature,' as Judith Shapiro has noted, reflecting 'an extreme case of the modernist conception of humans as fundamentally distinct and separate from nature': 'Mao's voluntarist philosophy held

---

[80] 'Reds Fail to Halt Epidemic in China; Communist Official Declares 10,000,000 Infected With an Intestinal Disease,' *New York Times* (April 3, 1952).

[81] Kawai Fan and Honkei Lai, 'Mao Zedong's Fight Against Schistosomiasis,' *Perspectives in Biology and Medicine*, vol.51, no.2 (Spring 2008): 176–187 (179–180).

that through concentrated exertion of human will and energy, material conditions could be altered and all difficulties overcome in the struggle to achieve a socialist utopia.' The people were pitted 'against the natural environment in a fierce struggle' with mass mobilization campaigns envisaged in adversarial terms as a battle against the defiant forces of nature.[82]

The anti-schistosomiasis campaign involved the widespread promotion of information about snails to the public. All means were co-opted for this purpose: 'broadcasting, wall newspapers, blackboards, exhibits of real and model objects, lantern-slide shows, and dramatic performances.' Citizens were encouraged to hark on the grim pre-Communist past and to help build a resplendent future.[83] On a more practical front, the campaign entailed the construction of new latrines to avoid the seepage of contaminated waste, as well sinking wells for clean water. Collectivized night-soil centers were established to prevent the application of untreated excrement as a crop fertilizer. Treatment units were set up, along with field stations for research. There was also an ambitious snail control strategy that targeted high-transmission areas. In early 1958, Mao launched the Great Leap Forward to accelerate industrialization and collectivization and in the same year the All-China Conference on Parasitic Diseases resolved to eradicate malaria, schistosomiasis, filariasis, hookworm, and kala-azar in a year. Disease eradication merged with a political program that sought to transform China's agrarian society.

Thousands of farmers took part in the grueling mission to eliminate the fluke-carrying snails around the waterways of the Yangtze. They waded through marshes, rivers, and lakes, extracting the snails with sticks or collecting them by hand (Figure 3.3). New drainage canals were opened and existing dykes filled in to bury the snails. As one Western observer noted: 'In between large-scale campaigns, regular anti-snail patrols are maintained by trained snail-spotters who cruise along the rivers in canoes, scrutinizing the banks for snails.'[84] Metaphors of warfare framed the campaign, which was envisaged as a fight against a stealthy 'enemy.' Workers were 'soldiers' who deployed military stratagems to defeat the parasite, operating in 'platoons' and 'brigades.' Such military metaphors inferred a security rationale and, from the outset, the anti-schistosomiasis drive was closely linked to military concerns. Some 40,000 troops stationed in

---

[82] Judith Shapiro, *Mao's War Against Nature: Politics and the Environment in Revolutionary China* (Cambridge: Cambridge University Press, 2001), pp.xii, 3.

[83] Victor W. Sidel and Ruth Sidel, *Serve the People: Observations on Medicine in the People's Republic of China* (New York: Josiah Macy Jr. Foundation, 1973), p.105.

[84] Joshua S. Horn, *'Away With All Pests . . .' An English Surgeon in People's China* (London: Paul Hamlyn, 1969), pp.94–106 (96).

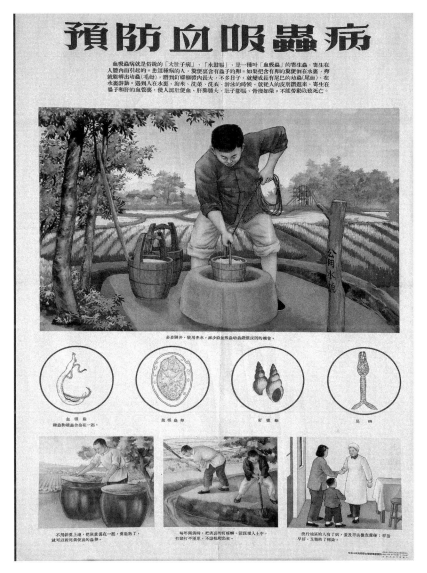

Figure 3.3. 'A Chinese public health poster on schistosomiasis prevention and control (ca. 1954).' Courtesy: US National Library of Medicine.

Anti-schistosomiasis public health posters

Figure 3.3 shows a farmer drawing water from a well. Smaller images in circles depict the lifecycle of the schistosome parasite: from adult worms that lay eggs in the bladder or intestine, to the eggs that are passed in feces and urine, releasing *miracidia* that infect snails, culminating in the release of free-swimming *cercariae*, which infect humans by penetrating the skin. At the bottom of the poster, three further images depict a farmer killing off the eggs by placing human feces in lidded compost containers, burying the snails while digging water channels, and finally a woman taking a child to a health center for a check-up. Schistosomiasis remains a challenge in China today, with over 800,000 people reportedly infected and a further 6.5 million at risk in 2011. An anti-schistosomiasis drive, launched in 2004, made use of public health posters that drew on Mao's earlier campaign, not only reiterating the importance of hygiene and clean water, but also re-emphasizing the need to collect and destroy snails.

Ka-wai Fan, 'Schistosomiasis Control and Snail Elimination in China,' *American Journal of Public Health*, vol.102, no.12 (2012): 2231–2232.

Shanghai for an amphibian invasion of Taiwan – which was held by Chiang Kai-shek's Nationalists – succumbed to the disease after they had taken swimming lessons in preparation for the assault. As a journalist in *Harper's Magazine* quipped, it was 'the blood fluke that saved Formosa': 'A tiny, arrow-shaped parasite turned out to be a precious ally of America and Nationalist China, stopping a Communist invasion that might have changed the history of the Pacific.'[85]

The Korean War (1950–1953) was another critical context for the mass elimination of infectious disease hosts. During the winter of 1951 and 1952, at the height of the conflict, large numbers of pests were recorded in North Korea, as well as in Manchuria and Qingdao, a port-city in eastern Shandong province. It was alleged that swarms of mosquitoes, fleas, flies, and rats were being deliberately introduced by the United States to spread infection in a subterfuge war against the PRC and North Korea. US warplanes were also purported to have dropped the smallpox virus

[85] Frank Algerton Kierman, 'The Blood Fluke That Saved Formosa,' *Harper's Magazine*, vol.218, no.1307 (April 1959): 45–47 (45); Gross and Fan, 'Schistosomiasis.' In: Andrews and Bullock, eds., *Medical Transitions*, p.121.

over Korea. Premier Zhou Enlai (1898–1976) accused the United States of perpetrating a war crime. In response, the PLA was ramped up for anti-bacteriological warfare and a Patriotic Health Campaign was initiated, involving the mass mobilization of citizens to assist in the war effort by eradicating pests and forestalling disease. Health posters promoted the fight against germs. Official newspapers reported the discovery of exploded germ bombs and contaminated material dropped over China to spread infection. Bombs were allegedly filled with tarantulas in Liaoning, while feathers impregnated with anthrax were identified in Shenyang. In what was undoubtedly one the most bizarre episodes of the war, an infestation of voles in Gannan county, on the Chinese–Korean border, was viewed as a planned attack; it was claimed that the rodents had been weaponized by the United States (Figure 3.4).[86]

The PRC leadership set up a committee to supervise epidemic prevention measures that would ensure the war effort was not derailed. These included rounding up and destroying infected animals, imposing strict quarantine measures, and establishing centers for the treatment of patients. As noted above, this countrywide anti-epidemic drive merged with a campaign for social change. Even those in unaffected areas were recruited to the cause as the state became increasingly embedded in citizens' lives, its intrusive operations normalized. By 1958, when Mao penned his poem 'Farewell to the Plague Spirit,' the Korean anti-imperialist campaign had been transformed and scaled up into a hygiene campaign to exterminate the so-called four pests: flies, mosquitoes, rats, and sparrows. The masses were recruited for this patriotic mission of pest control. Hygiene contests were held and rewards were given to those who had collected the greatest number of rats' tails, dead flies, mosquitoes, or sparrows.[87]

According to the British physician Joshua Horn, who spent 15 years as a teacher and medical worker in China and fully embraced Mao's 'gigantic campaign against snails,' it appeared likely that China would be 'the first country in the world to bring this disease under effective control.'[88]

---

[86] Ruth Rogaski, 'Nature, Annihilation, and Modernity: China's Korean War Germ-Warfare Experience Reconsidered,' *Journal of Asian Studies*, vol.61, no.2 (2002): 381–415 (383); Liping Bu, 'The Patriotic Health Movement and China's Socialist Reconstruction: Fighting Disease and Transforming Society, 1950–80.' In: Liping Bu and Ka-che Yip, eds., *Public Health and National Reconstruction in Post-War Asia: International Influences, Local Transformations* (Abingdon and New York: Routledge, 2015), pp.34–51.

[87] Nianqun Yang, 'Disease Prevention, Social Mobilization and Spatial Politics: The Anti-Germ Warfare Incident of 1952 and the "Patriotic Health Campaign,"' *Chinese Historical Review*, vol.11, no.2 (2004): 155–182.

[88] Horn, *'Away With All Pests . . .'*, pp.96, 94.

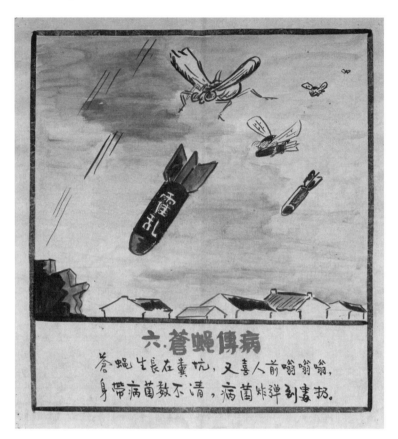

六. 蒼蠅傳病

蒼蠅生長在糞坑, 又喜人前嗡嗡嗡,
身帶病菌數不清, 病菌炸彈到處扔。

Figure 3.4. '"Flies Spread Disease": Public health and germ warfare during the Korean War (ca. 1952).' Courtesy: US National Library of Medicine.

Germ warfare: Epidemic invasions

Figure 3.4 – reproduced on the cover of this book in color – depicts cholera bombs, which were purportedly dropped on civilian homes during the Korean War. The text under the title ('FLIES SPREAD DISEASE') reads: 'Flies like to live in cesspools and like to sing in front of people too; they carry countless germs and throw germ bombs everywhere.' The bombs are envisaged both literally as a vehicle of US bacteriological warfare, but also metaphorically in that flies are imagined as 'throwing' germ bombs. The British scientist and sinologist Joseph Needham (1900–1995), who headed an international commission to investigate the allegations, was convinced that the United States had made use of insects and animals to spread diseases, such as anthrax, smallpox, typhus, and plague. Although Needham's report has long since been discredited, the overtly political nature of anti-disease campaigns in the 1950s was not unique to China. In the United States during the McCarthy era (1950–1956) – named after Republican Senator Joseph McCarthy – anxieties about Communist infiltration were linked to fears of infectious disease. This identification of foreign invasion with epidemic threat was evident in public health campaigns and extended to popular culture. For J. Edgar Hoover (1895–1972), the director of the Federal Bureau of Investigation (FBI), Communism itself was 'a condition akin to disease that spreads like an epidemic and like an epidemic, a quarantine is necessary to keep it from infecting the Nation.' In this tense atmosphere of paranoia, 'red scare' conspiracy theories abounded, alleging nefarious Communist plots to undermine the United States. A flyer produced by the 'Keep America Committee' in the 1950s, for example, identified polio vaccination, water fluoridization, and 'mental hygiene' as foreign plots to poison Americans.

Liping Bu, 'Anti-Germ Warfare Campaign Posters.' In: Michael Sappol, ed., *Hidden Treasure: The National Library of Medicine* (Bethesda and New York: National Library of Medicine/Blast Books, 2012), pp.198–199.

Alexandra Minna Stern and Howard Markel, 'The Public Health Service and Film Noir: A Look Back at Elia Kazan's *Panic in the Streets* (1950),' *Public Health Reports*, vol.118, no.3 (2003): 178–183.

Indeed, Mao's historic anti-schistosomiasis campaign is widely considered by the Chinese government to be one of the country's most successful anti-disease crusades. It occupies a near mythic status in popular memory, exemplifying patriotic participation and common cause in the face of great odds. To be sure, it did represent an epic attempt to eliminate an endemic disease. And yet, this version of the anti-schistosomiasis campaign ignores popular resistance and partial assimilation. It also ignores the fact that schistosomiasis was not eliminated in 1958. Since 2001, the incidence of schistosomiasis has been rising, with the construction of the

Three Gorges Dam (1994–2006) identified as one cause of the disease's re-emergence.[89]

Mao's anti-schistosomiasis campaign may therefore be viewed within the context of political efforts in the newly established PRC to reorganize economic production and reshape society through a material re-engineering of the land – a project symbolized by the much-publicized photograph of Mao wielding a shovel with members of the CCP as he inaugurated the works on the Ming Tombs Reservoir outside Beijing in 1958. Disease elimination and treatment formed an integral part of the war against nature. A Maoist 'annihilationist rhetoric' connected the conquest of nature with the defeat of germs and the fight against an imperialist enemy. Mao wrote his poem 'Farewell to the Plague Spirit' after having read about the successful annihilation (*xiaomie*) of the snails that harbor the disease. As Ruth Rogaski has argued of the Patriotic Health Campaign: 'The germ-warfare allegations combined two motifs that were central to the identity of New China: China as a victim of imperialism, and China as a victim of nature.' The campaign launched in 1952, 'embodied an enduring solution to China's dual victimization: the need to eradicate, to exterminate, or to annihilate (*chu, xiaomie*) perceived enemies, whether political or natural, in order to achieve a state of modernity.'[90]

So far in this chapter, I have been emphasizing the interconnections between environment and infectious disease, bringing into focus a number of issues. First, that environmental changes have their roots in social, political, and economic transformations. Second, that health and illness, as biological and cultural conditions, cannot be untethered from historical changes to the land – its organization, management, and exploitation. Third, and relatedly, that scientific and public health approaches to environmental issues are shaped by political and economic concerns, just as political and economic projects are often rationalized in terms of their health benefits. In the final section of this chapter, I consider the after-life of these colonial and modernizing efforts in postcolonial Asia, showing not only how epidemics of 'new' diseases may be produced through anthropogenic impacts on the environment, but how they may also reactivate historical social and political tensions.

Nipah virus: Bats, pigs, and ethnic politics

In September 1998, an outbreak of febrile encephalitis occurred in the Kinta district of Perak in northwest Malaysia, affecting pig farmers. Identified as Japanese encephalitis (JE), a mosquito-borne viral disease that

---

[89] Fan and Lai, 'Mao Zedong's Fight Against Schistosomiasis,' p.185; Gross and Fan, 'Schistosomiasis.' In: Andrews and Bullock, eds., *Medical Transitions*, pp.123–124.

[90] Rogaski, 'Nature, Annihilation, and Modernity,' p.382.

is endemic to the country, vaccination efforts against JE were stepped up and vector control intensified. However, distinctive features of the disease's epidemiology, specifically the clustering of cases around farms with sickness identified in pigs, as well as humans, suggested another cause. By early 1999, infection had spread from Perak to other areas and in March of that year, 11 workers came down with respiratory illness and encephalitis in an abattoir in Singapore, where pigs had been exported from Malaysia. In the event, there were 265 reported cases, with 105 fatalities. Meanwhile, the economic fallout for Malaysia was significant, posing a particular challenge in the wake of the 1997 Asian financial crisis. Domestic and export markets crashed, resulting in an estimated loss of US$244 million in revenue. The cost of the control program, lost tax revenue, and compensation for the 1.1 million pigs culled (close to half of the country's domestic pig population), amounted to a further US$338 million.[91] In April 1999, a novel virus was isolated and named Nipah (NiV) after the place in which the initial outbreak had occurred. Pteropid fruit bats – or flying foxes – were identified as the pathogen's natural host. Soon the focus shifted to other contributory environmental factors that may have influenced the disease's epidemiology.[92]

In 1997 and 1998, extensive areas of tropical rainforest in Indonesia were destroyed by fire, the result of a combination of factors, including land clearance activities associated with the preparation for industrial plantations. A drought attributed to the El Niño Southern Oscillation (ENSO) – fluctuating ocean temperatures in the equatorial Pacific that result in extreme weather patterns – allowed the conflagration to spread. Although the fires primarily affected the islands of Sumatra and Borneo, NASA satellite images showed an expansive belt of smoke stretching across Southeast Asia, enveloping neighboring Malaysia and Singapore. Smog also pushed westwards across the Indian Ocean, driven by high-altitude winds. While the fires gave rise to concerns about the impact of the smoke on human health, there were also worries about the environmental fallout, with reports that crops were failing and flowering fruit trees had been affected.[93]

These environmental conditions, it is thought, may have led to the spillover infection: fruit bats, which serve as the reservoir hosts of the NiV, were driven from their natural forest habitat northwards to roost

[91] *Manual on the Diagnosis of Nipah Virus Infection in Animals* (Rome: UN Food and Agriculture Organization, January 2002), pp.5–6.

[92] Heng Thay Chong, Suhailah Abdullah, and Chong Tin Tan, 'Nipah Virus and Bats,' *Neurology Asia*, vol.14 (June 2009): 73–76.

[93] M. J. Wooster, G. L. W. Perry, and A. Zoumas, 'Fire, Drought and El Niño Relationships on Borneo (Southeast Asia) in the Pre-MODIS Era (1980–2000),' *Biogeosciences*, vol.9, no.1 (January 2012): 317–340.

in areas where there were piggeries and cultivated orchards, including mango trees. It has been argued that pigs became infected as a result of eating fallen fruit contaminated by bat saliva or urine. From the pigs, the virus jumped species to the piggery workers. The emergence of NiV in humans – closely related to the Hendra virus (HeV), which was isolated in 1994 following an outbreak of severe respiratory and neurologic disease among horses and humans near Brisbane, Australia – was thus the outcome of interconnected events, including anthropogenic deforestation, ENSO, and the organization of the pig industry.[94] The 1998 epidemic in Malaysia not only suggests the impact of climatic factors and human environment interactions on complex ecologies, but also indicates the multiple biological and social factors driving disease.[95]

In addition, the NiV epidemic revealed and intensified ethnic tensions, which in turn shaped responses to the crisis. Several months before the NiV outbreak and in the aftermath of the 1997 financial crisis, the Indonesian Chinese community had been targeted in widespread riots that led to President Suharto's (1921–2008) resignation in May 1998. Anti-Chinese sentiments were to flare up in Malaysia, too. According to the 2000 census, out of a population of some 22 million, Malays and other indigenous groups comprise 65.1 percent of Malaysia's population, with the Chinese accounting for 26 percent, and Indians for 7.7 percent. Of the total population, 60.4 percent are Muslims, while most Chinese are Taoist-Buddhists. Although Malaysia is a multiethnic state, under Article 153 of the Constitution, Malays are granted 'special rights' in designated sectors, including education, business, and public service. This institutional privileging of one ethnic group over the others is in part a legacy of colonial rule. To manage the different ethnic communities, and in particular the mass migration of Chinese and Indians to the Federated Malay States in the nineteenth century, the British categorized the population according to occupation and ethnicity with Malays identified with agriculture, the Chinese with commerce, and Indians with plantations. Britain sought to rule through the Malay sultans and, in so doing, 'assumed the role of self-proclaimed protector of Malay interests and rights in various spheres of society' – interests and rights that were supposedly under threat from a surging non-Malay

[94] K. B. Chua, B. H. Chua, and C. W. Wang, 'Anthropogenic Deforestation, El Niño and the Emergence of Nipah Virus in Malaysia,' *Malaysian Journal of Pathology*, vol.24, no.1 (June 2002): 15–21; K. B. Chua, et al., 'Nipah Virus: A Recently Emergent Deadly Paramyxovirus,' *Science*, vol.288, no.5470 (May 26, 2000): 1432–1435.
[95] L. M. Looi and K. B. Chua, 'Lessons from the Nipah Virus Outbreak in Malaysia,' *Malaysian Journal of Pathology*, vol.29, no.2 (December 2007): 63–67 (65).

population.[96] Since Malaya's independence from Britain in 1957 and the establishment of Malaysia in 1963, there have been recurrent tensions between the Chinese and Malay communities. In the aftermath of the May 1969 general election, all-out violence erupted in the Malaysian state of Selangor. According to official estimates, the 'race riots' left 196 people dead with some 400 injured in clashes between Chinese and Malays. Other sources put the numbers much higher. A national emergency was declared and a country-wide curfew imposed by the military. Parliament was suspended until 1971 and an affirmative action program, known as the New Economic Policy (NEP), was adopted to achieve 'equity and balance among Malaysia's social and ethnic groups.' However, ethnic and racial issues, and community-specific grievances, continue to shape politics in peninsular Malaysia.[97]

Piggeries and abattoirs in Malaysia are largely owned and run by the Chinese, since the majority Malay population is predominantly Muslim and does not eat pork. As a result, pigs are considered to be 'Chinese.' The identification of NiV with pigs and through pigs with the Chinese led to a highly charged political situation. The government was accused by some of playing down the epidemic initially, since it was deemed to be a problem only affecting the minority Chinese. Even when evidence suggested that the disease was not JE, the Ministry of Health persisted in cautioning about the dangers of JE and its mosquito vector. Malays tended to lay the blame squarely on the Chinese, holding unscrupulous Chinese pig farmers liable for ignoring health regulations and handling pigs without taking due precautions, such as wearing protective masks and gloves. Following the outbreak, thousands of pig farmers and workers fled their homes and farms, jeopardizing the health of the wider community, and provoking anger. Castigated by some for being anti-Chinese, others alleged that the government had ignored earlier Malay protests about the unsanitary condition of the piggeries. According to more extreme Malay views, the outbreak was '[God's] warning.'[98] NiV thus disclosed a fragile socio-political ecology in an ethnocratic state founded on preferential policies that favor one community over others. Historic tensions erupted that highlighted the multifaceted relationship between labor, capital, and the state.

---

[96] M. Shamsul Haque, 'The Role of the State in Managing Ethnic Tensions in Malaysia: A Critical Discourse,' *American Behavioral Scientist*, vol.47, no.3 (November 2003): 240–266 (243, 244).

[97] Lian Kwen Fee and Jayanath Appadurai, 'Race, Class and Politics in Peninsular Malaysia: The General Election of 2008,' *Asian Studies Review*, vol.35, no.1 (2011): 63–82.

[98] Tuong Vu, 'Epidemics as Politics with Case Studies from Malaysia, Thailand, and Vietnam,' *Global Health Governance Journal*, vol.4, no.2 (April 2011): 1–22 (9).

Conclusion: Technologies of hope and despair

This chapter has examined the interconnections between anthropogenic environmental change and epidemic disease: from the Federated States of Malaya, to Japanese Taiwan, the PRC, and Malaysia. The creation of industrial-scale plantations in Southeast Asia from the 1890s involved the felling of vast tracts of rainforest. The construction of a transport infrastructure opened up the land, influencing patterns of human settlement. Together with the mass influx of laborers from India, these multiple human activities had far-reaching ecological effects in the twentieth century. In particular, they created conditions for the malaria host – the female *Anopheles* mosquito – to thrive. At the same time, plantations became sites of medical intervention, where the bodies of laborers could be studied and remedied. In this sense, the plantation became the model of a political economy – the colonial state in miniature – just as the Empire might be understood as the expansion of 'planted' colonies.[99] Examining the plantation complex in relation to epidemic disease highlights the linkages between land, capital, and the state. As the environmental historian Linda Nash has suggested, 'placing the stories of colonization and capitalist development alongside stories of health and disease creates a more complicated environmental history, one in which we can perhaps begin to see ourselves.'[100]

Attempts to check the threat of malaria epidemics induced other kinds of interventions. In Japanese Taiwan, the colonial state adopted different stratagems for fighting malaria. While the local population was initially targeted for blood testing and treatment, in the 1920s there was a sanitarian drive to eliminate the pathogenic properties of the natural environment through vector control. These parallel public health methodologies reflected different, sometimes incompatible, political notions of how colonized cultures were to be managed: on the one hand, through segregationist tactics that appropriated local institutions for state ends, where the priority was safeguarding the colonial population from the threats posed both by the colony's inauspicious environment; on the other hand, through an assimilationist program, where the object was to transform Taiwan though a process of enculturation – in effect, making Taiwan Japanese.

The importance of political contexts in determining state-directed environmental interventions and public health campaigns is

[99]   Robert K. Home, *Of Planting and Planning: The Making of British Colonial Cities*. Second edition (Abingdon and New York: Routledge, 2013).
[100]   Nash, *Inescapable Ecologies*, p.2.

exemplified in Mao's campaign against schistosomiasis in the PRC during the 1950s and 1960s. Efforts to 'annihilate' disease might be viewed as part of the Great Leap Forward – a project to reconfigure the environment in order to maximize productivity and fast-forward development. This mass mobilization against disease co-opted local networks into a national mission. The rhetoric of annihilation, which characterized the Patriotic Health Campaign during the Korean War, and explicitly linked disease with enemy infiltration, provided an ideological context for subsequent epidemic campaigns. However, while Mao's concerted disease prevention efforts were certainly ambitious, they were only temporarily successful. It could be argued that the war against nature and the destruction of ecosystems that it entailed ultimately created the very conditions that would facilitate the emergence and spread of disease. Today, schistosomiasis continues to be endemic, particularly in marsh and lake areas of southern China.

A concern throughout the chapter, then, has been with the ideological dimension of human–environment relations. Across much of Asia, land has been exploited by large-scale agri-industrial enterprises dependent on imported labor. Debates about the environment have pivoted on a racial politics, where the exigencies of the state become intertwined with the demands of capital. Moreover, efforts to change land use have often been inseparable from endeavors to regulate the behavior of migrant labor and reform indigenous practices. In this context, health is conceived as a precondition for productivity.

The emergence of NiV in Malaysia in the late 1990s underlined the effects of human-induced ecological change on the epidemiology of infectious disease. It also suggested the extent to which the legacy of the colonial world continues to shape postcolonial Southeast Asia. The epidemic of a 'new' disease became entangled in historic ethnic and racial tensions, as the pig farms, which were at the epicenter of the epidemic, were owned and run by members of the Chinese community, a minority in a predominantly Muslim non-pork eating state.

In this chapter, the concern has been with colonialism and modernization as deeply disruptive and coercive processes. However, if they are viewed exclusively in these terms as top-down impositions, it is easy to slip into an over-simplified binary, wherein modernizing projects are viewed as intrinsically alienating and unsustainable in contrast to indigenous, 'traditional' practices. Yet, as Anna Tsing has shown in her study of the controversies over Kalimantan rainforest conservation in Indonesia, the relationship is more complex than such a dichotomy would suggest. As she demonstrates, the rainforest is a site where different groups interact and often come into conflict through misunderstandings born of

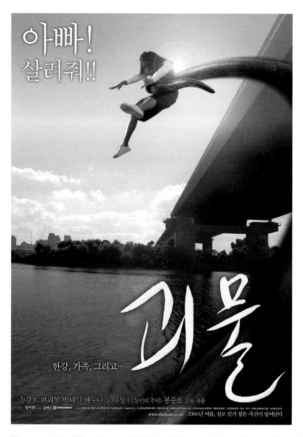

Figure 3.5. *The Host* (2006). Directed by Bong Joon-ho. Courtesy: Chungeorahm Film.

Contagious pollution: East Asia and the Cold War legacy

Documentaries and feature films can provide insights into how epidemics are imagined. If Hollywood movies, such as *Contagion* (2011), depict Asia as the locus of 'hot' viruses that crash into sub-urban America, Asian movies are increasingly exploring the socio-political contexts of disease emergence. One such example is the Korean movie *Flu* (2013), directed by Kim Sung-su, in which a highly pathogenic strain of avian influenza H5N1 is brought to

Seoul by immigrants illegally smuggled from the Philippines inside a shipping container. Another is the satirical Korean movie *The Host* (2006), directed by Bong Joon-ho. In the opening scene, set in Seoul in late 2000, a US military pathologist orders his Korean assistant to dispose of formaldehyde by pouring it down the sink, thereby contaminating the Han River. Over the next few years, rumors of a fish-like monster circulate in the city. It turns out that the chemicals have precipitated a mutation, creating a beast that lives in the river and preys on the city's population (Figure 3.5). What is more, the monster is the host of a lethal SARS-like virus. Soon, the US military get involved and enforce a quarantine on those who have been in contact with the creature. Meanwhile, the Korean government resolves to kill the marauding beast by releasing the toxic chemical 'Agent Yellow' into the river. Drawing on the recent past, *The Host* explores a number of critical themes: the US presence in South Korea and the legacy of the Cold War; the link between environmental degradation and disease emergence; the heavy-handed approach of bureaucratic government; and the fundamental disconnect between citizens and the peremptory state. The movie suggests that the monster and the deadly pathogen it hosts are the by-product of political processes, just as the outbreak itself reveals and exacerbates social divisions.

profound cultural differences: indigenous communities, local and international environmentalists, scientists, foreign investors, UN agencies, and many others. The outcome of these contestations is far from inevitable, however. In this 'zone of awkward engagement' there is, in other words, no preordained trajectory for the future of neoliberal globalization. As Tsing articulates it, 'hope and despair huddle together, sometimes dependent on the same technologies.'[101]

Today, rapidly changing environments across Asia are producing similar tensions and conflicts to those in Kalimantan. The construction of the Three Gorges Dam across the Yangtze in Hubei province, which began in 1992 and was completed in 2006, provoked controversy. This is the largest hydroelectric facility in the world, which reached full capacity in July 2012. The project created a 370-mile-long reservoir, submerging numerous cities, towns, and villages, and displacing an estimated 1.3 million people, with significant ecological impact on the region. The pace of

---

[101] Tsing, *Friction*, p.269.

urbanization in the PRC, fueled by the influx of rural migrants to large cities (including those uprooted to build the Three Gorges Dam), is evident in other Asian countries, too, where expanding cities are producing new pressures: slums, lack of water, and inadequate waste management systems (Chapter 2). Changes in land use and the development of large corporate agribusinesses across Southeast Asia are reshaping societies, economies, and natural environments. And all of these interlinked transformations, as we shall see in Chapter 5, have major implications for disease emergence. As human societies encroach on wild lands and industrial farming intensifies, the risk of cross-species spillovers increases.

Of course, natural processes have also played an important role in inducing environmental change with implications for disease. Floods and droughts alter ecosystems. The forest fires in Sumatra and Borneo in 1997 and 1998, which we discussed in the context of NiV, were exacerbated by the effects of the ENSO. In June 2015, the haze returned across Southeast Asia, again the result, not only of slash-and-burn activities, but also of the exceptionally dry conditions produced by the El Niño phenomenon. Natural disasters, such as earthquakes and tsunamis, may create conditions that facilitate outbreaks of communicable disease: crowded refugee camps, broken health infrastructures, the collapse of water and sanitation systems. The 1994 outbreak of plague in Surat, India, was preceded by flooding. The 2004 Indian Ocean earthquake and tsunami raised the specter of epidemics – cholera, hepatitis, and typhoid fever – as did the Sichuan earthquake in 2008, the Tohoku earthquake and tsunami in 2011, and Typhoon Haiyan in the Philippines in 2013.

Yet these natural disasters are increasingly viewed as being, in part, anthropogenic. Reliant on coal for its energy, the PRC is the largest emitter of greenhouse gas, which is understood to drive global warming. In 2013, China was responsible for approximately 30 percent of the world's carbon dioxide emissions. Scientists and officials in the PRC are becoming progressively vocal in speaking out about the consequences of climate change and ecological degradation. In 2014, President Xi Jinping announced an ambitious commitment to cutting emissions and boosting non-fossil fuel capacity. Given the scale of the challenge, along with issues of vested interest and corruption, many remain skeptical that these goals will be achieved. Aside from more extreme weather patterns, food scarcity could become an issue, with floods and protracted droughts, while coastal cities are threatened by rising sea levels. There is likely to be a health impact, particularly through the spread of vector-borne diseases, including malaria and dengue.

Some commentators have gone as far as to argue that the scale of this human impact on the environment heralds a new geological epoch. The Dutch atmospheric chemist Paul J. Crutzen and the biologist Eugene F. Stoermer coined the term 'Anthropocene' to define this new era. From the industrial revolution at the end of the eighteenth century, they argued, the global effects of human activities have intensified to an unprecedented degree.[102] The analysis of glacial ice cores, for example, suggests climate instability with an increasing atmospheric concentration of greenhouse gases, notably carbon dioxide and methane. The planetary effects of this human-induced activity may be understood as a geological process.[103]

Should we view the emergence of new diseases as a feature of a nascent geological epoch? Particularly as a result of the so-called 'Great Acceleration' after 1945, evidence suggests that population growth, resource depletion, changes in land-use, and loss of biodiversity are all factors driving epidemics.[104] Scientists have also intimated a connection between higher temperatures due to climate change and the occurrence of vector-borne and water-borne diseases, such as chikungunya, cholera, dengue, and malaria.[105] Low-lying countries, such as Bangladesh, are particularly vulnerable, with some attributing increases in cholera there to more extreme weather patterns. Climate influences the complex ecological relationships that determine infectious disease transmission. Population density and faster travel have also provided contexts for pathogens to spread more easily. In the age of the Anthropocene, no place is unconnected.

However, informing the Anthropocene is an assumption about the inevitability of the planet's ecological deterioration – at least, from a human perspective. To attribute epidemics to a geological force renders any preventive action redundant. Like an earthquake, epidemics may be anticipated but never forestalled. While such a view may fuel an apocalyptic environmentalism, it also obscures the anthropogenic determinants of many epidemics, such as inequality, poverty, and political failure. Conversely, acknowledging that epidemics are in part human-produced,

---

[102] Will Steffen, Paul J. Crutzen, and John R. McNeill, 'The Anthropocene: Are Humans Overwhelming the Great Forces of Nature?' *Ambio*, vol.36, no.8 (2007): 614–621.

[103] Simon L. Lewis and Mark A. Maslin, 'Defining the Anthropocene,' *Nature*, vol.519, no.7542 (March 12, 2015): 171–180 (173).

[104] Mark J. Hudson, 'Placing Asia in the Anthropocene: Histories, Vulnerabilities, Responses,' *Journal of Asian Studies*, vol.73, no.4 (2014): 941–962.

[105] Emily K. Shuman, 'Global Climate Change and Infectious Diseases,' *New England Journal of Medicine*, vol.362, no.12 (March 25, 2010): 1061–1063.

reinforces the notion that preventing disease requires changing human behavior. To be sure, recognizing the complexity of the determinants that produce and drive epidemics may not offer immediate, actionable policy, but it may redraw the balance to suggest that 'hope and despair huddle together, sometimes dependent on the same technologies.'

4 War

War and infectious disease are often viewed as 'fatal partners.'[1] On the face of it, the connection between conflict and disease appears self-evident. Conflicts amplify disease risks by creating conditions conducive for disease to spread; as military personnel move and as non-combatant populations get displaced, the likelihood of epidemic outbreaks increases. The destruction of infrastructure and disruption to services, including vector control, may produce environments where diseases are more likely to take hold. It has been argued that dengue fever became hyper-endemic in regions of Southeast Asia during and in the aftermath of the Second World War, not only due to the spread of genus *Aedes* mosquitoes (notably *Aedes aegypti*), which are vectors of the dengue virus, but as a result of urbanization and environmental degradation, which created mosquito breeding grounds. Epidemics of dengue hemorrhagic fever were conse-quences of this changing ecology.[2] Wars have also been crucial in the spread of plague (Chapter 1). Defoliation in southern Vietnam as a result of US herbicide spray missions to destroy agricultural land and forest cover in enemy held territory during the Vietnam War (1964–1975), cou-pled with the collapse of local infrastructure, are thought to have led to increased contact between humans and wild (so-called 'sylvatic') sources of the disease.[3]

War has also been a spur to migration. Those displaced may lack acquired immunity to diseases that are endemic in the areas they move to (Chapter 3), and they may introduce new diseases. Migrants may be physically and emotionally traumatized, and war may produce food inse-curity and malnutrition. In crowded refugee camps, the interplay of all

[1] Ralph H. Major, *Fatal Partners: War and Disease* (Garden City, NY: Doubleday, Doran & Co., 1941).
[2] Duane J. Gubler, 'Dengue/Dengue Haemorrhagic Fever: History and Current Status.' In: Gregory Bock and Jamie Goode, eds., *New Treatment Strategies for Dengue and Other Flaviviral Diseases* (Chichester and Hoboken, NJ: John Wiley/Novalis Foundation, 2006), pp.3–16 (6).
[3] M. Anker and D. Schaaf, *WHO Report on Global Surveillance of Epidemic-Prone Infectious Diseases* (Geneva: World Health Organization, 2000), pp.5–6.

these factors may lead to epidemics. Often different diseases are inter-twined and their co-emergence and co-transmission are associated with specific socio-political conditions: for example, discrimination, poverty, and violence. The term 'syndemic' has been used to describe the inter-action of two or more co-existent diseases, as well as the social and eco-nomic inequities that drive them.[4]

Some historians, however, have taken a more skeptical view of this straightforward correlation between war and epidemics, calling attention to changing ideas about war epidemics over time. The war–epidemic relationship is often treated as self-explanatory and has become so entrenched and taken for granted that there has been relatively little criti-cal attention paid to the dynamics of their co-evolution. As Roger Cooter has observed: 'Many, perhaps most, epidemics are not rooted in war.'[5] One of the issues, here, is the distinction often assumed between war as an exceptional situation and peacetime as a 'normal' condition, as well as the separation between endemic and epidemic diseases. While war con-ventionally refers to an armed conflict between states (or groups within states involved in a 'civil war'), it may also be understood as a more inte-gral cultural process, with the spaces of war and peace far more indistinct than classical definitions of war would suggest.[6] Our understanding of war is 'mediated through competing efforts to shape representations' of violence.[7] The routine dichotomization of war as a rupture or deviation from the normalcy of peace ignores the frequently blurred boundaries that separate 'the violent and the non-violent, the conjectural and the structural, the legal and the illegal, the physical and the psychological, the quotidian and the exceptional, the public and the private, the state and civil society.'[8]

This chapter explores how specific forms of violence have shaped epi-demics and how epidemics, in turn, have helped to produce particular forms of conflict. Rather than providing a list of major conflicts with a comprehensive description of wartime-associated epidemics, the aim is to show how epidemics can help us better understand the violent con-tinuities between war and peacetime. A further issue is how inter-state and intra-state struggles have provided a context for the development of

[4] Merrill Singer, *Anthropology of Infectious Disease* (Walnut Creek, CA: Left Coast Press, 2015), pp.220–222.
[5] Cooter, 'Of War and Epidemics,' p.285.
[6] John Keegan, *A History of Warfare*. Second edition (London: Pimlico, 2004), pp.1–60.
[7] Jenna M. Loyd, '"A Microscopic Insurgent": Militarization, Health, and Critical Geogra-phies of Violence,' *Annals of the Association of American Geographers*, vol.99, no.5 (2009): 863–873 (864).
[8] Julie Skurski and Fernando Coronil, 'Introduction: States of Violence and the Violence of States.' In: Fernando Coronil and Julie Skurski, eds., *States of Violence* (Ann Arbor: University of Michigan Press, 2006), pp.1–31 (2).

public health control measures, as well as the role of humanitarian medical assistance during conflicts. What have the consequences been of this belligerent history for health policies and practices today?

We begin with a discussion of the Philippine–US War (1899–1902), investigating how a military campaign functioned not only as a driver of infectious disease but also how, in responding to epidemic threats, a military logic shaped the priorities of a colonial health system with implications for the supervision of populations in peacetime. In so doing, we draw on a growing scholarship concerned with the interrelationship between war, medicine, and modernity to consider how a critical legacy of the war in the Philippines was the militarization of public health, which influenced the evolving institutions and apparatuses of twentieth-century international health. This convergence of biomedical, political, and military agendas in the late nineteenth and twentieth centuries is a key theme connecting each of the subsequent cases discussed. While biomedical and public health developments in the early twentieth century dramatically reduced mortality rates in many parts of the world, these advances, in conjunction with novel communication technologies and an expansion of state institutions, led to a new emphasis on defining and standardizing populations – a transformative biopolitical process that was, in turn, dependent on exclusionary and often coercive practices.

The second case focuses on the Manchurian plague of 1910 and 1911, and considers the military and geopolitical contexts of the epidemic. While disease heightened international divisions, it also highlighted the increasingly international culture of modern medical science and public health. Manchuria was a strategic geopolitical space and a prehistory of inter-state rivalry shaped responses to the outbreak of pneumonic plague there. The experience of the US-occupied Philippines and the expansion of Qing public health in Manchuria were in fact connected through the advisory role played by US scientists with long experience working for the colonial services in the Philippines – including the head of the Philippine Biological Laboratory, Richard Pearson Strong (1872–1948). While biomedicine and public health were political technologies forged in conflict, they subsequently played an important role in the state's management of its citizens in peacetime. These state-sponsored technologies effected a form of 'internal colonialism' to the extent that we should, perhaps, understand 'modernity' itself 'as a colonialist project in the special sense that both the societies internal to Western nations, and those they possessed, administered and reformed elsewhere, were understood as objects to be surveyed, regulated and sanitized.'[9]

---

[9] Nicholas Thomas, *Colonialism's Culture: Anthropology, Travel, and Government* (Cambridge: Polity, 1994), p.4.

Russians had established a settlement on the Pacific coast at Okhotsk in the 1640s, but it was not until the nineteenth century that the Russian Empire substantially extended and consolidated its East Asian territories, bringing it into conflict with China and Japan. The third section deals with an epidemic of typhus in Siberia during the Russian Civil War (1918–1921), specifically in relation to US-led humanitarian assistance to combat the spread of disease in the Russian Far East. American Red Cross (ARC) relief work became bound up with an ideological mission to support the anti-Bolshevik faction in a conflict that threatened the balance of power in East Asia. War opened up a humanitarian space that functioned as a way of advancing political interests through non-military means.

Next, we shift to an altogether different species of conflict: the so-called 'war on terror' initiated by President George W. Bush in 2001. Here, we consider how a polio eradication campaign on the Afghan–Pakistan border has become caught up in a counter-insurgency drive. Although the incidence of polio has been reduced by 99 percent globally since the inauguration of the Global Polio Eradication Initiative (GPEI) in 1988, the disease remains endemic in Pakistan, Afghanistan, and Nigeria. The killing of health workers in Pakistan has prompted a rethink of the polio eradication campaign, even though the threat posed by the poliovirus remains real and urgent. As Margaret Chan, director general of the WHO, declared in 2012, the anti-polio initiative has reached 'a tipping point between success and failure.'[10] Why has an anti-polio program become politicized to the degree that aid workers are being killed and the worldwide eradication of polio is now in jeopardy? In answering this question, we place the polio campaign within a number of interrelated contexts: that of post-Second World War eradication efforts; the 'war on terror' initiated after the al-Qaeda inspired terrorist attacks on the World Trade Center and the Pentagon in 2001; histories of resistance to colonial vaccination campaigns on the subcontinent; as well as opposition to the assimilationist drive of the modern secular state. In particular, we explore how a narrative of emerging terror has been re-contextualized to fit the plot line of emerging infection.

Both of these cases – the entwinement of an anti-typhus humanitarian mission to the Russian Far East with civil war and the equation of a polio immunization program in Pakistan with a counter-insurgency – reflect a similar 'global logic of intervention.' Epidemic crises and the military operations with which they are embrangled are conceived in political and

---

[10] 'Ending Polio, One Type at a Time,' *Bulletin of the World Health Organization*, vol.90, no.7 (July 2012): 477–556 (482).

moral terms and serve 'to justify a state of exception,' wherein foreign powers may admissibly infringe on another state's sovereignty in the name of humanity. What both cases highlight is the way in which disease control missions and military operations have been – and continue to be – closely connected.[11] If military interventions are promoted as humanitarian undertakings, humanitarianism itself often assumes the modality of militarized governance in health 'campaigns' fighting to 'eradicate' disease.

By way of conclusion, we consider state-sponsored violence in Burma directed at minority groups. Since independence from the British in 1948, the country's central government has sought to quell numerous ethnic rebellions. As a result of internal conflicts, hundreds of thousands have become internally displaced persons (IDP) and been forcefully relocated into new settlements. Over the last decade, many Karen refugees from Karen State in the south and southeast of Burma have fled their homes to Thailand, leading to a high prevalence of disease, including HIV/AIDS, TB, as well as neglected tropical diseases (NTDs). More recently, the plight of the Rohingya population in Burma's northern Rakhine State has been widely reported, as thousands have sought to evade persecution by crossing the border into neighboring Bangladesh, Thailand, and Malaysia, resulting in a refugee crisis.

Historically, conflict has played a critical role in the diffusion of infectious disease in and across Asia. In the nineteenth and twentieth centuries, wars were the result of inter-imperial rivalry and the territorialization of sovereignty associated with colonization. The process of Asia's 'opening up' to Western interests provoked regional skirmishes, which then produced further internal divisions with violent after-effects that often rippled out across the wider region. The Opium Wars in China, for example, became entangled with the catastrophic Taiping Rebellion (Chapter 1). Technological developments in the nineteenth and twentieth centuries transformed the scale of warfare, as well as its destructive potential. Military technology became more lethal and in these increasingly total wars, Asian soldiers fought outside Asia. Chinese and Indians, for example, took part in the First World War, while Asia was a critical theater in the Second World War and during the subsequent Cold War.

The Second Sino-Japanese War (1937–1945) led to the occupation of Manchuria by the Japanese, resulting in millions of casualties. The Japanese established a special biological and chemical warfare research division, known as Unit 731, in Harbin. Experiments were carried

[11] Didier Fassin and Mariella Pandolfi, 'Introduction: Military and Humanitarian Government in the Age of Intervention.' In: Didier Fassin and Mariella Pandolfi, eds., *Contemporary States of Emergency: The Politics of Humanitarian Interventions* (New York: Zone Books, 2010), pp.9–25 (10, 13).

out on captives who were infected with epidemic diseases, including anthrax, plague, and cholera. Bacteriological weapons were developed and deployed on the Chinese population. The Imperial Japanese Army Air Force dropped bombs with plague-contaminated fleas, causing outbreaks (Chapter 3).[12] From China, conflict expanded across Southeast Asia and, in September 1940, Japan invaded French Indochina, followed by Thailand. The war escalated further in December 1941, when the Japanese attacked Pearl Harbor, drawing the United States into the conflict. Japanese forces occupied Hong Kong, the Philippines, Singapore, and Malaya. Burma and the Dutch East Indies were subsequently seized. Throughout the Pacific campaigns, malaria posed a major challenge to military authorities, affecting 500,000 US servicemen, for example, and resulting in a new emphasis on malaria research.[13]

During the Korean War (1950–1953), an outbreak of a hemorrhagic fever among US troops was later identified as the first recorded case of a hantavirus infection, which was isolated by the South Korean virologist Lee Ho-Wang in the 1970s. Hantaviruses are spread by rodents and it is thought that ecological disturbances and habitat disruption caused by the conflict may have been responsible for the epidemic. During the decade-long Vietnam War (also known as the Second Indochina War), in which an estimated three million Vietnamese died, chloroquine-resistant *Plasmodium falciparum* malaria and insecticide-resistant fleas led to an upsurge in infections. As noted earlier, chemicals were used to defoliate vegetation and deprive the enemy of food crops and forest cover, thereby changing the ecology of vectors and the epidemiology of vector-borne diseases. The years after the war saw the re-emergence of malaria, hemorrhagic fever, cholera, plague, and other parasitic diseases – with possible connections identified between the use of herbicides, such as the controversial Agent Orange, and chronic diseases including sarcomas and malignant lymphomas.[14]

Epidemics in a 'howling wilderness': The Philippine–US War

By the mid nineteenth century, as we saw in Chapter 1, the United States, vying with other Western powers, had become involved in efforts to 'open

---

[12] Daniel Barenblatt, *A Plague Upon Humanity: The Hidden History of Japan's Biological Warfare Program* (New York: HarperCollins, 2004).

[13] Mary-Ellen Condon-Rall, 'Malaria in the Southwest Pacific in World War II, 1940–1944.' In: Roy M. MacLeod, ed., *Science and the Pacific War: Science and Survival in the Pacific, 1939–1945* (Dordrecht: Kluwer, 2000), pp.51–70.

[14] Myron Allukian, Jr. and Paul L. Atwood, 'Public Health and the Vietnam War.' In: Barry S. Levy and Victor S. Sidel, eds., *War and Public Health*. Revised edition (Washington, DC: American Public Health Association, 2000), pp.215–237 (222–223).

up' East Asia for new markets. It was not until the turn of the century, however, that the United States acquired an Asian colony. In the mid 1890s, a revolt had broken out in Cuba, which had been colonized by the Spanish in the early sixteenth century. In 1898, ostensibly in response to the sinking of the battleship *USS Maine* in Havana Harbor, the United States had intervened on the side of the rebels. War in Cuba soon escalated into a global conflict, with US forces deployed against Spain in other theaters, notably the Spanish Philippines. This was the first overseas war fought by the United States and one that established it as an imperial power in Asia.

Commodore George Dewey's scuppering of the Spanish fleet in Manila Bay on May 1, 1898, and the seizure of the city a few months later by US troops under the command of Major General Wesley Merritt, brought an effective end to Spanish rule. Yet by early 1899, the United States was at war with nationalist Filipino forces headed by Emilio Aguinaldo (1869–1964), who had proclaimed an independent republic. As US President William McKinley (1843–1901) conceded, the United States opposed Philippine independence on the grounds that Filipinos were 'unfit for self-government.' The underlying reason for the United States' annexation of the archipelago, however, was a quest for Asian markets, investment opportunities, and the exploitation of raw materials. In the US popular press, the Philippines was depicted as a strategic bridgehead for spreading American values and offloading American consumer goods into the vast and lucrative Chinese market. An illustration in the March 1900 issue of the satirical magazine *Judge* by the political cartoonist Emil Flohri, for example, was captioned: 'And, after all, the Philippines are only the stepping-stone to China.' A giant Uncle Sam, with one foot on the Philippines, carries a sack of industrial goods – steel rails, trains, sewing machines, bridges, and bicycles – to an open-armed Chinaman. Although massive in territorial and population terms, China is pictured as undeveloped and in its craving for modern commodities it is readily dominated by a colossal United States. Consumerism and Orientalism in Flohri's cartoon go hand in hand. As the American journalist Henry Watterson proclaimed in 1898, while overseas expansion offered a way out of an economic depression, it also 'announced the arrival upon the scene of the world's action of a power which would have to be reckoned with by the older powers in determining the future of civilization.'[15]

Invariably downplayed by US officials as an 'insurrection,' the Philippine–US War officially began in February 1899 and ended in July 1902. An estimated 80,000 to 100,000 Filipinos fought in the

[15] Henry Watterson, *History of the Spanish–American War: Embracing a Complete Review of Our Relations with Spain* (New York: The Werner Co., 1898), pp.vii–viii.

conflict.[16] While over 16,000 combatants died, perhaps 200,000 civilians succumbed to cholera, typhoid, smallpox, TB, and plague – as well as famine. These figures remain elastic, however, with some historians estimating the death toll at well over these numbers. In May 1901, the *New York Times* reported Brigadier General James Montgomery Bell's claim that 'one-sixth of the natives of Luzon have either been killed or have died of the dengue fever in the last two years.'[17] Given that the population of Luzon was over 3.5 million, this would put the figure at approximately 600,000. By contrast, US fatalities numbered 4,234, with 2,818 wounded.[18] Often relegated to the status of a 'small' war against Filippino 'bandits,' the conflict revealed aspects of a 'total war' associated with European conflicts in the twentieth century.[19] Despite McKinley's declaration in 1898 that the United States' objective was 'benevolent assimilation, substituting the mild sway of justice and right for arbitrary rule,' historians have pointed to the brutal character of the US pacification campaign: the use of concentration camps and torture, arson, and the indiscriminate killing of civilians. In November 1899, after suffering heavy losses in conventional battles, Aguinaldo's army disbanded and Filipino forces resorted to guerilla combat. Insurgency efforts intensified in 1900 as the rebels attempted to influence the outcome of the US elections in which McKinley was up against the anti-imperialist Democrat William Jennings Bryan (1860–1925).[20] In the event, however, McKinley was re-elected and Brigadier General Arthur MacArthur took control of US operations, imposing martial law and pursuing insurgents with renewed vigor. In March 1901, Aguinaldo was captured by US forces.

Allegations of atrocities committed by occupying forces against civilians were becoming publicized in the United States by late 1900. Anti-imperialist newspapers and magazines seized upon reports of military misconduct to agitate for an end to the colonial misadventure.[21] The violence was reciprocated. In September 1901, 48 US infantrymen were

---

[16] Brian McAllister Linn, *The Philippine War, 1899–1902* (Lawrence: University of Kansas Press, 2000), p.325.

[17] 'How Filipinos Meet Death: Bullets and Fever Have Killed One-Sixth of Luzon Natives in Two Years, Gen. Bell Says,' *New York Times* (May 2, 1901), p.1.

[18] Max Boot, *The Savage Wars of Peace: Small Wars and the Rise of American Power* (New York: Basic Books, 2002), p.125.

[19] Glenn Anthony May, 'Was the Philippine–American War a "Total War"?' In: Manfred F. Boemeke, Roger Chickering, and Stig Förster, eds., *Anticipating Total War: The German and American Experiences, 1871–1914* (Cambridge: Cambridge University Press, 1999), pp.437–457.

[20] John Morgan Gates, *Schoolbooks and Krags: The United States Army in the Philippines, 1898–1902* (Westport, CT: Greenwood Press, 1973), p.160.

[21] Richard E. Welch, Jr., 'American Atrocities in the Philippines: The Indictment and the Response,' *Pacific Historical Review*, vol.43, no.2 (1974): 233–253 (233–235).

butchered by insurgents in the town of Balangiga on Samar, an island in the Visayas. The perpetrators had allegedly disguised themselves as women, hiding their *bolos* (large, machete-like knives) in the coffins of cholera victims. In retaliation, General Jacob H. Smith – who had fought in the Civil War and subsequently in the Indian campaigns – infamously ordered his officers 'to kill and burn' and reduce the island to 'a howling wilderness.'[22]

The areas that suffered worst in the war were the densely inhabited regions of central Luzon, home to half of the Philippines' estimated 7.4 million population, as well as the southern province of Batangas. The widespread destruction inflicted by the conflict led to social and economic breakdown, creating an environment for disease to spread.[23] An epidemic of rinderpest killed an estimated 90 percent of draft cattle and water buffalo.[24] Historian Ken De Bevoise has gone as far as to argue that the Americans disrupted the country's ecological equilibrium and in this sense served as 'agents of apocalypse.'[25] With the collapse of agriculture, rural communities suffered from malnutrition and were susceptible to concurrent vector-borne infections, such as malaria and dengue. Mass population displacements, forced relocations, and the so-called 'recon-centration' of rural communities facilitated the spread of cholera.[26]

Endemic infections erupted into epidemics. The movement of troops and inter-island naval operations spread disease to hitherto isolated Filipino populations. During the war, the annual death rate rose to 50 per thousand between 1899 and 1902. Although the United States had intervened in Cuba in part to stop the internment of civilians in guarded camps, similar incarceration strategies were used by the US military in the Philippines. Civilians were increasingly targeted in an anti-guerrilla offensive, exemplified by Brigadier General J. Franklin Bell's ruthless treatment of the population of Batangas and, in particular, his order to

---

[22] Stanley Karnow, *In Our Image: America's Empire in the Philippines* (New York: Random House, 1989), pp.189–191.

[23] Reynaldo C. Ileto, 'Cholera and the Origins of the American Sanitary Order in the Philippines.' In: David Arnold, ed., *Imperial Medicine and Indigenous Societies* (Manchester: Manchester University Press, 1988), pp.125–148.

[24] Paul A. Kramer, *The Blood of Government: Race, Empire, the United States, and the Philippines* (Chapel Hill: University of North Carolina Press, 2006), p.170.

[25] Ken De Bevoise, *Agents of Apocalypse: Epidemic Disease in the Colonial Philippines* (Princeton, NJ: Princeton University Press, 1995).

[26] Glenn Anthony May, *Battle for Batangas: A Philippine Province at War* (New Haven, CT: Yale University Press, 1991), pp.270–275; Matthew Smallman-Raynor and Andrew D. Cliff, 'The Epidemiological Legacy of War: The Philippine–American War and the Diffusion of Cholera in Batangas and La Laguna, South-West Luzón, 1902–1904,' *War in History*, vol.7, no.1 (2000): 29–64.

establish concentration camps in December 1901.[27] In late 1901, shortly before the outbreak of cholera in Manila, Bell had entered Batangas with 4,000 troops to quash Filipino guerrilla forces. The campaign decimated the area, as Bell set fire to villages, rounded up natives, and executed suspects. As one US correspondent acknowledged, this was 'not civilized warfare' – adding: 'We are not dealing with a civilized people. The only thing they know is force, violence and brutality, and we give it to them.'[28] The policy of 'reconcentration' created a lethal concoction: conditions of poor hygiene, overcrowding, and malnutrition – as food became increasingly scarce – were conducive to infections. Panic was also a contributory factor. According to De Bevoise, Batangas had one of the highest mortality rates in the Philippines, with over 10 percent of the province's population dying. Figures remain estimates, however, and based on a re-evaluation of the parish records and 1903 census, one study suggests that the population of Batangas declined by some 34,000 in 1902.[29]

Although the conflict was declared officially over on July 4, 1902, Filipino resistance continued after this and became embroiled in the cholera epidemic of 1902–1904, during which thousands perished. As Reynaldo Ileto has suggested, in 1902 it was difficult to differentiate the anti-cholera campaign from the pacification of Filipinos since 'medico-sanitary measures and popular resistance to such, were continuing acts of war.'[30] Drastic counter-insurgency strategies conflated in the minds of many Filipinos with the regime's increasingly authoritarian health policing.

The colonial view was exemplified by Dean Conant Worcester (1866–1924) in his survey of cholera in the Philippines published in 1908. A zoologist and graduate of the University of Michigan who served as Philippine secretary of the interior between 1901 and 1913, Worcester ascribed the 1902–1904 epidemic to the importation of infected produce from southern China via Hong Kong. He vindicated US actions and resolutely condemned any criticism of the regime's response. 'Energetic measures,' he professed, had been adopted to prevent the spread

[27] De Bevoise, *Agents of Apocalypse*, p.13; Iain R. Smith and Andreas Stucki, 'The Colonial Development of Concentration Camps (1868–1902),' *Journal of Imperial and Commonwealth History*, vol.39, no.3 (2011): 417–437 (423–425).

[28] Karnow, *In Our Image*, p.188.

[29] De Bevoise, *Agents of Apocalypse*, p.181; Glenn Anthony May, '150,000 Missing Filipinos: A Demographic Crisis in Batangas, 1887–1903,' *Annales de Démographie Historique* (1985): 215–243 (241).

[30] Ileto, 'Cholera and the Origins of the American Sanitary Order in the Philippines.' In: Arnold, ed., *Imperial Medicine*, p.127.

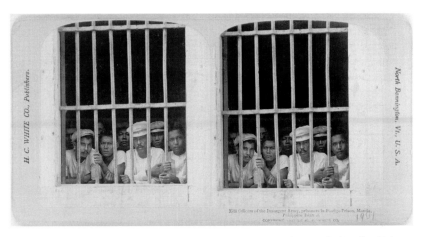

Figure 4.1. 'Officers of the Insurgent Army, Prisoners in Postigo Prison, Manila, Philippine Islands (H. C. White Co., 1901).' Courtesy: US Library of Congress.

of the disease and these stood in stark contrast to the ineffective Spanish handling of the 1882 cholera epidemic. At the same time, while Worcester noted that 'not a few evil-intentioned persons' had used the war as a pretext for violence, he attributed the disease's spread across the archipelago squarely to native defiance:

Visualizing violence

From the 1880s, innovations in photography, and in particular the development of film roll by Kodak, made photography easier and cheaper, bringing it to a wider audience. During the Philippine–US War, many photographs were taken for different reasons (Figure 4.1). Soldiers took photographs, which they enclosed in letters. Images were reproduced on postcards for commercial distribution. The camera also functioned as an instrument of military surveillance, while colonial officials used documentary photographs in their push for public health. At the same time, journalists illustrated their reportage with photographs and politicians sought to buoy a war-weary American public by exploiting edifying images of American military prowess. Photographs from the Philippines, however, also revealed the dark side of Western progress. Depictions of the horrors of the campaign, including executions, mass graves, and disease-ravaged communities, were a stark reminder of the brutality of the conflict and its human cost. As David Brody has suggested, how Americans looked (or visualized) was integral to the machinery that ran the colonial engine.

Christopher Capozzola, 'Photography & Power in the Colonial Philippines I: The US Conquest & Occupation (1898–1902),' *MIT Visualizing Cultures* (2014): http://visualizingcultures.mit.edu

David Brody, *Visualizing American Empire: Orientalism and Imperialism in the Philippines* (Chicago, IL: University of Chicago Press, 2010).

The people, entirely unaccustomed as they were to any sanitary restrictions, believing as many of them did that the disease was not cholera and firm in their conviction that they had a right to do whatever they liked so long as they kept on their own premises, bitterly resented the burning or disinfection of their houses and effects and the restriction of their liberty to go and come as they pleased, and, in spite of the fact that the number of cases was kept down in a manner never before dreamed of at Manila, there arose an increasingly bitter feeling of hostility toward the work of the Board of Health.[31]

The cholera epidemic underscored the differences that officials such as Worcester perceived between retrograde Filipino beliefs and a colonial sanitary policy, underpinned by modern science, which focused on decontaminating native bodies, understood to be carriers of disease. US troops were ordered to close off the slum district of Farola in Tondo, at the epicenter of the epidemic. Natives were placed in detention camps, while the area was burned to the ground.

Photographs of indigenous nipa huts in US newspapers and books were used 'to inscribe the Philippines as a geographic locale where the primitive population could not be trusted.'[32] It was represented as an occluded locale, where infectious diseases were ubiquitous and threatened the social order. As Warwick Anderson has observed: 'All the fauna in the archipelago, whether human or nonhuman, seemed increasingly duplicitous, ready at any moment to come into focus, to sting, to infect, to shoot.'[33] When US atrocities against Filipinos were acknowledged in the US media, they were often construed as an effect of the

---

[31] Worcester, *A History of Asiatic Cholera*, pp.3–27 (17).
[32] Brody, *Visualizing American Empire*, p.140.   [33] Anderson, *Colonial Pathologies*, p.60.

country's unhealthy environment, which induced atavistic behavior in US soldiers.[34]

Cholera and the burning of Farola

Victor George Heiser (1873–1972) was appointed quarantine officer and later director of the Bureau of Health in Manila before joining the Rockefeller Foundation as director for the East of the International Health Board. 'Large parts of the population,' Heiser observed, 'were ignorant and inaccessible.' Although he stressed the need for compromise and recognized that US officials should 'not ride roughshod over the customs and the religion of the people,' he also acknowledged that in seeking to manage the cholera epidemic, the US 'was guilty of discourtesy and even abuse of power.' According to Heiser, many Filipinos viewed 'the dictation and ruthlessness' of American public health interventions as akin to military occupation. Responding to the threat of cholera in the Farola district of Tondo, a place 'covered with warehouses, coal piles, and a crowded mass of small filthy nipa huts,' Dean C. Worcester ordered the evacuation of residents to the San Lazaro and Santa Mesa detention camps and the burning of the district on March 27, 1902:

Under the blazing sky, the terrified and resentful owners watched the shooting sparks as shack after shack crackled and collapsed. The report spread about the homes of the poor burned to make room for future dwellings and warehouses of rich Americans. Further rumors that the foreign doctors had poisoned the wells were also widely credited; it was even said the American aim was to annihilate the Filipino Race.

Victor Heiser, *An American Doctor's Odyssey: Adventures in Forty-five Countries* (New York: W. W. Norton & Co., 1936), pp.105, 111, 114, 291.

Tensions between the colonizers and the colonized over sanitary interventions intensified. Filipino resistance took the form of the non-reporting of cases and the illegal burial of the dead. According to the local colonial press, the corpses of those who had perished from cholera were disposed of in the Pasig River or hastily buried in shallow graves. Such defiance of US sanitary decrees triggered more stringent counter-measures, summed up in Captain C. F. de Mey's injunction that

---

[34] Brody, *Visualizing American Empire*, p.71.

health officers ought to 'rule with a rod of steel.'[35] Quarantine, rigorous house-to-house inspections, and the removal of suspected cholera cases to isolation camps, provoked panic and disrupted economic life. Outside Manila, in the provinces, the destruction of infected dwellings continued.[36] Although President McKinley had declared that the United States would not interfere with Filipino customs, the newly constituted Bureau of Health extended its scope to a degree that interference became inevitable.[37] As Anderson has observed, 'the strategies and tactics of colonial warfare against guerilla forces favored a rapid extension of military hygiene into Philippine social life.'[38] Filipino customs were scorned for their insalubrity: the layout of their cramped and fetid shacks, their pollution of the rivers, and their religious superstitions.[39]

The spread of disease among local communities, however, was not the main concern of the medical corps of the US army. Their priority, as Anderson has suggested, was protecting Americans by preventing and managing disease in tropical conditions (Figure 4.2). A policy of pacification, and the administrative logic that drove it, influenced disciplinary structures, including military hygiene. Under these circumstances, bacteriology and parasitology assumed political significance. To meet the threat of insurgency, the US adopted new methods of coercion 'marked by clandestine penetration, psychological warfare, disinformation, media manipulation, assassination, and torture.' Many of these innovative strong-arm tactics, it has been argued, were repatriated to the United States around the time of the First World War for domestic legislation.[40]

'The involvement of the military in the medical interventionism of the imperial period is one of its most striking features,' Arnold has observed in the context of South Asia.[41] The development of state medicine was inextricably bound up with the military. As disciplinary regimes, the army and the penal system provided ways of ensuring order. Hospital and other medical institutions were also 'perceived as models of how Western medical and sanitary practices might – in theory, at least – be deployed in the

---

[35] Willie T. Ong, 'Public Health and the Clash of Cultures: The Philippine Cholera Epidemics.' In: Milton J. Lewis and Kerrie L. MacPherson, eds., *Public Health in Asia and the Pacific: Historical and Comparative Perspectives* (London: Routledge, 2008), pp.206–221 (209).

[36] De Bevoise, *Agents of Apocalypse*, p.181.

[37] Heiser, *An American Doctor's Odyssey*, p.64.   [38] Anderson, *Colonial Pathologies*, p.8.

[39] Bantug, *A Short History of Medicine in the Philippines*, pp.34–36.

[40] Alfred W. McCoy, *Policing America's Empire: The United States, the Philippines, and the Rise of the Surveillance State* (Madison: University of Wisconsin Press, 2009), pp.5, 8.

[41] David Arnold, 'Introduction: Disease, Medicine and Empire.' In: Arnold, ed., *Imperial Medicine*, pp.1–26 (19).

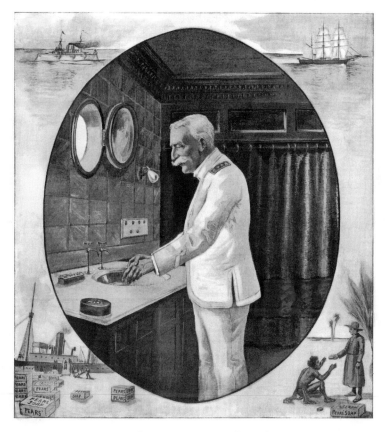

The first step towards lightening

The White Man's Burden

is through teaching the virtues of cleanliness.

Pears' Soap

is a potent factor in brightening the dark corners of the earth as civilization advances, while amongst the cultured of all nations it holds the highest place—it is the ideal toilet soap.

Figure 4.2. 'Pears' Soap advertisement featuring Admiral Dewey.' *Harper's Weekly* (September 30, 1899), p.968.

Hygiene and imperial politics

The 'White Man's Burden' is taken from the title of a poem by the English writer Rudyard Kipling, which was published in the monthly periodical *McClure's Magazine* in February 1899, just as conflict was breaking out between Filipino and US forces in Manila. The role of empire, envisaged by Kipling as a 'burden,' is to spread 'civilization' to the 'savage' populations of the world. Figure 4.2 is a Pears' Soap advertisement. The accompanying text claims that Pears' Soap is an agent of civilization, bringing light to 'the dark corners of the earth.' Hygiene and imperial politics are inextricably linked; cleanliness is viewed as a facet of enlightenment. Admiral George Dewey (1837–1917) is pictured in the advertisement washing his hands in a sink aboard the protected cruiser *USS Olympia*. The year before this advertisement appeared, Dewey had led the US navy to a victory over the Spanish in Manila Bay aboard the flagship. In 1918, the vessel was dispatched to the Russian port of Murmansk as part of the Allied response to the civil war there, discussed in the final section of this chapter.

Rudyard Kipling, 'The White Man's Burden,' *McClure's Magazine*, vol.12, no.4 (February 1899), pp.290–291.

wider society.'[42] In a similar way, military and medical operations were closely connected in the Philippines. As US forces defeated the Spanish and strove to quell a native 'insurrection,' they found themselves dealing with an epidemic that had, at least in part, been produced by the conditions of war. Given the fraught context of counter-insurgency, the military assumed a leading role in medical and health institutions with consequences for their subsequent development and deployment as key apparatuses of colonial control.

War, diplomacy, and international health: The Manchurian plague epidemic

Advances in biomedicine and public health in the nineteenth century were closely linked to the expanding operations of the modern state. Epidemic crises provided state institutions with opportunities to extend and consolidate their authority. This was certainly the case in China, when pneumonic plague erupted in Manchuria, killing an estimated 60,000

---

[42] David Arnold, *Colonizing the Body: State Medicine and Epidemic Disease in Nineteenth-Century India* (Berkeley: University of California Press, 1993), pp.62, 114.

people in the sixth months between October 1910 and March 1911. In many histories, this catastrophic event is viewed as a critical turning point: the juncture when modern science and Western medicine demonstrated their unchallenged superiority in relation to traditional Chinese customs and practices.[43] It is a transformation often associated with Wu Lien-teh (1879–1960), the British-educated, Malaysian-born Chinese physician who took a lead role in anti-plague efforts. Wu himself was instrumental in promoting this view of the Manchurian plague epidemic as the moment in which Chinese state officials seized the initiative and mobilized Western public health as a crucial tool of government and a means of keeping rival powers in check:

> The terrible epidemic of pneumonic plague which invaded Manchuria and North China in 1910–11, though it exacted a toll of 60,000 lives and caused monetary losses estimated at 100 million dollars, definitely laid the foundation for systematic public health work in China. Those in authority from the Emperor downwards, who had formerly pledged their faith to old-fashioned medicine, now acknowledged that its methods were powerless against such severe outbreaks. They were thus compelled to entrust the work to modern-trained physicians and to give their consent to drastic measures, such as compulsory house-to-house visitation, segregation of contacts in camps or wagons, and cremation of thousands of corpses which had accumulated at Harbin and elsewhere.[44]

Manchuria is named after the Manchu people and as a geographical area it has been defined in different ways at different times. In China, it is taken to comprise the three Northeastern provinces of Fengtian (Liaoning), Kirin (Jilin), and Heilongjiang. Rich in natural resources and with a strategic Pacific coastline, this was a contested region of 'entangled histories.'[45] By 1910, it had been carved up as a result of war and international treatises into different spheres of influence: Chinese, Japanese, and Russian. The plague threatened this fragile political arrangement and the national interests that it accommodated, holding out the prospect that tensions might reignite into outright conflict. As different foreign powers – namely the Russians and the Japanese – threatened to encroach further onto Chinese territory and assume responsibility for managing the epidemic, the Chinese were forced to respond to

---

[43] Carl F. Nathan, *Plague Prevention and Politics in Manchuria, 1910–1931* (Cambridge, MA: East Asian Research Center, Harvard University, 1967), p.6.

[44] Wu Lien-teh, 'A Short History of the Manchurian Plague Prevention Service by Wu Lien-teh, Director, Manchurian Plague Prevention and National Quarantine Services.' In: *Manchurian Plague Prevention Service Memorial Volume, 1912–1932* (Shanghai: National Quarantine Service, 1934), pp.1–12 (1).

[45] Dan Ben-Canaan, Frank Grüner, and Ines Prodöhl, 'Entangled Histories: The Transcultural Past of Northeast China.' In: Dan Ben-Canaan, Frank Grüner, and Ines Prodöhl, eds., *Entangled Histories: The Transcultural Past of Northeast China* (Dordrecht: Springer, 2014), pp.1–11.

a crisis that was both medical and political. It was in this fraught context that anti-plague measures were implemented. In other words, a complex prehistory of war and inter-state rivalry shaped anti-plague responses there.

Russia had expanded across Siberia to the Pacific coast in the seventeenth century, establishing a presence on the Kamchatka peninsula. Further south there were Russian settlements at Okhotsk and Nikolayevsk on the Amur River, opposite the island of Sakhalin, the northern portion of which served as a Russian penal camp from the late 1850s. In the nineteenth century, against the backdrop of great power rivalries and the weakening of the Qing Empire, Russia began a more concerted drive to acquire and consolidate possessions in the Far East. By the Treaty of Peking concluded with the Qing in 1860 after the Second Opium War, Russia was ceded a strip of Pacific coastline south of the Amur and founded the naval base of Vladivostok on the Sea of Japan.

The Russian Far East

The area between Lake Baikal in Siberia and the Pacific Ocean is commonly referred to as the Russian Far East. The Far Eastern Federal District, as it is officially designated, makes up one-third of the territory encompassed by the Russian Federation and contains major natural resource deposits, although its population is sparse: less than seven million inhabitants. In the mid nineteenth century, the annexation of land from the Amur River to the Pacific pushed the frontiers of the Russian state to the extreme southeastern tip of the Eurasian landmass. These new frontiers in the East, which abutted China, Korea, and Japan, were celebrated as Russia's version of the American West: a land of opportunity, where agriculture and commerce could be developed. Russia's incorporation of these new Asian regions spurred a colonizing mission to bring 'civilization' to the region's indigenous peoples. The influx of Russian colonizers into the remoter regions of Siberia and the Russian Far East also helped to spread smallpox, typhus, typhoid, and syphilis – epidemic diseases that decimated indigenous communities. The construction of the Trans-Siberian Railway, begun in 1891, provided a further route for epidemics to disperse westwards from Asia and eastwards from Europe.

Yuri Slezkine, *Arctic Mirrors: Russia and the Small Peoples of the North* (Ithaca, NY: Cornell University Press, 1994).

Russia was also intent on obtaining an ice-free port that could be used throughout the year for its navy, as well as for boosting maritime trade. These expansionist policies in East Asia were to bring it into conflict with Japan, particularly over rival claims to southern Manchuria and Russia's acquisition of Port Arthur at the tip of the Liaodong peninsula. With the restoration of the Meiji Emperor in 1868, Japan became an emerging industrial power, and its military status was affirmed with its victory over China in the First Sino-Japanese War (1894–95), when large portions of southern Manchuria were ceded to it. The war exposed the Qing government's failure to modernize and overhaul the military, and marked a significant geopolitical shift: Japan now emerged as the dominant power in the region. The devastating loss of Korea, a Qing vassal state, triggered an outcry in China, leading to political upheaval and calls for reform that would culminate in the 1911 Revolution and the establishment of the Republic of China under Sun Yat-sen.

A key to Russia's policy in the East, promoted by the Tsar's modernizing prime minister Sergei Witte (1849–1915), was the construction of the Trans-Siberian Railway. This would connect Moscow to the Russian Far East across Siberia, passing through the city of Chita, east of Lake Baikal, and then on to Vladivostok. The writer Anton Chekhov had undertaken the taxing 11-week journey to Sakhalin in 1890 and was dismayed to find that the only route from Europe to the East was along a rutted, 'foul smallpox of a road,' which turned into a quagmire when it rained. 'The Siberian Highway,' he asserted, 'is the longest, and, I should think, the ugliest road on earth.'[46] In August 1895, Russian surveyors crossed into Manchuria to explore options for a strategic shortcut from Chita to Vladivostok across Chinese territory.[47] The Qing had recently suffered defeat in a war with Japan and would soon be caught up in the Boxer Rebellion (1900–1901). In no position to rebuff the Russians, the Chinese granted them a concession to construct the Chinese Eastern Railway (CER). Work was begun in 1897 and the line was open to regular traffic by 1903.[48] This extension of Russian influence into China threatened Japanese interests, resulting in the Russo-Japanese War of 1904–1905, which was fought over control of the Liaodong peninsula. Japan had

---

[46] Anton Chekhov, *A Journey to Sakhalin*. Translated by Brian Reeve (Cambridge: Ian Faulkner Publishing, 1993), pp.53–55.

[47] David Wolff, 'Russia Finds Its Limits: Crossing Borders into Manchuria.' In: Stephen Kotkin and David Wolff, eds., *Rediscovering Russia in Asia: Siberia and the Russian Far East* (Armonk, NY: M. E. Sharpe, 1995), pp.40–54 (44–45).

[48] S. C. M. Paine, 'The Chinese Eastern Railway from the First Sino-Japanese War until the Russo-Japanese War.' In: Bruce A. Elleman and Stephen Kotkin, eds., *Manchurian Railways and the Opening of China: An International History* (Armonk, NY: M. E. Sharpe, 2010), pp.13–36 (16).

offered to recognize Russian dominance in Manchuria in exchange for Russia acknowledging that Japan's sphere of influence extended to Korea. Russia rejected this overture, insisting on its retention of Port Arthur, and demanding that a line be drawn across the north of the Korea peninsula as a neutral buffer zone between Russia and Japan. In the ensuing war, the principal theaters were around the Liaodong peninsula and Mukden (Shenyang) in southern Manchuria, with naval operations in the Sea of Japan and the Yellow Sea.

By the terms of the Portsmouth Peace Treaty (1905), Russian concessions in Manchuria were handed over to Japan, including the South Manchurian Railway (SMR) from Changchun to Dairen (Dalian). The SMR, which by 1910 employed 35,000 Japanese and 25,000 Chinese, served in effect as an agency of the Japanese state and underpinned the military administration of the Japanese sphere in Manchuria. As the British journalist Lancelot Lawton noted, 'the wide political influence exercised by the Japanese in Southern Manchuria is derived from their possession of the railway, and the peculiar interpretation which they place upon the rights and privileges attached thereto.'[49] Gotō Shinpei, erstwhile Japanese governor of Taiwan (Chapter 3) and first president of the SMR Company, was to observe more bluntly that in Manchuria Japanese imperialism 'chose to assume the form of a railroad company.'[50] Like the Russians, the Japanese administered extensive territory contiguous with the railway and stationed troops along the lines to protect their interests.

Meanwhile, the Russians retained control of the CER, while the Chinese oversaw the Chinese Imperial Railway, which ran south from Mukden. It was in the context of this knotty and 'damned inheritance' that the epidemic of pneumonic plague occurred.[51] If the railway served as a vehicle for Japanese and Russian territorial aspirations, it also proved to be a critical pathway for disease. Concerns about safeguarding strategic and commercial interests conflated with anxieties about the plague's diffusion through Russian and Japanese territories and settlements abutting the lines. The first reported plague outbreak occurred in the fall of 1910 in the vicinity of Manzhouli on the CER bordering the Russian Trans-Baikal. From there, plague spread south along the railway lines to Harbin and Changchun, reaching Beijing by mid January 1911 and the provinces

---

[49] Lancelot Lawton, *Empires of the Far East: A Study of Japan and of Her Colonial Possessions, of China and Manchuria and of the Political Questions of Eastern Asia and the Pacific*, 2 vols. (London: G. Richards, 1912), II, p.1254.

[50] Itō Takeo, *Life Along the South Manchurian Railway: The Memoirs of Takeo Itō*. Translated by Joshua A. Fogel (New York: M. E. Sharpe, 1988), p.5.

[51] George Alexander Lensen, *The Damned Inheritance: The Soviet Union and the Manchurian Crises, 1924–1935* (Tallahassee, FL: Diplomatic Press, 1974).

of Jilin and Shandong by February. As Carl Nathan has observed, 'the exceptional communicability, fatality, and novelty of the disease inspired terror.'[52]

Thousands of Chinese laborers and seasonal agricultural workers had migrated to Manchuria from northern China to take advantage of the opportunities that the new railways offered as they 'opened up' the region. Trappers had migrated there in search of skins and furs for sale on the European market, including the fur of the *tarbagan*, a species of large Siberian marmot (*Marmota sibirica*), which was later found to harbor the plague. The onset of Chinese New Year in late January 1911, when many Chinese returned south to their homes by train, further spread infection. Unlike bubonic plague, which is transmitted via rat fleas, pneumonic plague is airborne, spreading through human-to-human contact. 'The complexity of the railway administration,' notes William Summers, 'their paramount political importance, and their crucial role in transporting people infected with plague ensured that the railroads in Manchuria became the focus of plague control efforts as well as the main locus of contention.'[53]

From the outset, the Chinese were concerned that Russia and Japan would seize the opportunity and assume control of anti-plague measures in order to impinge on Chinese sovereignty. The United States, Britain, France, and Germany were also apprehensive that Russia and Japan would use the epidemic as a ploy to extend their territorial claims in Manchuria, destabilizing the region. As news of the plague reached foreign diplomats, flurries of dispatches reflected a foreboding that the epidemic might presage war. The US 'Open Door' policy advocated by Secretary of State John Hay (1838–1905) in 1899, recognized China's territorial integrity along with the need for equitable trading access for all countries. As tensions mounted over the plague, the US consul in the Russian-controlled city of Harbin – the headquarters of the CER – worried that there was now a danger that Chinese authority could be undermined and a 'pretext for aggression may be found at any moment.' According to the British acting consul general in Harbin, force alone would prevent a Japanese offensive.[54] After all, two months previously, Japan had annexed Korea.

Wu Lien-teh conveyed this charged political atmosphere in the opening pages of his autobiography, *Plague Fighter*, describing his arrival in snow-bound Harbin, which by 1910 had a population of some 65,000, including 15,000 Chinese. The Russians, noted Wu,

---

[52] Nathan, *Plague Prevention*, p.1.
[53] William C. Summers, *The Great Manchurian Plague of 1910–1911: The Geopolitics of an Epidemic Disease* (New Haven, CT: Yale University Press, 2012), p.17.
[54] Nathan, *Plague Prevention*, p.4.

were all powerful here and controlled the strategic northern trunk line known as the Chinese Eastern Railway, with its multifarious military, political, and economic interests. In a similar way the Japanese, after their successful war against Russia in 1904–05, had secured control of the southern half of the great line from Dairen to Changchun, 150 miles to the north.

Between the Russians and the Japanese, there had been an unceasing struggle for more rights and control over this huge recently opened-up country known to the world as Manchuria and to the Chinese as the Three Eastern provinces comprising Fengtien, Kirin and Heilungkiang. When it is realised that in size Manchuria is equal to Germany, France and Switzerland put together and that it occupies the whole southern half of the basin of one of the world's largest rivers, the Amur, including that of its main tributary the Sungari, the reason for this struggle is not difficult to explain. Moreover, the output of such vital foodstuffs as wheat, soya bean and millet, as well as such minerals as coal, iron, and gold is immense, and only awaits peace and continuity of policy to reach full development and benefit not only itself but the world at large.[55]

Plague fighter: Dr. Wu

Born in Penang, British Malaya, Wu Lien-teh or Wu Liande studied medicine at the University of Cambridge and spent time at the Institut Pasteur in Paris and at Robert Koch's Institute for Infectious Diseases in Berlin. Wu became vice-director of the Imperial Army Medical College in Tientsin (Tianjin) and on instruction from Peking left for Manchuria in December 1910 to investigate the plague epidemic. Wu sought and was granted imperial approval to cremate plague victims, even though cremation violated Chinese custom. He subsequently chaired the International Plague Conference in Mukden in April 1911 and became director of the North Manchurian Plague Prevention Service (1911–1931), the first president of the China Medical Association (1916–1920), and the head of the National Quarantine Service (1931–1937). An effective self-promoter, Wu was instrumental in defining the Manchurian plague as the moment when modern public health was effectively introduced in China. In his autobiography, *Plague Fighter: The Autobiography of a Modern Chinese Physician* (1959), and in other publications, Wu Lien-teh invariably refers to himself imperiously in the third person as 'Dr. Wu.'

---

[55] Wu Lien-teh, *Plague Fighter: The Autobiography of a Modern Chinese Physician* (Cambridge: W. Heffer & Sons, 1959), p.3.

The Scottish medical missionary Dugald Christie (1855–1936), who had opened the Shengjing Clinic in Mukden in the 1880s, similarly described the wild rumors that swirled around the city during the plague. Japanese agents were alleged to have contaminated the drinking water with poison: 'The Japanese were credited with encouraging or even causing the epidemic in order to destroy the people and possess the land.' When Christie was handed a sample of the 'poison' to analyze – discovered by a policeman beside a locked well – he found it contained nothing but 'a harmless mixture of naphthalin and a white powder used in preparing Chinese pork for the market.'[56]

Medical and public health concerns became intertwined with mounting political and military pressures. The Chinese had long been suspicious of the CER's commercial activities, including its lumbering and mining operations. As the Russian community expanded, so did the infrastructure required to service it: churches, schools, and administrative institutions. The retention of troops to ensure the security of the railway was another point of contention. Russian railroad guards had been incorporated with Trans-Amur forces to protect the Russian zone along the trunk line.[57] The Chinese thus viewed Russian anti-plague measures, particularly those aimed at the Chinese population, with increasing apprehension. William J. Calhoun (1847–1916), the US minister to China, made this political dimension explicit when he stressed 'the necessity for active and effective work upon the part of the Chinese, in order to prevent any excuse for interference by either Russia or Japan, or both, under pleas of necessity for the protection of their respective local interest, or for the prevention of the spread of the plague to Korea or Siberia.'[58] There were, in fact, direct links between the Manchurian plague and the US health campaigns in the Philippines. Calhoun had played a key role in persuading President McKinley to enter the Spanish–US War in 1898, and the chief US delegate to the International Plague Conference in 1911 was Richard Pearson Strong, a scientist who had taken a lead role in the supervision of infectious disease in the newly established colony of the Philippines. A medical graduate of Johns Hopkins, Strong was instrumental in establishing the Biological Laboratory of the Philippine Bureau

[56] Dugald Christie, *Thirty Years in Moukden, 1883–1913: Being the Experiences and Recollections of Dugald Christie, C.M.G.* (London: Constable and Co., 1914), p.247.
[57] R. Edward Glatfelter, 'Russia, the Soviet Union, and the Chinese Eastern Railway.' In: Clarence B. Davis and Kenneth E. Wilburn, Jr., eds., *Railway Imperialism* (Westport, CT: Greenwood Press, 1991), pp.137–154 (143).
[58] Carl F. Nathan, 'The Acceptance of Western Medicine in Early 20th-Century China: The Story of the North Manchurian Plague Prevention Service.' In: John Z. Bowers and Elizabeth F. Purcell, eds., *Medicine and Society in China* (New York: Josiah Macy Jr. Foundation, 1974), p.58.

of Science, which he headed for over a decade.[59] It was Strong who had verified the first case of cholera in Manila in March 1902, and together with Dean C. Worcester – who had recommended Strong to Calhoun – he had been an outspoken critic of the Filipinization of the US colony's health service. In his collaboration with the Chinese, then, Strong brought not only technical knowledge of infectious disease, but a familiarity with 'emerging techniques of population management' that had been shaped by the military logic of US colonialism (Figure 4.3).[60]

Japan, meanwhile, had demonstrated the way in which medical and public health systems could function as critical mechanisms of state control. In Korea, public health administration formed an integral part of the colonial regime's military apparatus. Russian anti-plague measures, including the disinfection of Chinese residential areas and the destruction of 'plague' homes, elicited objections from the Chinese who balked at Russian interference. By the same token, the Russians complained of a lack of Chinese cooperation, alert to the danger that the wider spread of disease might pose to their interests. Epidemics in the Far East could threaten Russians at 'home.' A few years previously, in 1904 during the Russo-Japanese War, an epidemic of cholera had incited panic among Russian authorities who feared that the disease might spread into Russia from Manchuria. As one medical official noted from the city of Saratov, a port on the Volga: 'Obviously, the unfortunate war with its outrageous mass of victims is not confined to those who die in the fields of Manchuria; most likely, it also brings in its wake tens and hundreds of thousands of deaths here, in the heart of Russia, which is helpless to organise the fight against cholera.'[61]

It was at this juncture that Wu Lien-teh was summoned to coordinate plague prevention duties in Harbin on behalf of the Chinese. This was a war fought through medicine and public health: 'Political complications were also feared because Russia and Japan had both threatened to send their own medical staff and military into the infected areas unless more radical measures were adopted by the Chinese.' Autopsies were performed on unclaimed plague victims. Pits were dug and corpses cremated, measures 'that still conjure up in the native mind all that is repulsive and contrary to natural feeling.'[62] The police were recruited for

[59] Eli Chernin, 'Richard Pearson Strong and the Manchurian Epidemic of Pneumonic Plague, 1910–1911,' *Journal of the History of Medicine and Allied Sciences*, vol.44, no.3 (1989): 296–319.

[60] Anderson, *Colonial Pathologies*, pp.2, 61, 190.

[61] Charlotte E. Henze, *Disease, Health Care and Government in Late Imperial Russia: Life and Death on the Volga, 1823–1914* (Abingdon and New York: Routledge, 2011), p.141.

[62] 'Appendix: Wu Lien-teh – A Short Autobiography.' In: *Manchurian Plague Prevention Service Memorial Volume, 1912–1932* (Shanghai: National Quarantine Service, 1934), pp.459–469 (462–463).

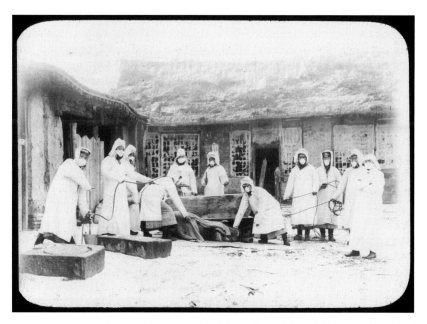

Figure 4.3. 'Encoffining body, Changchun (1911).' Papers of Richard P. Strong [GA82.3, B-31]. Courtesy: Harvard Medical Library in the Francis A. Countway Library of Medicine.

Face masks

The wearing of gauze face masks had become routine in surgery by the end of the nineteenth century. At the beginning of the twentieth century, masks were used as a prophylaxis in epidemic situations. During the Manchurian plague epidemic, the wearing of cloth face masks was advocated by Wu Lien-teh (Figure 4.3). In 1918, face masks were widely used as a precaution against influenza. Since the 1990s – and particularly the 2003 SARS outbreak – the face mask has become an enduring emblem of East Asia. During SARS, people sought out the best quality medical air-purifying respirators they could find, including the 'N-95' respirator, which was deemed superior to other, cheaper varieties and came recommended by the US Centers for Disease Control and Prevention (CDC).

sanitary inspections, disinfecting dwellings and isolating the sick in hospitals. Cordons were established along transport routes, while schools and theaters were closed. A team of 20 doctors trained in Western medicine supported Wu's efforts, along with a contingent of 29 medical student volunteers from medical schools across China. Hundreds of laborers were contracted to dig pits and cremate bodies, while local police were recruited and over a thousand soldiers drafted in from Changchun to conduct house-to-house searches and impose a military cordon.

There was widespread local opposition to these public health interventions that targeted 'coolies' – interventions that were, in many ways, more heavy-handed than those undertaken by the British in response to the 1894 outbreak of bubonic plague in Hong Kong (Chapter 1). Chinese migrant laborers to northern Manchuria, notably those from the Shandong peninsula who were involved in hunting marmots for their skins, became the particular object of the state's sanitary drive. These unskilled and deracinated coolies were pitted against the skill of Mongol and Buryat marmot hunters, who were native to northern Manchuria.[63] Coolies were viewed as ignorant and superstitious; a recalcitrant force that was deemed largely responsible for the vicious excesses of the Boxer Rebellion in 1900. They were taken to exemplify the failings of the imperial regime and, in the opprobrious writings of reformers such as Wu Lien-teh, they were customarily linked to disease, slum-living, and opium addiction. The proceedings of the First International Plague Conference in Mukden characterize the coolie settlement of Fuchiatien (Fujiadian) as a locus of dirt and crime that stokes virulent infection: 'Almost all the buildings of this town represent inns, eating houses, opium dens, low-roofed, dirty, half-tumbled-down dwellings swarming with insects and parasites.' This invasive pathogenic life is soon conflated by Wu with the teeming coolies who overrun every nook of the slum city, propagating disease with their polluting habits. Vector and victim are transposable: 'Although opium smoking is prohibited both by the Russian and the Chinese authorities, there are a great many secret opium dens in Fuchiatien as well as in Harbin. During the night these dens are invaded by a large number of coolies, who fill every available space in them. If by chance a plague-infected person gets into such a crowded house the disease is most readily conveyed to the others (as has been proved several times by the night patrols), especially by means of the opium pipe, which passes from mouth to mouth.'[64]

[63] Christos Lynteris, 'Skilled Natives, Inept Coolies: Marmot Hunting and the Great Manchurian Pneumonic Plague (1910–1911),' *History and Anthropology*, vol.24, no.3 (2013): 303–321.
[64] Lynteris, 'Skilled Natives, Inept Coolies,' p.326.

Chinese plague interventions marked a new degree of state control and, it is often suggested, laid the ground for post-crisis state involvement in the oversight of health. Photographs of the epidemic, depicting abandoned Chinese corpses and plague pits heaped with bodies and rubble, reflect the scale of the catastrophe, as well as the unrelenting response. Although the Chinese had reason to be mistrustful of Russian intentions, given the latter's ambitions in Manchuria and the recent history of conflict in the region, they tacitly supported Russia's draconian sanitary measures. Mark Gamsa has gone as far as to argue that 'the coercive policy which Russia was applying within its railway zone was carried out with the consent and active participation of the Chinese state.'[65] In the aftermath of the crisis a new organization, the North Manchurian Plague Prevention Service, was set up and became, in effect, China's first public health service. As Nathan has remarked: 'When epidemics swept Manchuria, Plague Prevention Service hospitals attended exclusively to infectious disease control. In the lulls between epidemics, however, the hospitals were thrown open as a free, general medical service for North Manchuria, representing the service's major extra-epidemic activity.'[66]

The Manchurian plague epidemic highlights a number of critical issues in relation to our theme of epidemics and war. First, it reveals the extent to which a prehistory of conflict shaped responses to an epidemic crisis. Second, it demonstrates how Chinese officials were able to use Western science and public health as tools for promoting international diplomacy and averting inter-state aggression. Third – and relatedly – it suggests how the 'breakthroughs' in modern medicine and public health, with which Wu Lien-teh is identified, were also political breakthroughs: science legitimated the extension of state services into social and cultural spaces that had hitherto been considered out of bounds. As Sean Hsiang-lin Lei has noted, central to this process of legitimation was the microscope and the practice of modern bacteriology. The Qing government's emphasis was on 'scientific investigation rather than administrative maneuvering.'[67] In order to forestall intervention by the Russians and Japanese, the Chinese sought to frame the epidemic as a scientific crisis, calling on the international community – above all the United States – for technical assistance. This was the context for the International Plague Conference, convened in Mukden in April 1911 at Chinese insistence (Figure 4.4).

---

[65] Mark Gamsa, 'The Epidemic of Pneumonic Plague in Manchuria, 1910–1911,' *Past & Present*, vol.190, no.1 (2006): 147–183 (183).

[66] Carl F. Nathan, 'The Acceptance of Western Medicine in Early 20th Century China: The Story of the North Manchurian Plague Prevention Service.' In: John Z. Bowers and Elizabeth F. Purcell, eds., *Medicine and Society in China* (New York: Josiah Macy, Jr. Foundation, 1974), pp.55–75 (68).

[67] Lei, *Neither Donkey nor Horse*, pp.21–44; Summers, *The Great Manchurian Plague*, p.89.

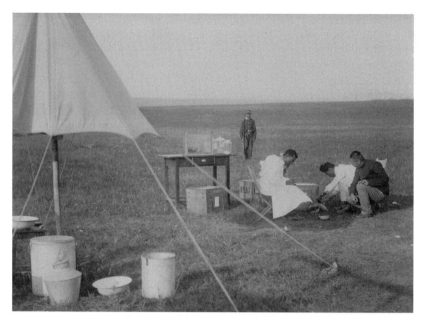

Figure 4.4. 'Taking the temperature of the tarbagan (June 1911).' Courtesy: Special Collections, University of Hong Kong.

The North Manchurian Plague Prevention Service

Figure 4.4. is a photograph from an album presented to the University of Hong Kong by Wu Lien-teh and shows a field laboratory with researchers from the North Manchurian Plague Prevention Service taking the rectal temperature of the *tarbagan*, understood to be the vector of the pneumonic plague. Wu served as director of the North Manchurian Plague Prevention Service, which was founded in 1911, following the Mukden International Plague Conference, and placed under the oversight of the Chinese Ministry of Foreign Affairs. The Revolution of 1911, which overthrew the Qing dynasty and established a republic, delayed the Service's operations until 1912. Headquartered in Fuchiatien, the Service ran research and clinical laboratories, supervised the construction and management of hospitals along the Chinese Eastern Railway and the Siberian border, and conducted epidemiological surveys. Although the Service was intended to deal with the prevention and control of epidemics, it assumed a more general remit in non-crisis periods.

The Service has been viewed as the first concerted attempt to create a modern, science-based public health infrastructure in China. For several decades after its inception, it constituted the only organized Chinese-run medical system in China. However, the Service was dependent for its existence on foreign funds and its jurisdiction was limited to Manchuria. In 1931, following the Japanese invasion of Manchuria, the Service was disbanded and its staff absorbed into the new National Quarantine Service in Shanghai.

'A Short History of the Manchurian Plague Prevention Service by Wu Lien-teh, Director, Manchurian Plague Prevention and National Quarantine Services.' In: *Manchurian Plague Prevention Service Memorial Volume, 1912–1932* (Shanghai: National Quarantine Service, 1934), pp.1–12.

The interconnections between Chinese bacteriology, medicine, and politics – as well as the importance of the struggle over Manchuria in their formation – can be illustrated by comparing two well-known events in the lives of two of China's celebrated 'modernizers.' The first involves a critical moment in the life of Lu Xun (1881–1936), undoubtedly China's most famous modern writer, who was to assume canonical status as a cultural leader in the PRC, and was fêted by no less a figure than Mao. In 1906, Lu had been studying at the Sendai Medical School in Japan. One day, for the amusement of his students and to fill the remaining time at the end of a bacteriology lesson, Lu's lecturer had shown the class a magic lantern image (the 'magic lantern' was a device for projecting images on sheets of glass), which depicted an incident from the Russo-Japanese War of 1904–1905 in Manchuria. A crowd of Chinese bystanders looked on passively as the Japanese executed a fellow Chinese citizen branded as a Russian spy. Surrounded by jubilant Japanese classmates, Lu was shocked by the apathy of the Chinese crowd on the projected image and experienced a moment of epiphany: he would abandon his medical studies and devote himself to literature.

Microbes, politics, and reform

Lu Xun – the pen name of Zhou Shuren – described his conversion from aspiring doctor to writer in the Preface to his collection of short stories *Outcry*, completed in December 1922 and published the following year:

I have no idea what progress has been made in the teaching of microbiology since my time, but back then we were shown the outlines of microbes as images on lantern slides. Because lectures sometimes finished early, the teacher would make up the remaining minutes by entertaining students with slides depicting picturesque landscapes or current affairs. As it so happened that the Russo-Japanese War was ongoing at the time, our lectures were often concluded by scenes from this conflict. In this classroom setting, I found myself obliged to echo – with my own claps and cheers – my classmates' jubilation. There came a day, though, when I suddenly found myself staring at a great mass of my fellow Chinese – a people I had long been deprived the pleasure of encountering. One stood in the middle, tied up, surrounded by a crowd of his countrymen. Though they were all of them perfectly sturdy physical specimens, every face was utterly, stupidly blank. The man tied up, the caption informed us, had been caught spying for the Russians and was about to be beheaded by the Japanese as a public example to the appreciative mob.

Before the academic year was out, I had left for Tokyo. For I no longer believed in the overwhelming importance of medical science. However rude a nation was in physical health, if its people were intellectually feeble, they would never become anything other than cannon fodder or gawping spectators, their loss to the world through illness no cause for regret. The first task was to change their spirit; and literature and the arts, I decided at the time, were the best means to this end. And so I reinvented myself as a crusader for cultural reform.

Lu Xun, *The Real Story of Ah-Q and Other Tales of China. The Complete Fiction of Lu Xun.* Translated by Julia Lovell (London: Penguin, 2009), pp.15–20 (16–17).

The second event took place at the end of 1910 in Fuchiatien, the ramshackle Chinese coolie town that had sprung up opposite Harbin on the CER in Manchuria and became the object of radical public health interventions. Wu Lien-teh had just arrived to direct the anti-plague campaign there. On the morning of December 27, Wu and his assistant, responding to a telephone message, collected their medical equipment and drove to a house in a poor part of town where they had been informed that a Japanese woman innkeeper 'had died during the night showing symptoms of coughing and spitting of blood.' They found the dead woman in a cheap cotton kimono prostrate on a soiled tatami mat that was placed on planks above the floor. In this dingy setting, Wu and his colleague proceeded to perform a post-mortem. 'It was under such strange and unusual circumstances,' Wu wrote, 'that the first post-mortem upon a pneumonic plague patient was made in Fuchiatien, perhaps in Manchuria.' Returning to their quarters, Wu examined the specimens he had taken from the victim in an improvised laboratory, which had been set up in a room requisitioned from the Chamber of Commerce. He observed how 'all the specimens from blood, heart, lungs, liver, and spleen, when seen under a high-powered microscope, showed swarms of the characteristic oval-shaped plague bacilli with bipolar staining at the ends. Further confirmation of plague was established in the growths in the agar tubes.'

What connects these moments of epiphanous breakthrough? For one, both involve forms of violence: the execution by the Japanese of a Chinese 'spy' during the Russo-Japanese War in Manchuria, and the dissection of a Japanese woman by a Chinese physician in Harbin. Indeed, Wu gives a particularly visceral description of the medical procedure conducted in the plague victim's dwelling:

Next, the surface of a lung and the spleen were scarified, and a platinum needle was inserted into the substance of each organ and the necessary cultures and films made. Pieces of the affected lungs, spleen, and liver, each two inches by two inches, were removed and placed in glass jars containing 10 percent formalin. Owing to the need of preserving secrecy, as little time as possible was wasted on the proceedings. The parts were replaced, the skin was sewn up and the body dressed properly, before being carted to the burial ground in a government-supplied coffin.[68]

Second, both breakthroughs take place in improvised spaces: a provisional screening room in a bacteriological classroom in Sendai, and a makeshift laboratory in the Chamber of Commerce in Fuchiatien. Third, both events center on a visual experience: the projected image on the lantern slide where microbes are usually shown, and the confirmation, looking through a microscope, that the plague bacterium is in fact present in the specimens. As the cultural critic Rey Chow has observed, Lu Xun's 'magic lantern' incident suggests how an emerging modernity was grounded in a 'technologized visuality.'[69] The same, too, might be claimed of Wu Lien-teh's revelations through the microscope.

Read together in this way, these texts suggest a paradoxical convergence. The moment of epiphany in which Lu Xun grasps the limitations of science and lights out into the world for a career as a political writer, turns out to be the same moment that Wu Lien-teh banishes the extraneous world of politics for the incontestable truth revealed by the microscope: the plague bacterium. Responses to the Manchurian plague epidemic demonstrate that modern science and public health acquired their

[68] Wu, *Plague Fighter*, p.11.
[69] Rey Chow, *Primitive Passions: Visuality, Sexuality, Ethnography, and Contemporary Chinese Cinema* (New York: Columbia University Press, 1995), pp.4–12.

political force precisely from their claims to be apolitical. These claims are explored more thoroughly in the next case, specifically in relation to US humanitarian efforts aimed at containing a typhus epidemic in Siberia during the Russian Civil War. There, the focus is on the interrelationship between epidemics and the way in which US military and humanitarian interventions were justified in terms of their neutrality. How and with what consequences did humanitarian efforts to relieve suffering and treat disease become intertwined with a political agenda that strove to promote US interests by showcasing American medical technology and the civilizing values it embodied?

Typhus and humanitarianism in Russia's Far East

Russia, as we have seen, had become an Asian power by the end of the nineteenth century, with territorial aspirations in Manchuria and along the Pacific coast. A revolution in Petrograd (St. Petersburg) in February 1917, however, created a power vacuum that was to destabilize East Asia. On March 2, 1917, in the midst of the First World War, Tsar Nicholas II (1868–1918) abdicated and a provisional government was set up. Law and order soon deteriorated, and the economic situation worsened. Setbacks in the war led to increasing disillusionment and social unrest. In October 1917, Bolshevik revolutionaries under the leadership of Vladimir Lenin (1870–1924) overthrew the provisional government and seized power. In March 1918, the Bolshevik leadership agreed terms with Germany and signed the Treaty of Brest-Litovsk, pulling Russia out of the First World War.

For the next five years, Russia was to remain caught up in a bloody civil war. The Red Army of the Bolsheviks clashed with disparate anti-socialist forces, the so-called White Army, in a conflict that extended from Europe to the furthest reaches of the Russian Far East. The Reds were eventually to defeat the Whites in the Ukraine and in 1919 they crushed the forces of Admiral Alexander Kolchak (1874–1920), who had established an anti-Communist government at Omsk in southwest Siberia. However, the war persisted in Asia with skirmishes between the Bolshevik army and the remnants of the Whites. The geopolitical maneuverings that we have just explored in connection with the pneumonic plague in Manchuria, were also crucial in determining events in East Asia after the Bolshevik seizure of power in the fall of 1917. Early on in the First World War, Japan had occupied the German treaty port of Qingdao in Shandong. Japan's expansionist aspirations in Manchuria and its demands on China worried other Allied Powers, notably Britain and the United States, who were at war with the Central Powers, Germany and Austria. These

concerns came to a head following the removal of the provisional government in Petrograd and the spread of revolution to eastern Siberia.

The extended border between Russia and China became a flashpoint
of conflict as thousands of Russians streamed into northern China and
Manchuria, seeking refuge from the Bolsheviks.[70] The CER comprised
a crucial stretch of the Trans-Siberian line under Russian authority.
The Bolshevik Revolution introduced a period of chaos in the Russian-
controlled zone of the CER, particularly in the cities of Changchun and
Harbin, where General Dmitri Horvath (1858–1937), manager of the
CER since 1902, sought to establish a conservative Russian government
in exile – a move strongly opposed by the Chinese.

In unilaterally withdrawing from the First World War, the Bolsheviks
had given new impetus to Germany's war effort, freeing up over two million troops that had been fighting Russia on the Eastern Front. Britain,
France, and Japan began extending financial aid to anti-Bolshevik groups
in the East, apprehensive about the radical phase of the revolution for
their war efforts and for the long-term security of the region. They also
feared that once the Bolsheviks had secured control of Siberia, the provisions that had piled up in Vladivostok for Russia's war effort would fall
into the hands of the Germans. As Henry Pomeroy Davison, the banker
philanthropist and chairman of the War Council of the ARC, noted in
1919: 'On the wharves of Vladivostok were lying millions of dollars' worth
of supplies for the Russian soldiery which should have been delivered
three years before.'[71] The Allies considered the possibility of sending an
expeditionary force to Siberia to reinstate an Eastern Front. Allied ships
had been monitoring events off the coast of Vladivostok since the winter
of 1917. In the spring of 1918, the first Japanese troops disembarked at
Vladivostok to protect Japanese interests in the city. In August, a small
British force arrived from Hong Kong, the first of the Allied participants
in an intervention designed to influence the outcome of the Civil War
and reinstate the Eastern Front, as well as to assist some 70,000 troops
of the Czechoslovak Legion who had been fighting for the Allies. As
the Japanese boosted their presence in the port, an American contingent
was dispatched from the Philippines, with other military support arriving from China, French Indochina, Italy, Serbia, and Romania. Canadian
expeditionary forces disembarked in October 1918 and January 1919.[72]

[70] Betty Miller Unterberger, *America's Siberian Expedition, 1918–1920: A Study of National
Policy* (New York: Greenwood Press, 1969), p.13.

[71] Henry P. Davison, *The American Red Cross in the Great War* (New York: Macmillan Co.,
1919), p.238.

[72] Benjamin Isitt, *From Victoria to Vladivostok: Canada's Siberian Expedition, 1917–19* (Vancouver: UBC Press, 2010), pp.64–65.

A priority was maintaining control of the Trans-Siberian Railway. In what was known as the Inter-Allied Railroad Agreement, concluded in August 1919, supervision of the railways was divided up amongst the Allies.[73]

While this was a political and military crisis, it was also an epidemic crisis. Of the 10 million Russians who died from the First World War to 1921, 800,000 perished in battle; the rest were victims of typhus, cholera, influenza, and famine.[74] Typhus, an acute febrile disease caused by the bacterium *Rickettsia prowazekii* that is transmitted by the human body louse, is estimated to have caused three million deaths during the First World War in Russia alone. Symptoms of the disease include severe fever and delirium, with a mortality rate of between five and 40 percent or higher. The role of the louse in the transmission of typhus was discovered in 1909 by the French bacteriologist Charles Nicolle (1866–1936) in Tunisia, although the pathogen was not identified until 1916. While typhus had been endemic in Russia for centuries, the breakdown of social order acted as a driver of infection. The railroad network, in particular, facilitated the dispersal of infection as refugees fled the conflict.[75] The chaos of revolution and civil war fostered new 'lethal mobilities,' which helped drive the country to the brink of collapse.[76] Civilian refugees, along with demobilized soldiers and deserters, clogged the railways and roads. Troops spread disease, while the upheavals of war led to a shortage of food and the disintegration of law and order. In 1921, a famine across tracts of Russia resulted in further social convulsions, with refugees expanding the radius of infection.

Typhus was to be a significant factor in the Civil War between the Bolsheviks and the Whites. From Western Russia, the disease spread to Siberia and Central Asia. The city of Omsk, east of the Urals, saw an outbreak of typhus in the summer of 1919 and from there it reached Irkutsk in September of the same year. As one officer remarked, incidents of armed revolt in 1919 resembled 'the rapid progress of a case of typhus when plotted with dots on a map' at high command.[77] War refugees and counter-revolutionary forces fleeing the Bolshevik offensive carried typhus along the Trans-Siberian Railway southeast from Tomsk

[73] William S. Graves, *America's Siberian Adventure, 1918–1920* (New York: Peter Smith, 1931), pp.177–178.

[74] Jonathan D. Smele, *Civil War in Siberia: The Anti-Bolshevik Government of Admiral Kolchak, 1918–1920* (Cambridge: Cambridge University Press, 1996), p.1.

[75] George Stewart, *The White Armies of Russia: A Chronicle of Counter-Revolution and Allied Intervention* (New York: Macmillan Co., 1933), p.31.

[76] Robert Argenbright, 'Lethal Mobilities: Bodies and Lice on Soviet Railroads, 1918–1922,' *Journal of Transport History*, vol.29, no.2 (2008): 259–276.

[77] Smele, *Civil War in Siberia*, p.384.

to Lake Baikal, and then along the Amur to the Pacific: some 50,000 of Kolchak's soldiers had succumbed to typhus by the beginning of 1920.[78]

Francis McCullagh, a British war correspondent captured by Bolsheviks in Siberia in January 1920, provided a bleak account of epidemic typhus there. Naked corpses were flung callously from the doors of a train 'with as little ceremony as the stoker threw out ashes.' Bodies were stacked in warehouses or piled up 'like logs of wood' since the ground was too frozen for pits to be dug. Infected clothes were stolen from corpses, furthering the spread of disease. Refugees streamed into Vladivostok by train, seeking a safe haven from the chaos. As McCullagh expressed it, these were 'death trains' – 'that is, trains in which nearly everybody aboard was sick, dying, or dead, the dead lying among the living.' Since station masters refused to let these typhus trains stop at their stations, they were forced on to Vladivostok. On arrival, the condition of their human cargo was 'so frightful that no description of them is possible.'[79] 'Refugees in Siberia Dying in Trains – Typhus and Hunger Take Terrible Toll,' declaimed the *New York Times* on August 11, 1919, in a report filed by the Associated Press. Authorities were overwhelmed by the sick and dying who clogged the railways: 'There have been instances where entire trains have been side-tracked with typhus victims, many of them in a dying condition. Every night numbers of dead are removed from trains, some of them having perished from starvation.'

It was in response to this catastrophe that humanitarian missions were dispatched to East Asia. The ARC was at the forefront of this humanitarian effort.[80] As Clara Noyes, director of the US Department of Nursing, noted in 1919: the Red Cross (RC) had prepared 'for an intensive fight in Siberia against the typhus.'[81] Under the direction of the American physician Rudolf Bolling Teusler (1876–1934) – a missionary doctor based in Japan who happened to be a cousin of President Woodrow Wilson's (1856–1924) wife, Edith – the ARC Commission to Siberia linked up with regional branches of the RC and set up its base in Vladivostok in September 1918.

This was a sizeable operation and in the course of its 20-month duration, the ARC oversaw the running of hospitals with several hundred American doctors, nurses, and other personnel. The Peking chapter of

---

[78] K. David Patterson, 'Typhus and its Control in Russia, 1870–1940,' *Medical History*, vol.37, no.4 (1991): 361–381 (373–375).

[79] Francis McCullagh, *A Prisoner of the Reds: The Story of a British Officer Captured in Siberia* (London: John Murray, 1921), pp.31–35, 320–323.

[80] Julia F. Irwin, 'The Great White Train: Typhus, Sanitation, and U.S. International Development during the Russian Civil War,' *Endeavour*, vol.36, no.3 (2012): 89–96.

[81] Clara D. Noyes, 'The Red Cross,' *American Journal of Nursing*, vol.20, no.2 (1919): 134–138 (134).

the RC sent supplies, while funds were donated by expatriates in Shanghai, Tianjin, and Harbin. A hospital was established on Russian Island in the harbor of Vladivostok. As refugees poured into the port city, the RC sought to relieve the acute housing situation, setting up refugee barracks where the emphasis was on hygiene. At the same time: 'Two sewing rooms, a weaving establishment and a tailor shop were operated by the Red Cross at Vladivostok to furnish employment for refugees. In the sewing rooms 6,500 garments had been turned out to December 31, 1918.' The RC also ran schools for refugee children.

The RC were active along the entire stretch of the Trans-Siberian Railway from Vladivostok to Omsk in the West – a distance of over 4,000 miles. In 1919, the organization's work in Siberia 'involved equipping and operating hospitals and dispensaries, the distribution of drugs and other medical supplies, the establishment and operation of baths and disinfecting plants, and the equipping and maintenance of an anti-typhus sanitary train.' Aside from running hospitals directly, they also 'furnished equipment and supplies to a large number of Siberian hospitals, including such items as beds, mattresses, blankets, operating tables, instruments, drugs, surgical dressings and food.'[82]

One of the ARC's first initiatives on its arrival in Siberia in 1918 was to cooperate with the other RC chapters to finance a mobile treatment clinic, known as the 'Inter-Allied Typhus Train.'[83] This was 'a train of seventeen cars equipped for bathing and delousing purposes which can be rushed to the point where the plague is most severe.'[84] As an ARC report put it: 'An important part in the fight against typhus was taken by a complete Red Cross sanitary train made up of bath, boiler, tank, sterilizing, dressing, hair-clipping and other cars. This train, manned by RC workers, went into infected districts applying modern sanitary methods.'[85] The train spearheaded the anti-typhus campaign along the Trans-Siberian Railway. Shuttling between Vladivostok and Perm, the train bathed 105,000 people, disinfected one million items of clothing, issued 500,000 articles of new clothes, and operated a free clinic and drug dispensary. In addition, there was also a dental clinic and a 'hospital on wheels,' which covered a distance of 18,000 miles. As Davison noted: 'Sanitary trains were equipped to accompany the Czech army into the interior and a rolling canteen and a station canteen were set up between Harbin and the

---

[82] *The Work of the American Red Cross During the War: A Statement of Finances and Accomplishments for the Period July 1, 1917 to February 28, 1919* (Washington, DC: American National Red Cross, 1919), pp.83–86.
[83] Irwin, 'The Great White Train,' p.90.   [84] Noyes, 'The Red Cross,' p.134.
[85] *The Work of the American Red Cross During the War*, p.85.

forward Units, in which many American women cheerfully volunteered their services.'[86]

Political neutrality: The Great White Train

The article below on the 'Great White Train' celebrates the role of the ARC's mobile sanitary unit as a 'weapon in fighting typhus.' This military language, however, is countered by an emphasis on the humanitarian nature of the mission, 'its work of aid and mercy.' The train has an educational assignment, which is to spread professional know-how and expertise. The symbolism of the 'Great White Train' is clear: the color white encapsulates the idea of neutrality and purity, at the same time as it points to the ongoing civil war that is pitting Whites against Reds – a war in which the United States unambiguously favors the Whites. The hue of the Red Cross is clearly wholly different from the red of Bolshevism.

After covering thousands of miles and caring for thousands of victims of typhus the train known throughout Siberia as 'The Great White Train,' is now at Perm where the doctors and nurses are combatting a recent outbreak of typhus among the soldiers and civilians of that district.

The reputation of the train as an effective weapon in fighting typhus has spread far and wide. Built by the American Red Cross for the Allies, it was originally intended to be used first in the maritime provinces of Siberia. Then came the tremendous epidemics of typhus out west in the heart of winter – epidemics that ran the number of hospital cases up into the tens of thousands and the unreported cases into the twenties of thousands. From military camp and concentration point; from soldier and prison barracks; from hospitals and orphanages and refugee colonies; from railroad trains crowded with homeless people and stations even more crowded, came reports of the spread of the 'spotted fever.'

So the Great White Train went west – long cars for bathing men, women and children unwashed for months; cars for cutting the hair and sterilizing the clothes; cars laden with medicaments and clothing, and began its work of aid and mercy – and prevention of even worse epidemics... About 20,000 men have been handled by the personnel in the six months the train has been out. These men have been bathed, their heads clipped, their clothes disinfected, and in many cases they have received underwear and medical treatment. Side by side with the purely physical aspect of the anti-typhus expedition went the work of education. In every city or town visited the train officers arranged conferences with the leading officials, military

---

[86] Davison, *The American Red Cross in the Great War*, p.276.

and civilian, of the district who were in charge of sanitary, medical or surgical work.

'The "Great White Train" in Siberia,' *Public Health Nurse*, vol.11, no.19 (October 1919): 842–843.

'On the surface,' observes historian Julia Irwin, 'the purpose of the Inter-Allied (and later ARC) Typhus Train appeared clear cut: to improve the wellbeing of soldiers and civilians by overcoming the scourge of typhus. To be sure, many of the Typhus Train's personnel understood this as their principal goal and saw their work as overwhelmingly beneficent.'[87] As Davison of the ARC declared: 'From the beginning, the purpose of the Red Cross was to help the people of Russia without regard to political situations, and with utter indifference to the policies of the political party that happened to be in power. Its aim was to keep clearly before the Russians the fact that the United States, through the Red Cross, wanted to help them.'[88] However, whatever benevolent motivations may have driven humanitarian workers, they operated in an environment that was intensively political as the US sought to promote its interests and push back against the Bolshevik threat.

From the outset, the Japanese were uneasy at the presence of the ARC. President Wilson had been keen to dispatch a business delegation 'to carry on America's economic program in Russia.' An aide-memoire from the office of the US Secretary of State, Robert Lansing (1864–1928), to the Allied ambassadors, confirmed the US government's intention to send out 'a commission of merchants, agricultural experts, labor advisers, Red Cross representatives, and agents of the Young Men's Christian Association' in order to promote education and assist in economic development in Siberia. 'To many in the Japanese Foreign Ministry,' notes James William Morley, 'this was a virtual declaration of the economic war they had feared.'[89] Even on the US side, there were reservations about the ARC's neutrality. Given Teusler's presidential connection, his views were influential amongst the military, diplomats, and reporters. The head of the US military in Siberia, Major General William Graves complained: 'The American Red Cross ran hospitals exclusively for Kolchak people and acted in practice as Kolchak's supply agent as long as Dr. Teusler was in Siberia.'[90] Graves admonished Teusler for his partisanship and warned

---

[87] Irwin, 'The Great White Train,' p.93.
[88] Davison, *The American Red Cross in the Great War*, p.275.
[89] James William Morley, *The Japanese Thrust into Siberia, 1918* (New York: Columbia University Press, 1957), p.294.
[90] Graves, *America's Siberian Adventure*, p.206.

that he would cease to protect ARC trains if Teusler continued to favor the Whites. As Jamie Bisher writes: 'Controversy – and peril – swirled around foreign benevolent representatives for the duration of their missions in Siberia.'[91]

Humanitarian aid had other objectives. It sought 'to win hearts and minds, to persuade Russians of the legitimacy of both the US intervention and of the White Russian (anti-Bolshevik) government.' As Irwin observes: 'Beyond the clear propaganda value of such assistance, officials believed that tackling disease was essential to maintaining social order and stability and to counteracting the influence of Bolshevism.'[92] The 'Great White Train' was promoted as an exemplar of Western sanitary technology. Yet its role was undermined by the confused situation in Siberia. Railway lines were blown up in acts of sabotage and, as Davison acknowledged, the Trans-Siberian was not 'a perfectly running, perfectly managed road. Far from it. To begin with, the rolling stock was old and dilapidated, the engines badly in need of repair and fuel was scarce; nor did they run on schedule time, breakdowns being the rule rather than the exception.'[93]

With the death of Kolchak in February 1920, and the collapse of White forces in Siberia, the rationale for foreign intervention evaporated. US troops withdrew in April, leaving the Japanese to retain a presence in the unruly Russian Far East. From an Allied point of view, the Siberian intervention had been a disaster and its legacy would be profound. First, the escapade would help to project an image of the United States in the Soviet Union as a warmongering nation with expansionist designs. Second, while the Allies had interceded to ensure stability, the outcome achieved was precisely the opposite: Japanese hegemony in East Asia, exemplified by the annexation of Manchuria in 1931.[94]

The US-led humanitarian relief work in Siberia was hardly impartial. In helping to control typhus from spreading among the population, the ARC assumed a political function: the success of a humanitarian mission would make the benefits of a US social and political system self-evident in contrast to Bolshevism. This ideological dimension of modernization and development was to drive US foreign affairs for much of the twentieth century. Beyond this, the Allied intervention in the Russian Far East during the Civil War, and the humanitarian efforts that accompanied it,

---

[91] Jamie Bisher, *White Terror: Cossack Warlords of the Trans-Siberian* (Abingdon and New York: Routledge, 2005), p.153.

[92] Irwin, 'The Great White Train,' p.89.

[93] Davison, *The American Red Cross in the Great War*, p.273.

[94] Carl J. Richard, *When the United States Invaded Russia: Woodrow Wilson's Siberian Disaster* (Lanham, MD: Rowman & Littlefield, 2013), pp.26–29.

suggest the extent to which humanitarian actions, despite their pro-claimed impartiality, are always enmeshed in political contexts.[95] The emphasis on infrastructural development was predicated on a discourse of progress. It is precisely these ethical ambiguities and the legacy of imperialism in the project of global health and humanitarianism that are considered in the next section.

Pre-emptive strike: Polio in the tribal lands

The examples above from the Philippines, Qing China, and the Russian Far East, have illustrated how war and disease prevention are inter-twined operations. Both involve the strategic management of populations through the deployment of technologies that target the human body. At the same time, armed conflicts – or the threat of conflict – create the space for military-style approaches to disease control as belligerent states assume responsibility for health and launch quasi-military-style public health campaigns.

It was in the post-Second World War period that 'eradication' gained traction: the notion, as defined by the US CDC, that the worldwide incidents of a specific disease might be 'reduced to zero as a result of deliberate efforts.' Eradication or 'eradicationalism' – faith in a disease-free world – was not a new concept.[96] Earlier in the twentieth century, the Rockefeller Foundation had launched campaigns to eliminate hook-worm, yellow fever, and malaria, with a particular focus in Asia on Java and Malaya.[97] As opposed to eradication, however, the goal of elimi-nation entailed reducing the prevalence of disease in targeted regional populations.[98] After the Second World War, there was a fresh impetus for dealing with infectious disease on a global scale. The newly established WHO launched unprecedented eradication campaigns against yaws, yel-low fever, malaria, and smallpox. The WHO's smallpox eradication cam-paign, which had begun in 1958, was re-launched in 1967. An Intensi-fied Smallpox Eradication Program (INSEP) targeted those regions of the world, including Indonesia, where the disease was endemic. While smallpox had been virtually wiped out in Indonesia by 1939, the Second World War and the ensuing upheaval of the revolutionary period that

---

[95] Michael Barnett, *Empire of Humanity: A History of Humanitarianism* (Ithaca, NY: Cornell University Press, 2011).

[96] Nancy Leys Stepan, *Eradication: Ridding the World of Diseases Forever?* (Ithaca, NY: Cornell University Press, 2011), p.16.

[97] John Farley, *To Cast Out Disease: A History of the International Health Division of the Rocke-feller Foundation (1913–1951)* (Oxford: Oxford University Press, 2004), pp.65–66.

[98] Walter R. Dowdle, 'The Principles of Disease Elimination and Eradication,' *Bulletin of the World Health Organization*, vol.76, Supplement 2 (1998): S22–S25.

followed saw a recrudescence of the disease as routine vaccination was disrupted.[99] The WHO officially declared the world free of smallpox in 1980, an event that appeared to vindicate eradication as a feasible public health objective. This was the first time in history that a disease had been eradicated. The only other disease to have since been eradicated is rinderpest in 2010, a viral disease affecting cattle.

Another disease singled out for eradication was poliomyelitis, a highly contagious intestinal viral infection, which mainly affects children under the age of five and invades the central nervous system, destroying motor neurons and causing paralysis with a five to 10 percent risk of mortality when a patient's breathing muscles become immobilized. While there is no cure for the disease, an inactivated poliovirus vaccine (IPV) was pioneered by Jonas Salk (1914–1995) in the early 1950s, and a live attenuated oral polio vaccine (OPV) was developed by Albert Sabin (1906–1993) and licensed in 1962. OPV is considered the vaccine of choice in developing countries since it is less expensive and more effective at achieving herd resistance in populations with no history of immunization. While IPV is given by injection and requires trained health workers to administer, OPV is given orally. By 1979, polio had been eliminated from the United States and in 1988, the WHO spearheaded a Global Polio Eradication Initiative (GPEI), which has been highly successful. According to the WHO, there has been a decrease of over 99 percent globally from an estimated 350,000 cases in 1988 to 359 reported cases in 2014.

Despite the efforts of the GPEI, the wild poliovirus remains endemic in three countries: Nigeria, Afghanistan, and Pakistan. In May 2014, the WHO declared a global health emergency as the virus spread from infected countries into adjacent states. War-damaged health infrastructures and the anti-vaccination stance adopted by fundamentalist Islamic groups such as Islamic State of Iraq and the Levant (ISIL) in Syria and Iraq, al-Shabaab in Somalia, Boko Haram in northern Nigeria, and the Taliban in Afghanistan and Pakistan, have contributed to concerns about the re-emergence of polio across Asia and Africa. A UN agency report described a polio outbreak in Syria in early 2014 as being 'the most challenging outbreak in the history of polio eradication.'[100] Such examples suggest that the success of an eradication campaign is not simply a matter of scientific advances and financial resources: political circumstances are also crucial.

---

[99] Vivek Neelakantan, 'The Eradication of Smallpox in Indonesia.' In: Tim Harper and Sunil S. Amrith, eds., *Histories of Health in Southeast Asia: Perspective on the Long Twentieth Century* (Bloomington and Indianapolis: Indiana University Press, 2014), pp.149–153.

[100] Sam Jones, 'UN Brands Polio Outbreak in Syria and Iraq "Most Challenging in History",' *Guardian* (March 28, 2014).

Pakistan – one of the three countries where polio remains endemic – was established as an independent, predominantly Muslim state in 1947, as a result of the partition of India that followed independence from Britain. In 1956, it became an Islamic republic and after a civil war in 1971, East Pakistan broke away to become Bangladesh. The polio immunization program was launched in Pakistan in 1994 as part of the GPEI campaign with the support of WHO, Rotary International, the US CDC, and the UN Children's Fund (UNICEF). While the campaign in India has been overwhelmingly successful, the polio immunization campaign in Pakistan has met with opposition among some communities, notably the Taliban, adherents of a fundamentalist Islamic political movement (the word *taliban* in Arabic means 'student'). The center of this resistance has been in the province of Khyber Paktunkhwa (KP) and the country's Federally Administered Tribal Areas (FATA), a semi-autonomous region of Pakistan that borders Afghanistan in the northwest and includes the 'agencies' or districts of North and South Waziristan. Those involved in the anti-polio campaign are faced with mounting security challenges, while there are concerns that the influence of the Taliban may spread more widely through the region, undermining the ultimate success of the GPEI itself.[101]

The Taliban opposition to immunization has a number of causes: first, it is deemed *haram* or proscribed by Islam; second, it is widely believed to be a concerted Western strategy to sterilize Muslims; and third, the anti-polio campaign is considered a US ploy to gather intelligence. As we shall see, the use by the United States of unmanned aerial vehicles (UAVs) or 'drones' for counter-insurgency surveillance and targeted strikes has become associated in the eyes of some with the immunization program. Conventional explanations of local resistance to the immunization program in Pakistan, however, have tended to emphasize the Taliban's hostility to modernity and the group's rejection of the authority of the secular nation-state. The WHO's eradication initiative has been understood, from this perspective, as a significant push for 'hygienic modernity' in the face of pockets of antagonistic and recalcitrant 'backwardness,' epitomized by the war-torn 'tribal' areas of the subcontinent. Those in the developing world who resist the immunization drive are viewed as anti-progressive, fanatical, and refractory forces allied to 'terrorists.' In this way, the Taliban-dominated tribal areas of Pakistan have become emblematic for many Western commentators of a descent into what Bauman has called the 'no man's land' of the post-Cold War future.

---

[101] Dermot Maher, 'The Human Qualities Needed to Complete the Global Eradication of Polio,' *Bulletin of the World Health Organization*, vol.92, no.4 (2013): 283–289.

In these borderlands of the failing modern state, convictions in President George H. W. Bush's 'new world order' have given way to anxieties about the 'haphazard' emergence of a precarious, post-national global environment.[102]

While the Afghan–Pakistan border has long been viewed as a strategic zone, the ambiguous space of the borderland may itself be understood as a product of colonial rule. The FATA, which consists of seven tribal agencies and six frontier regions, was annexed from the Sikh Empire by the British as a bulwark against Afghanistan in the nineteenth century.[103] The imposition by the British of a formal border between Pakistan (then part of the British Raj) and Afghanistan (an independent emirate) in 1893, known as the Durand Line, sought to demarcate spheres of influence and reflected British concerns about Russia's expansion in Asia.[104] The formal imperial border was buttressed by tribal lands so that, in effect, the British 'created a bifurcated frontier, with an administrative one marking the end of colonial rule, and a political one marking the end of imperial rule. The space between these boundaries, though ruled by the colonial state, was in fact an imperial space. Consequently, the inhabitants of this space were not colonial subjects like the Indians of the South Asian plains, but rather were imperial objects.' The British governed there by co-opting native institutions, an arrangement set out in the Frontier Crimes Regulation (FCR) of 1901. As Benjamin Hopkins has observed, while this substantially reduced the cost of developing 'the expensive apparatus of the colonial state,' such indirect rule was also considered 'more effective, as it mediated colonial control through local institutions and personnel with embedded legitimacy in indigenous society.'[105] The FCR was critical in producing a form of 'frontier governmentality,' which was undergirded by assumptions about the inherent lawlessness of the 'tribal' lands and the belligerence of its Pashtun population.[106] The lawlessness of the borderland legitimated the colonial state's often violent interventions in the name of the law. In 1919, during the Third

---

[102] Alasdair Spark, 'Conjuring Order: The New World Order and Conspiracy Theories of Globalization.' In: Jane Parish and Martin Parker, eds., *The Age of Anxiety: Conspiracy Theory and the Human Sciences* (Oxford: Blackwell, 2001), pp. 46–62 (46–47).

[103] Sana Haroon, *Frontier of Faith: Islam in the Indo-Afghan Borderland* (New York: Columbia University Press, 2007), pp.4–6.

[104] Bijan Omrani, 'The Durand Line: History and Problems of the Afghan-Pakistan Border,' *Asian Affairs*, vol.40, no.2 (2009): 177–195.

[105] Benjamin Hopkins, 'The Frontier Crimes Regulation and Frontier Governmentality,' *Journal of Asian Studies*, vol.74, no.2 (2015): 369–389 (371, 369).

[106] Magnus Marsden and Benjamin D. Hopkins, *Fragments of the Afghan Frontier* (New York: Columbia University Press, 2011), pp.51–73.

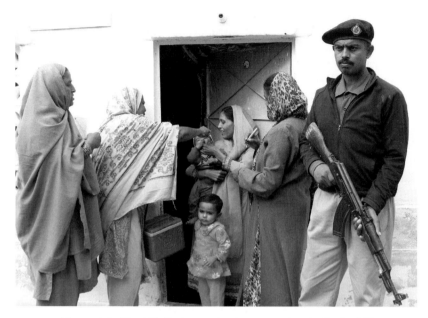

Figure 4.5. 'Anti-Polio immunization campaign in Surjani Town area in Karachi, Pakistan' (January 20, 2015). Courtesy: ppiimages/Demotix/Corbis.

Culture, belief, and immunization

Opposition to the polio immunization program in certain areas of Pakistan has demonstrated the suspicion and mistrust felt by some members of the community towards Western-led public health campaigns (Figure 4.5). It has also underlined the importance of deep-seated beliefs, cultural viewpoints, and value systems in shaping attitudes to vaccination. Controversies over the efficacy, safety, and morality of immunization are not confined to Asia or Africa. In Western countries, there has been opposition to vaccination since mandatory vaccination was first introduced in the mid nineteenth century. In 1853, a Vaccination Act in Britain made smallpox vaccination compulsory for infants. Religious arguments were advanced to contest vaccination. As the educator and diplomat Andrew Dickson White noted in 1910 in the United States, 'vague survivals of theological ideas' significantly impeded the advance of immunization, amounting to 'one of the most singular struggles of medical science during modern times.' In recent years, there has been resistance to vaccination initiatives on religious and other grounds. Opposition to a combined measles, mumps, and rubella vaccine (MMR), which was allegedly linked to autism, led to a drop in vaccination rate and a reported increase in incidence in Britain.

Paul A. Offit, *Bad Faith: When Religious Belief Undermines Modern Medicine* (New York: Basic Books, 2015).

Anglo-Afghan War, the Royal Air Force (RAF) bombarded Jalalabad and villages in Waziristan in order to establish effective 'air control.'[107]

Later in the twentieth century, the Afghan–Pakistan border area became a focal point during the Cold War. In 1979, the Soviet Union invaded Afghanistan, destabilizing the tribal lands. *Mujahideen*, or Muslim guerrilla fighters funded by the US Central Intelligence Agency (CIA), operated against the Soviets from across the border. After the Soviet withdrawal in 1989, a civil war ensued in Afghanistan, which saw the Taliban seize power. In the wake of the al-Qaeda initiated attacks on New York and Washington in September 2001, President George W. Bush declared a 'war on terror.' A US-led coalition force toppled the Taliban regime, which was giving safe refuge to members of al-Qaeda, a militant Islamist group founded in the late 1980s by Osama bin Laden ('al-Qaeda' means 'the base' in Arabic). Taliban militants and al-Qaeda operatives began crossing the border into Pakistan, using KP and South Waziristan in FATA as bases for incursions into Afghanistan. The borderland region was targeted in intensifying counter-insurgency operations by both the United States and Pakistan aimed at crushing the armed militancy and stemming the 'Talibanization' of the area.

Today, the 'tribal' areas of Pakistan are thus associated with a double-threat: that of terrorism and infectious disease. Since the late 1980s, the two have in fact been increasingly viewed as intertwined. Commentators in the West have warned of the global threat posed by destabilizing social, economic, and biological forces unleashed from the spaces of former colonial states. As the preface to the report *Emerging Infections: Microbial Threats to Health in the United States*, commissioned by the Institute of Medicine, noted in 1992,

---

[107] Brandon Marsh, *Ramparts of Empire: British Imperialism and India's Afghan Frontier, 1918–1948* (Basingstoke: Palgrave Macmillan, 2015), p.198.

in the context of infectious diseases, there is nowhere in the world from which we are remote and no one from whom we are disconnected. Consequently, some infectious diseases that now affect people in other parts of the world represent potential threats to the United States because of global interdependence, modern transportation, trade, and changing social and cultural patterns.[108]

Emerging infections are defined in relation to proliferating global inter-dependencies that imperil national security (Chapter 5). While transna-tional relations are recognized as underpinning the nation, generating its wealth and influence, they are simultaneously construed as pathways for 'foreign' toxic reverse-flows. The logic underpinning the 'battle against disease' formulated in the Institute of Medicine's report was pred-icated on the development of evermore innovative 'weapons' in the form of drugs, vaccines, and pesticides to beat off infection. Disease and war were conceived as cause and response to the spillover of global virulence. In 2000, the link between security and pandemic threat was made explicit when the UN Security Council adopted Resolution 1308, effectively framing HIV/AIDS in security terms. While the 9/11 attacks spurred the establishment of the Global Health Security Initiative (GHSI) – an international collaboration that sought to boost global security against imminent bio-terrorist threats – the remit of the GHSI was extended in 2002 to encompass pandemic influenza. Subsequent outbreaks of SARS and avian influenza also underscored the security challenge that pan-demics represent, not only to Southeast Asia, but to countries around the world.[109]

In Pakistan, the drive to contain and eliminate forms of militant Islam, which threaten to diffuse across the wider region, has coincided with a concerted campaign to eradicate virulent disease, which likewise endan-gers Asia and the world. This conflation has not been one sided. If US politicians and officials have linked the campaigns, emphasizing the secu-rity dimension of both missions, opponents of the US counter-insurgency operation have also viewed the immunization program as an extension of the military conflict. In the eyes of many US critics, this connection seemed borne out by the assassination of Osama bin Laden, leader of al-Qaeda, in an assault on his secret compound in Bilal Town, Abbot-tabad, northern Pakistan, by US Navy SEALs in May 2011 – an episode portrayed in the 2012 US movie *Zero Dark Thirty* directed by Kathryn Bigelow.

---

[108] Joshua Lederberg and Robert E. Shope, 'Preface.' In: Lederberg, Shope, and Oaks, eds., *Emerging Infections*, pp.v–viii (v).

[109] Yanzhong Huang, 'Pandemics and Security.' In: Rushton and Youde, eds., *Routledge Handbook of Global Health Security*, pp.83–91.

A Pakistani physician had been recruited by the CIA to head a spurious hepatitis B immunization campaign, which was part of a covert operation to confirm bin Laden's presence in the compound. The fake program was even started 'in a poorer part of town to make it look more authentic,' with posters put up that featured a vaccine made by Amson Vaccines & Pharma (Pvt) Ltd, a Pakistani pharmaceutical company. Local government health workers were paid to participate in the operation.[110] The disclosure of the Pakistani physician Shakil Afridi's involvement in tracking down bin Laden under the aegis of the CIA (and, in his own admission, through the intercession of the NGO Save the Children Fund) led to international concerns that public health campaigns in the region – and in particular the polio immunization program – were now jeopardized through their association with US intelligence agencies and the military.[111] In light of the anti-vaccine conspiracy theories circulating in the developing world, the CIA plot involving a sham vaccination program exacerbated tensions and played into the hands of the anti-polio campaign's detractors. Following the 9/11 attacks, rumors had circulated in Pakistan that the United States was using immunization as a cover to sterilize the local population. Opposition to immunization on religious grounds gathered momentum. In 2007, Abdul Ghani Marwat, the director of a government vaccination program in the FATA's Bajaur Agency, was killed.[112] After the assassination of bin Laden, however, this opposition intensified as Taliban leaders issued *fatwas* (Islamic religious decrees) against vaccination, and incidents of kidnapping and violent attacks on health workers and their security increased sharply.

In the aftermath of bin Laden's killing, Pakistan's anti-polio campaign came under pressure as communities in KP and other areas became reluctant to immunize their children, prompting a message of reassurance from the WHO. In early June 2012, a key Pakistani Taliban commander, Hafiz Gul Bahadur, halted the vaccination campaign in North Waziristan until US drone strikes ceased, arguing that the health initiative could be used by Western forces as a cover for espionage.[113] A few weeks later, Mullah Nazir, another Taliban leader, banned polio vaccinations in South Waziristan. A link has repeatedly been made by critics of the immunization campaign between the Predator drone attacks and polio

[110] Saeed Shah, 'CIA Organised Fake Vaccination Drive to Get Osama bin Laden's Family DNA,' *Guardian* (July 11, 2011).
[111] Jeffrey Kluger, 'Polio and Politics,' *Time* (January 14, 2013).
[112] Haider J. Warraich, 'Religious Opposition to Polio Vaccination,' *Emerging Infectious Diseases*, vol.15, no.6 (June 2009): 978.
[113] Declan Walsh, 'UN Suspends Immunization Work in Pakistan,' *New York Times* (December 19, 2012).

vaccinations. Between 2004 – when George W. Bush launched the first covert drone strike inside Pakistan – and 2012, there were an estimated 307 drone attacks, with the number escalating markedly from January 2009 when Barack Obama assumed the US presidency.[114] As Donald McNeil has suggested, overlapping technologies and protocols connect both activities, including the fact that health workers carried global positioning system (GPS) devices, even as drones used GPS coordinates to target militants.[115] Western newspaper reports conflating drone surveillance and counter-insurgency activities with polio immunization reinforce local misgivings. Thus, Pakistan is described by *Time* magazine as 'the ground zero' of polio, while a language of 'surgical strikes' is employed in relation to the midwives who are equipped which GPS-enabled cellphones to 'target their efforts more precisely.'[116] In December 2012, the vaccination campaign in Pakistan, involving some 225,000 vaccinators, was suspended following the murder of nine vaccination workers, six of whom were young women. Since 2013, there has been a spate of attacks on polio vaccination teams. In February 2015, four members of a team were abducted and killed by Taliban militants in Baluchistan, while in March 2015 gunmen shot two female polio workers in KP.[117] In 2014, there were 306 reported cases of wild polio in Pakistan, the highest in 14 years. However, in 2015, there was a marked fall in cases, as a consequence of a military push into Taliban-held territory, which allowed health workers to reach previously unvaccinated areas.

Viral chatter: Epidemic intelligence on the frontline

There is a close connection between epidemic surveillance technologies and military intelligence. Many technologies developed in a military context subsequently migrate into mainstream public health. The use of satellite imaging and Internet data trawling, for example, are now central to disease preparedness and prevention. Over the last decade, virologists have sought to develop

---

[114] Peter Bergen and Jennifer Rowland, 'CIA Drone Strikes and the Taliban.' In: Peter Bergen with Katherine Tiedemann, eds., *Talibanistan: Negotiating the Borders Between Terror, Politics, and Religion* (Oxford and New York: Oxford University Press, 2013), pp.229–236 (229–230).

[115] Donald G. McNeil, 'Fighting Polio, as well as Suspicion,' *International Herald Tribune* (December 26, 2012).

[116] Jeffrey Kluger, 'The Battle to Eradicate Polio in Pakistan,' *Time* (July 29, 2014).

[117] 'Gunmen Kill Health Workers From Pakistan Polio Drive,' *New York Times* (March 17, 2015).

a pre-emptive capacity, using bush hunters as sentinels for monitoring unusual intensities of 'chatter' between humans and wildlife viruses. The term 'viral chatter' has been used by the epidemiologist and virologist Donald S. Burke to describe this cross-species traffic. 'We're seeing lots of these cross-species interactions now in Southeast Asia,' Burke has remarked and he has been explicit about the term's military provenance: 'I call it "viral chatter" because it's like the terrorist "chatter" that goes on over the airwaves and suggests something serious is just around the corner.' The aim is to establish 'listening posts' or sentinels in hotspots around the world in order to identify unusual occurrences near their point of origin, analyze the data on site, and feed the information back to a central command, which would trigger an alarm for potential epidemic disease threats. Burke's former student and collaborator, Nathan Wolfe, has also been explicit about the military prehistory of the 'viral chatter' technology, noting that it seeks to monitor samples for early warnings of a pandemic, just as analysts 'at the National Security Agency (NSA) scour the Internet, listening for clues of impending terrorist attacks.' As Wolfe puts it, the goal 'is to find these new viruses before they make it through to the blood banks, airplanes, sexual networks.' What are the consequences of framing virology as a counter-insurgency operation, particularly in regions where viral and terrorist threats converge, such as the Taliban in Pakistan or Boko Haram in Nigeria? Today the biological and the social are being securitized through a newly reconfigured discourse of lethal emergence.

Nathan D. Wolfe, et al., 'Bushmeat Hunting, Deforestation, and Prediction of Zoonotic Disease,' *Emerging Infectious Diseases*, vol.11, no.12 (December 2005): 1822–1827.

Bush's 'war on terror' and a Cold War politics provide one context for the military conflict in northwest Pakistan. It was during the Cold War that the United States developed its counter-terrorism apparatus to meet the challenges of unconventional warfare and in particular to ensure a 'balance of terror' in the face of an existential nuclear threat. Given the prospect of nuclear annihilation, the focus shifted to pre-emption. The 'war on terror,' according to Joseph Masco, 'is thus the ideological fulfillment of the Cold War state project, creating an institutional commitment to permanent militarization through an ever-expanding universe of threat identification and response.' This pre-emptive anti-terror drive, which has extended to a 'planetary theater of operations,' is evident not only in anti-terrorist missions, but in the handling of every kind of emergent terror threat: from natural disasters to incipient pandemics.[118]

There is also a pre-Cold War context for the conflict in the borderlands. Anti-vaccination movements in the subcontinent have a deep colonial history. In the imperial world, mass-immunization programs targeting indigenous peoples often assumed a coercive character. The colonial state's vaccinating drive in India was part of a distinctive 'civilizing mission' and as such belongs to what Gyan Prakash has called a 'grid,' which is 'a coherent strategy of power and identity underpinned by an ideology of modernity that is legitimated in the last instance by science.'[119] In the nineteenth century, the colonial state was faced with numerous difficulties in implementing policy and vaccination was slow to gain acceptance. There were conflicting interests between different government departments, and often glaring disparities between policies and their execution. Producing, storing, and delivering effective vaccines posed logistical challenges.[120] Colonial medicine was also faced with 'a rival prophylactic practice in inoculation and a rival agency in the indigenous variolators.'[121] Resistance to smallpox vaccination – as opposed to inoculation with 'variolous matter' taken from infected individuals, in a process known as 'variolation' – was grounded on cultural and religious convictions. Until the widespread use of calf lymph for vaccination, the arm-to-arm method was adopted, which 'transferred body fluids directly from one individual to another.' As Arnold has observed, 'for most Hindus this was offensively polluting, especially since lower-caste or Untouchable children were often the only vaccinifers available.' There were objections to the use of calf lymph, similarly on religious grounds during the 1870s and 1880s, given the sacred nature of the cow in Hinduism. Above all, vaccination was opposed for what Arnold has called its 'raw secularity.' Since there was no ritual associated with vaccination, it was deemed to be 'irreligious': 'It treated smallpox purely as a disease, stripped of any religious significance – if indeed it was seen to have any connection with disease at all and not to be merely the 'mark' the colonial state made on its subjects.' Rumors held that colonial vaccination was a strategy for undermining caste and religion and propagating Christianity. There was

---

[118] Joseph Masco, *The Theater of Operations: National Security Affect from the Cold War to the War on Terror* (Durham, NC: Duke University Press, 2014), pp.37, 187–189.

[119] Gyan Prakash, *Another Reason: Science and the Imagination of Modern India* (Princeton, NJ: Princeton University Press, 1999), p.3.

[120] Sanjoy Bhattacharya, Mark Harrison, and Michael Worboys, *Fractured States: Smallpox, Public Health and Vaccination Policy in British India, 1800–1947* (Hyderabad: Orient Longman, 2005).

[121] David Arnold, 'Smallpox and Colonial Medicine in Nineteenth-Century India.' In: Arnold, ed., *Imperial Medicine*, pp.45–65 (46).

also a belief that vaccination 'was a prelude to a new impost or forced labor overseas.' Yet, in the end, vaccination involved a 'tacit compromise' between colonized and colonizers with vaccination being combined with Hindu rituals hitherto associated with variolation and with the Hindu goddess Sitala Mata.[122]

Notwithstanding these challenges, however, the colonial anti-smallpox campaign 'entailed a degree of state medical intervention unparalleled until the anti-plague campaigns of the late 1890s.'[123] Moreover, resistance to vaccination in India did not end with colonial rule. There was opposition to the WHO's global smallpox immunization program, which had been instituted in the 1960s and intensified in the mid 1970s, when the Indian government launched the 'Operation Smallpox Zero' campaign. Healthcare workers led by foreign epidemiologists acting as 'advisors,' who were unfamiliar with local languages and customs, adopted increasingly invasive measures; in places where smallpox was detected, members of the entire community were vaccinated whatever their immune status.[124] Houses were searched, as were schools, markets, and Sitala Mata temples. 'At times,' one WHO publication conceded, 'the efforts in India looked like a military campaign. Occasionally WHO workers were called upon to use strong-arm tactics and forced vaccination, when there was resistance.'[125] As William Muraskin has argued, many of the 'eradicationists' involved in the smallpox program spearheaded the polio program in the 1980s, changing global priorities from primary healthcare to a vertical 'eradication' agenda. As such, the 'war' against polio could be said to represent 'an ideological project' with antecedents in the smallpox program.[126]

Eradication efforts are often described, at least by Western commentators, in relation to a grand narrative of closure. Yet the threat of bioterrorism has undermined many of the assumptions of final closure that have driven eradication programs. The framing of immunization by sections of Pakistani society as a political act needs to be understood, I suggest, within the broader context of a discourse of emergence that, at least

---

[122] Arnold, *Colonizing the Body*, pp.141–144.

[123] Arnold, 'Smallpox and Colonial Medicine in Nineteenth-Century India.' In: Arnold, ed., *Imperial Medicine*, p.45.

[124] Paul Greenough, 'Intimidation, Coercion and Resistance in the Final Stages of the South Asian Smallpox Eradication Campaign, 1973–1975,' *Social Science & Medicine*, vol.41, no.5 (1995): 633–645.

[125] *Bugs, Drugs and Smoke: Stories from Public Health* (Geneva: World Health Organization, 2011), pp.14–15.

[126] William A. Muraskin, *Polio Eradication and Its Discontents: An Historian's Journey Through an International Public Health (Un)Civil War* (Hyderabad: Orient Blackswan, 2012), p.35.

since the 1990s, has associated infection with conflict, and located the potential for global destabilization within former colonial spaces in Asia and Africa. At the same time, responding to disease emergence as a homeland security threat is fundamentally counter-productive since meeting the challenge of epidemic disease, like tackling climate change, ultimately requires 'a willingness to substitute global concerns for national interests.'[127]

Explanations of the polio controversy as a conflict between, on the one hand, a secular and progressive scientific worldview and, on the other hand, blinkered conviction and prejudice, ignore the overlaps and shared assumptions that underpin both perspectives. Both may be seen as responses to the contaminated reverse-flows of globalization. While the United States is intent on closing off the pathways of communicable disease and eliminating infectious radicalization, the 'militant' Taliban seek to oppose and eradicate an encroaching secular modernity. An analysis of the socio-cultural contexts of the polio controversy, and the framing of 'infection' in terms of a terror-menace, thus helps to illuminate deep-rooted and often unhelpful suppositions about disease and political order that continue to shape policy and mold local, national, and international perspectives on health and security in the contemporary world. It also points to the ways in which colonial and imperial histories continue to shape the present. As the historians Frederick Cooper and Jane Burbank have remarked,

imperial name-calling – invocations of the word *empire* or *colonialism* to discredit interventions by American, French, or other governments – does not provide means to analyze or improve today's world. But an exploration of the histories of empires, both old and recent, can expand our understanding of how the world came to be what it is and open a wider perspective on the organization of political power in the past, present, and, perhaps, future.[128]

Conclusion: State-making, conflict, and disease

In this chapter, we have explored the history of four different epidemics – of cholera, plague, typhus, and polio – in relation to four very different types of conflict: a campaign of colonization in the Philippines, epidemic prevention in the contested terrain of Manchuria, an RC humanitarian effort in the Russian Far East, and a US-led eradication program in the tribal border areas of Afghanistan and Pakistan, which is also the theater

---

[127] Masco, *The Theater of Operations*, p.110.
[128] Frederick Cooper and Jane Burbank, 'The Empire Effect,' *Public Culture*, vol.24, no.2 (2012): 239–247 (239).

of a US counter-insurgency operation. These four cases illustrate a number of key issues. Most obviously, they underline the political dimension of medical and public health technologies, which are deployed by state agencies to contain disease episodes through the management of populations. As we saw in Manchuria and the Russian Far East, these technologies – exemplified by the 'Great White Train' as an emblem of hygienic modernity – serve ideological ends, too. Wars are fought, not only on the battlefield, but through science and the proprietorial claims that it makes on the 'truth.' What is being contested by the opponents of the immunization campaign in Pakistan is precisely the claims made by science and modern biomedicine to neutrality.

War and infectious diseases are intertwined on numerous levels. Conflict places stress on state systems, reducing their capacity to deal with disease; the movement of troops and the displacement of civilians may facilitate the spread of infection; and the destruction wrought by war may create an environment for disease agents to flourish in the absence of vector control. The very language of epidemic prevention points to the militarization of health and epidemic prevention, with its emphasis on 'campaigns,' 'fights,' 'eradication,' and 'targeting.' The experience of war has shaped the ways in which infectious diseases have been understood and ultimately how they have been managed in peacetime, just as epidemic control measures have influenced the techniques of war.

In each of the four case studies, past contexts fed into and shaped present epidemics, best demonstrated perhaps in the Taliban's hostility to polio vaccination, which reprises earlier colonial campaigns of vaccination on the subcontinent. This colonial dimension of the war–epidemic matrix in Asia is an important theme: from the full-out US colonial war against Filipino nationalists at the turn of the nineteenth and twentieth centuries, to Japanese and Russian imperialist ambitions in Manchuria, and Western concerns about the balance of power in East Asia following the October Revolution in Russia in 1917. A coercive colonial agenda was integrated into science, medicine, and public health; state authority was thereby naturalized, coming to seem inevitable and therefore incontrovertible. Wu Lien-teh's anti-plague measures involved the employment of quasi-colonial technologies that extended the authority of the Qing state, even while this enlargement of power was justified on the grounds of being modern, progressive, and disinterested. A colonial legacy shaped non-state actors, as well, including peace-building and humanitarian agencies, such as the Red Cross, involved in relief and development work across Asia.

There is a tendency to think of wars as inter-state conflicts – in terms, that is, of invasion and defense. This is a border-centered view of conflict, which reaffirms the apportionment of the world into taken-for-granted sovereign states. While Asia is conventionally conceived as an aggregate of discrete nation-states, such a state-oriented view ignores minority populations and areas where allegiance to the state is weak and in many instances rejected. Large portions of mainland Southeast Asia, for example, are rugged and remote from central government and in this sense are only partially governed. The anthropologist James C. Scott has suggested that the vast mountainous region, which extends from China to the Central Highlands of Vietnam and northeastern India, across swathes of Cambodia, Laos, Thailand, and Burma, has historically been populated by peoples in search of self-determination. Rather than viewing the history of Asia from a lowland, state-centric perspective, Scott invites us to view this region from the standpoint of stateless peoples who have consciously sought to evade 'the oppressions of state-making projects': slavery, conscription, taxes, statute labor, warfare, and epidemics.[129]

The assimilationist drive of the modern state and the process of state-making itself may be thought of as a form of 'internal colonialism.' There are many examples of conflicts in Asia between state agencies pushing for assimilation and fugitive or marooned communities who have sought to elude state control and fight for their autonomy. Often such conflicts are fueled by ethnic or religious divisions, as is the case in the predominantly Muslim southern Philippines, where indigenous ethnic groups have long been at war with the central government in Manila. In Sri Lanka, where the majority of the population is Sinhalese, the government was involved in a 25-year campaign (which ended in 2009) to quash rebel forces of the Liberation Tigers of Tamil Eelam, known as the 'Tamil Tigers,' who were fighting for the independence of the Tamil minority in the northeast of the island state.

In the Cold War period, ideological divisions tore countries apart. In Cambodia, the Communist Party of Kampuchea – better known as the Khmer Rouge – seized power in 1975 after a civil war. Under the leadership of Pol Pot (1925–1998), Cambodia was effectively closed off from the world. Private property was abolished and citizens were 'evacuated' from cities and towns to the countryside, where they were forced to work on the land in rural cooperatives. Malaria and infectious diarrheal diseases took their toll. Over 1.5 million people are estimated to have died in this state-sponsored genocide – many from forced labor, starvation, and disease, as well as those executed in the notorious 'killing fields.' Following a Vietnamese invasion in 1979, the Khmer Rouge regime fell,

129 Scott, *The Art of Not Being Governed*, p.ix.

leading to a refugee crisis as people fled across the border into Thailand. There, epidemic disease afflicted the internees of crowded camps.[130]

The violence that stems from resistance to the centripetal pull of the modern state often drives epidemic disease. One such case is the conflict in Burma, a country that is characterized by considerable ethnic diversity and contains numerous minority groups. Like many sovereign states in Asia, Burma was formerly a colony, acquiring its independence from Britain in 1948. A military coup in 1962, however, overthrew a democratically elected government and installed a military dictatorship. The latest military junta, installed in 1988, was officially dissolved in 2011. Although power continues to be wielded by the military with a nominally civilian government, in general elections held in 2015, Aung San Suu Kyi's National League for Democracy (NLD) won a landslide victory.

Under military rule, the country's name was officially changed from 'Burma' (as it was known during colonial times) to 'Myanmar,' although political and ethnic opposition groups refused to recognize the change. While the resistance by ethnic minorities to integration into the Burmese state predated the military regime, intensified campaigns to quash ethnic movements from the 1990s to the early 2000s led to an escalation of violence, particularly along the country's eastern border, which is home to ethnic groups, including the Shan. There, the Burmese military adopted a strategy of concerted depopulation as part of a counter-insurgency drive, and the UN and other organizations have reported systematic human rights violations.

The conflict in Burma has led to the displacement of hundreds of thousands of ethnic peoples. Many have been forcefully relocated into new settlements, while thousands have fled their homes, crossing the border or retreating into the remoter interior regions of the country. In such settings, there is little access to essential healthcare, while the military have consistently blocked any foreign humanitarian assistance. The result has been a high prevalence of HIV/AIDS, TB, malaria, as well as neglected tropical diseases (NTDs) among refugee communities.[131]

The Muslim Rohingyas, who live in the northern Burmese state of Rakhine (formerly known as Arakan) on the border with Bangladesh, are a particularly discriminated ethnic group in Burma. Classified as 'resident foreigners' by the Burmese state, they are denied citizenship and as

---

[130] Ben Kiernan, *The Pol Pot Regime: Race, Power, and Genocide in Cambodia under the Khmer Rouge, 1975–79*. Third edition (New Haven, CT: Yale University Press, 2008), pp.236, 456–460.

[131] Chris Beyrer and Thomas J. Lee, 'Responding to Infectious Diseases in Burma and Her Border Regions,' *Conflict and Health*, vol.2, no.2 (2008): doi: 10.1186/1752–1505–2-2.

a consequence face numerous restrictions on basic rights, including the freedom of movement, ownership of property, access to healthcare and education. Their plight gained international attention following an escalation of sectarian violence and riots in 2012, when ethnic Buddhists targeted Rohingya communities and some 140,000 Rohingyas were forced into government-designated refugee camps, where access to humanitarian agencies is limited and subject to government approval. In the unsanitary conditions of these makeshift camps, malnourished refugees are susceptible to water-borne diseases, particularly during the monsoon months. Perhaps as many as 400,000 Rohingyas have fled to Bangladesh and Malaysia. In the summer of 2015, widespread media coverage of emaciated Rohingyas – many of whom were sick – left adrift on crowded boats by traffickers in the Andaman Sea and the Strait of Malacca, refocused attention onto their plight.

The interethnic strife in Burma reminds us of the complex ways in which violence can increase vulnerability to disease. Populations are displaced and relocated to refugee camps, where poor sanitation increases exposure to infections and drives transmission. Government obstruction and a lack of civil rights impede disease surveillance and research, incapacitating healthcare systems, and hindering humanitarian assistance. In an extreme form, the Burmese military's effort to subjugate minority groups lays bare the coercive dimension of all state-making projects that are predicated on assimilation.

This internal conflict in Burma has had repercussions on neighboring countries. In Malaysia and Thailand, undocumented people who have fled across the border from persecution in Burma are not considered to be legitimate refugees and live without the protection that a legal status would confer. Regarded as 'economic migrants,' they are cut off from healthcare services and often exploited. Research has shown that these displaced communities suffer from a disproportionate burden of disease, including HIV/AIDS and TB. The prevalence of undetected infections within Thailand also threatens to undermine Thailand's success in preventing and managing epidemics.[132]

The Burmese case underscores the shifting scales of violence and disease, as people and pathogens move across borders. While viruses and infection have long been considered 'apt metaphors for processes and objects of border crossing, travel, and migration,' today they have become a means of articulating concerns about the impact of globalization and, in

---

[132] Voravit Suwanvanichkij, 'Displacement and Disease: The Shan Exodus and Infectious Disease Implications for Thailand,' *Conflict and Health*, vol.2, no.4 (2008): doi:10.1186/1752–1505–2–4.

particular, about 'life in the contact zone' where containment becomes impossible.[133] As the philosophers Gilles Deleuze and Félix Guattari have noted, the terms 'contagion' and 'epidemic' indicate difference, heterogeneity, and the anomalous.[134] The 'battle' against polio, like the 'war against terror,' exemplifies the challenges posed to containment on the borderlands of the modern state. Or rather, the contestations over polio immunization expose the flip-side of state-making: 'terrorists' are those who have opted to live outside the mechanisms of modern statehood and strive to remain 'ungoverned.'

[133] Ruth Mayer, 'Virus Discourse: The Rhetoric of Threat and Terrorism in the Biothriller,' *Cultural Critique*, vol.66 (2007): 1–20 (1).

[134] Gilles Deleuze and Félix Guattari, *A Thousand Plateaus: Capitalism and Schizophrenia*. Translated by Brian Massumi (London and New York: Continuum, 2004), p.267.

5   Globalization

From the 1930s, Asia was at the forefront of an international push for development. Across the region, there was an emphasis on tackling infectious diseases, particularly in the period after the Second World War, which witnessed anti-colonial struggles in many Asian countries and the rise of ambitious global programs of disease prevention.[1] In April 1948, the Health Organization of the League of Nations was transformed into the WHO, reflecting an optimism about the prospect of controlling infectious diseases by deploying the tools of modern biomedicine and public health, especially antibiotics, vaccines, and drugs, as well as DDT (dichlorodiphenyltrichloroethane), an insecticide widely used to combat malaria. Eradication – the 'reduction of the worldwide incidence of a disease to zero as a result of deliberate efforts' – became the avowed goal of international health organizations and national governments. In 1972, the virologist and Nobel laureate Sir Frank Macfarlane Burnet (1899–1985) posed the question, 'On the basis of what has happened in the last thirty years, can we forecast any likely developments for the 1970s?' To which he answered: 'If for the present we retain a basic optimism and assume no major catastrophes occur and that any wars are kept at the "brush fire" level, the most likely forecast about the future of infectious disease is that it will be very dull.'[2]

Post-Second World War optimism was embodied in the Declaration of Alma-Ata, the outcome of an international conference convened in September 1978 in Kazakhstan. In the Declaration, WHO member-states along with numerous international organizations affirmed the UN's definition of health as a 'fundamental human right' and launched a global campaign of 'Health for All by the Year 2000.' As the science journalist Laurie Garrett has observed, 'The goal was nothing less than pushing

---

[1] Sunil S. Amrith, *Decolonizing International Health: India and Southeast Asia, 1930–65* (Basingstoke and New York: Palgrave Macmillan, 2006).
[2] Sir Macfarlane Burnet and David O. White, *Natural History of Infectious Disease.* Fourth edition (Cambridge: Cambridge University Press, [1940] 1972), p.263.

humanity through what was termed the "health transition," leaving the age of infectious disease permanently behind.'[3]

There was political significance in the decision to hold the conference in Kazakhstan, a Central Asian country with a common border with China, which was then part of the Soviet Union. Given global health disparities, the WHO had studied a number of developing countries that had successfully implemented local-level health campaigns. In particular, China's national 'barefoot doctors' policy from the late 1960s influenced WHO's global Health for All program.[4] So-called 'barefoot doctors' (*chijiao yisheng*) were farmers who had received rudimentary medical training and were dispatched to rural areas of the country, where there were no qualified physicians. The Rural Co-operative Medical System in the PRC, from the 1950s through the 1970s, provided the first comprehensive health coverage that extended from county level to commune and village.[5] The success of these community paramedics, whose focus was primarily on preventive care and health education, was extolled in movies such as *Spring Shoots* (1976). There, a young woman from the countryside is inspired to become a doctor after witnessing the death of an infant in a local hospital. Ironically, the Declaration of Alma-Ata took place precisely as Deng Xiaoping (1904–1997) launched his economic policy of 'reform and opening to the outside,' which was ultimately to lead to the dismantling of the PRC's health system.

On December 9, 1979, the year after the importance of primary healthcare was affirmed at Alma-Ata (today's Almaty), a WHO commission certified the eradication of smallpox. Both events appeared to represent critical milestones on the road to global health equity, holding out the prospect that other infectious diseases would follow smallpox and be consigned to history. This optimism, however, proved to be premature and soon faded. In 1976, an outbreak in Zaire (now the Democratic Republic of the Congo) and Sudan of Ebola, an acute febrile disease, marked the appearance of a lethal new viral infection. Ebola was to be one of an increasing number of such 'emerging diseases' that made their appearance from the 1970s. It has been estimated that over 60 percent of new emerging diseases are zoonotic and of the nearly 1,400 known

---

[3] Laurie Garrett, 'The Return of Infectious Disease,' *Foreign Affairs*, no.74, no.1 (January/February 1996): 66–79 (66).

[4] Sung Lee, 'WHO and the Developing World: The Contest for Ideology.' In: Andrew Cunningham and Bridie Andrews, eds., *Western Medicine as Contested Knowledge* (Manchester: Manchester University Press, 1997), pp.24–45.

[5] Xiaoping Fang, 'Barefoot Doctors and the Provision of Rural Health Care.' In: Andrews and Bullock, eds., *Medical Transitions in Twentieth-Century China*, pp.267–282.

human pathogens, 87 new species have been recognized since 1980.[6] They are 'new,' not in the sense that they have suddenly materialized, but rather in the sense that they have '"come into view" in the communities threatened by them.'[7] It would seem likely, for example, that there had been outbreaks of NiV before 1999 in the subcontinent, even though the virus was only formally identified as 'Nipah' in Malaysia in 1999.

Although the term 'emerging' had been applied to disease from the 1960s, the notion of 'emerging infections' and 'emerging viruses' gained currency after the May 1989 conference 'Emerging Viruses: The Evolution of Viruses and Viral Disease' convened in Washington, DC. The writer Richard Preston captured the dread provoked by the global spread of these novel hemorrhagic fevers – including the Ebola and Marburg viruses – in his quasi-fictional thriller *The Hot Zone: A Terrifying True Story*, published in 1994. 'Crashing' into the human race from faraway tropical rainforests, Preston describes how these biosafety level 4 (BSL-4) viruses endanger the developed world. They are, he argues, 'a natural consequence of the ruin of the tropical biosphere. The emerging viruses are surfacing from ecologically damaged parts of the earth.'[8] The 'damaged parts of the earth' from which this new viral menace is materializing are also, for the most part, struggling postcolonial states. Significantly, a discourse of 'emerging infections' overlaps with a discourse of 'emerging markets,' the latter term coined by the World Bank in 1981 as an alternative to 'Third World.'

Above all, it was HIV/AIDS in the early 1980s that focused attention back onto the global threat posed by infectious diseases. As the US Institute of Medicine's report *Emerging Infections* noted in 1992, 'there is nowhere in the world from which we are remote and no one from whom we are disconnected.' Writing in the foreword to the proceedings of the 1989 Washington conference, the microbiologist Richard M. Krause asserted: 'Like science, emerging viruses know no country. There are no barriers to prevent their migration across international boundaries or around the 24 time zones.'[9] In fact, a decade earlier, just as the HIV/AIDS epidemic was beginning in the United States, Krause had sounded a warning. The eradication of smallpox, the impact of antibiotics, and the development of vaccines against diseases, such as

---

[6] Mark Woolhouse and Eleanor Gaunt, 'Ecological Origins of Novel Human Pathogens,' *Critical Reviews in Microbiology*, vol.33, no.4 (2007): 231–242.

[7] D. Ann Herring and Stacy Lockerbie, 'The Coming Plague of Avian Influenza.' In: Herring and Swedlund, eds., *Plagues and Epidemics*, pp.179–191 (179).

[8] Richard Preston, *The Hot Zone: A Terrifying True Story* (New York: Random House, 1994), p.405.

[9] Richard M. Krause, 'Foreword.' In: Stephen S. Morse, ed., *Emerging Viruses* (New York: Oxford University Press, 1993), pp.xvii–xix (xvii).

diphtheria, measles, tetanus, typhoid, polio, and yellow fever may have been spectacularly successful, but according to Krause these advances had created a false sense of security.[10]

As medical research began to refocus onto chronic and degenerative diseases, HIV/AIDS served as a reminder that infectious diseases continued to present a real challenge. HIV/AIDs demonstrated how local events could rapidly amplify into global crises as a result of 'global interdependence, modern transportation, trade, and changing social and cultural patterns.'[11] At the same time, as Preston concluded, HIV/AIDS was arguably 'the worst environmental disaster of the twentieth century.'[12] It was against this background that the 1990s saw the formulation of an 'emerging diseases worldview,' along with an increasing emphasis on the need to understand the global processes driving microbial traffic.[13] Informing this new worldview was a preoccupation with preparing for a potentially catastrophic outbreak. The idea of 'preparedness' became central to planning and was linked to biosecurity concerns, particularly after the terrorist attacks against the US in September 2001. As Andrew Lakoff has observed, 'a norm of preparedness came to structure thought about threats to public health'; 'preparedness' called forth a set of responses that drew on military models of intelligence-gathering and counter-insurgency to combat epidemic disease through pre-emptive action (Chapter 4).[14]

HIV/AIDS also created a context for reappraising past pandemics. Although originally published in 1976, Alfred Crosby's account of the 1918–1919 influenza, *Epidemic and Peace*, was reissued in 1989 with a preface that drew connections between HIV/AIDS and the so-called 'Spanish Flu.' In a second 2003 edition, Crosby set the experience of 1918–1919 within an even more encompassing historical sweep: AIDS, antibiotic-resistant TB, Lyme disease, West Nile fever, Ebola, and SARS. 'The flu virus seems a poor choice for bioterrorism,' he noted, 'but our "globalized" transportation systems increase the probability of natural pandemics of influenza. In 1918 the fastest way to cross oceans was by steamship. In 2003, thousands of us daily and tens of millions of us annually make such trips in aircraft at speeds not far short of that of sound,

---

[10] Richard M. Krause, *The Restless Tide: The Persistent Challenge of the Microbial World* (Washington, DC: National Foundation for Infectious Diseases, 1981).

[11] Lederberg and Shope, 'Preface.' In: Lederberg, Shope, and Oaks, eds., *Emerging Infections*, p.v.

[12] Preston, *The Hot Zone*, p.407.

[13] Nicholas B. King, 'Security, Disease, Commerce: Ideologies of Postcolonial Global Health,' *Social Studies of Science*, vol.32, nos.5/6 (2002): 763–789.

[14] Andrew Lakoff, 'The Generic Biothreat, or, How We Became Unprepared,' *Cultural Anthropology*, vol.23, no.3 (2008): 399–428 (401).

carrying with us in our lungs and bowels, on our hands and in our hair, micro-organisms of all kinds, including pathogens. We are all, so to speak, sitting in the waiting room of an enormous clinic, elbow to elbow with the sick of the world.'[15]

This chapter explores the interrelationship between globalization and epidemics in Asia against the background of these late twentieth-century anxieties about emerging infections. Developing the themes from the last case studies, the chapter considers the tensions between an increasingly global disease ecology and the local contexts that shape how diseases are understood and responded to. Given that infections diffuse across national boundaries and populations, they call for coordinated global responses. Yet individuals and communities continue to inhabit institutional and social spaces defined predominantly by the operations of the territorial state. Globalization in this sense connotes not only the dissolution of borders but their re-inscription in state efforts to impose limits on a borderless world. To introduce this last theme, we consider the 1918–1919 influenza pandemic and the critical issues that it raises about Asia's integration into a world system, with a particular emphasis on India. The first case study examines epidemics of HIV/AIDS in the PRC, tracking connections between China's post-socialist market liberalization from the late 1970s, the social transformations that resulted from this process, and the spread of disease. The focus is on the links between HIV/AIDS and the sex work industry, the plasma economy, and intravenous (IV) drug users. HIV/AIDS provides a lens for examining the connections between modernity, capitalism, and globalization in relation to the evolving role of the state.

A particular concern in this chapter is with zoonotic diseases. Why is Asia a 'hotspot' for emerging infections of animal origin? I address this question directly in the second and third case studies by considering the effects of globalization across the region, specifically in relation to avian influenza from the mid 1990s and SARS in 2002–2003. This section also interrogates the links between influenza and the global forces transforming the environment. Focusing on the mass culling of poultry in Vietnam in 2004–2005 as a preventive measure against the spread of avian influenza, a further question is posed: Why have small-scale farms been targeted for radical anti-influenza measures, with less focus on large-scale agribusinesses, where the majority of H5N1 cases have been identified? In relation to SARS, this section also highlights how the globalization of disease is testing many entrenched assumptions about

---

[15] Alfred W. Crosby, *America's Forgotten Pandemic: The Influenza of 1918*. Second edition (Cambridge: Cambridge University Press, [1989] 2003), pp.xi–xiv (xiii).

the state's role in disease prevention. It considers the discrepancy between a viral infection, which has invariably been defined by its novelty (SARS as a 'new and emerging' disease), and the kinds of conventional public health measures adopted to stop its spread, including quarantine. The chapter concludes by briefly discussing China's 'humanitarian' interventions in Africa, namely the PRC's increasing involvement in disease prevention projects there, chiefly malaria, but most recently Ebola. What is driving China's new engagement with global health? What are the implications of this engagement for epidemic preparedness in the PRC and across Asia more generally?

Informing these three case studies – of HIV/AIDS, avian influenza, and SARS – are a number of interconnected concerns. First, to study the ways in which social and ecological developments associated with globalization may be determining patterns of infectious disease in Asia. Second, to investigate how globalization may be transforming the role of the state and its institutions in epidemic disease surveillance and prevention. And third, to explore the entanglement of social and ecological factors that have been produced by globalization. Given these entanglements, customary conceptualizations of the world based on sliding scales (from micro to macro) are no longer helpful. The concept of scale implies a fixed, linear relationship, whereas the globalized world today is constituted by multiple overlapping systems with myriad mobile connections (Chapter 1). In short, the aim is to outline some of the analytical challenges that this fluidity raises, while suggesting conceptual tools for grappling with complex global connections.

Globalization and the 1918–1919 influenza pandemic

The term 'globalization' has been used in many different and often contradictory ways. The political scientist Barry Gills has suggested that we speak of 'globalizations' in the plural, rejecting the 'idea that there can ever be a single theory or interpretation of globalization.'[16] Most commonly, perhaps, the term globalization is used to refer to increasingly rapid and intense flows of people, capital, and commodities around the globe. This extension of social connections between the local and the distant has eroded the borders of the nation-state, resulting in a form of 'supra-territoriality.'[17] A fundamental feature of globalization defined in this way is time–space compression: the shrinkage of the world as a result

---

[16] Barry K. Gills, 'The Turning of the Tide,' *Globalizations*, vol.1, no.1 (2004): 1–6 (1).
[17] Michael Lang, 'Globalization and Its History,' *Journal of Modern History*, vol.78, no.4 (2006): 899–931 (900).

of new technologies of transportation and communication. Globalization has also been identified with the deepening integration of local and national economies into global markets and a transnational division of labor. This process is characterized by four features: 'extensity (stretching), intensity, velocity, and impact.' Globalization may be understood in terms of 'spatial–temporal processes of change' that link together and expand human activity.[18] In relation to infectious disease, the effects of these processes are obvious enough: they serve to increase pathogenic dissemination through global trade, migration, and ecological disruption.

To what extent is globalization a new phenomenon? Should we think of globalization simply as the extension of earlier modernizing processes linked to the nation-state or, as the historian Arif Dirlik has argued, modernity gone global?[19] Most accounts of globalization proclaim its 'newness.' There has tended to be a 'temporal foreshortening of the global' with globalization located in the present and future, rather than in the past.[20] However, global interdependence should not be regarded as a condition unique to the twentieth and twenty-first centuries: Asia has long been connected. Before the arrival of Europeans, the territories of East Asia, Southeast Asia, and the subcontinent were linked by multiple networks of trade and migration. To be sure, European colonization from the sixteenth century expanded and deepened these networks, but it did not displace them. As we saw in Chapter 1, the diffusion of cholera across Asia from Bengal by 1820 revealed the proliferating route-ways of imperial trade and the likely role of troop movements in contagion. Towards the end of the century, this interdependence was being conceptualized explicitly as a process of 'shrinkage' enabled by novel technologies. Faster travel by means of steam power and near instantaneous communication via the telegraph and telephone were compressing time and space. Yet this 'onrush of modern globalization in the late nineteenth century was not just the story of the "new imperialism," as the West thrust itself into China by making use of new technologies.' New imperial networks 'also built upon and even gave a new vitality to older forms of globalization.'[21]

The consequences of this global compression and the convergence of old and new transnational networks were evident in the influenza

[18] David Held, et al., *Global Transformations: Politics, Economics and Culture* (Stanford, CA: Stanford University Press, 1999), pp.14–15.

[19] Arif Dirlik, *Global Modernity: Modernity in the Age of Global Capital* (Boulder, CO: Paradigm, 2007).

[20] David Armitage, 'Is There a Pre-History of Globalization?' In: Deborah Cohen and Maura O'Connor, eds., *Comparison and History: Europe in Cross-National Perspective* (New York: Routledge, 2004), pp.165–176 (167).

[21] Hans van de Ven, 'The Onrush of Modern Globalization in China.' In: A. G. Hopkins, ed., *Globalization in World History* (New York: W. W. Norton, 2002), pp.167–195 (175).

pandemic of 1889 to 1890, which spread around the world in some four months along intercontinental and transoceanic pathways of trade and mass transit.[22] Newspapers exploited cable networks to report the influenza's daily and inexorable progress from the Russian Far East to Europe and the United States, moving by road, rail, and steamer.

Two decades later, the influenza pandemic of 1918–1919 demonstrated with brutal starkness the global reach of disease and the speed at which it could now travel.[23] The precise mortality figures are unclear but one estimate puts the number at 100 million dead, when unreported cases are factored in – many more than those who perished in military action during the First World War. With an incidence rate of up to 50 percent in some places, the pandemic had an estimated case fatality rate of between two and 20 percent. According to the WHO, it may justifiably be regarded as 'the most deadly disease event in the history of humanity,' providing a worst-case scenario for contemporary fears about a future pandemic – a 'coming plague.'[24] Aided in its spread by the mobilization of troops on the Western Front during the First World War, the influenza dispersed across the globe with extraordinary rapidity. The name 'Spanish Flu,' by which the pandemic is most commonly known, derives from the fact that in Spain – a non-belligerent country during the First World War – the press was free to report the effects of the pandemic, unlike Germany, Britain, France, and the United States, where early reports were censored. In early June 1918, the *Times* of London referred to 'The Spanish Epidemic,' noting several weeks later: 'Everybody thinks of it as the Spanish influenza to-day [sic].'[25] Restrictions on the dissemination of information during the war hindered attempts to control the 1918 influenza pandemic: 'Censorship converged with the rapid abatement of the disease to bury many historical details of the 1918 influenza pandemic.'[26] Epidemic crises often prompt state authorities to close down information networks in the name of security, as illustrated by the example of SARS discussed later in this chapter. Yet a lack of information, particularly in the face

---

[22] Alain-Jacques Valleron, et al., 'Transmissibility and Geographic Spread of the 1889 Influenza Pandemic,' *Proceedings of the National Academy of Sciences of the United States of America*, vol.107, no.19 (May 11, 2010): 8778–8781.

[23] Niall P. A. S. Johnson and Juergen Mueller, 'Updating the Accounts: Global Mortality of the 1918–1920 'Spanish' Influenza Pandemic,' *Bulletin of the History of Medicine*, vol.76, no.1 (2002): 105–115 (105).

[24] *Avian Influenza and Human Health: Report by the Secretariat* (Geneva: World Health Organization, 2004), p.1.

[25] 'The Spanish Epidemic,' *Times* [of London] (June 3, 1918), p.5; 'The Spanish Influenza,' *Times* [of London] (June 25, 1918), p.9.

[26] Ron Barrett and Peter J. Brown, 'Stigma in the Time of Influenza: Social and Institutional Responses to Pandemic Emergencies,' *Journal of Infectious Diseases*, vol.197, Supplement 1(February 15, 2008): S34–S37.

of an unfamiliar infection, may give rise to a perceived lack of control, causing fear and panic.

The origin of the pandemic has been much debated. While the influenza has been traced back to a US Army base in Kansas, it has also been linked to the trenches in France, and to an influenza epidemic in China during the winter of 1917. According to this last hypothesis, Chinese coolies who worked behind the British and French lines on the Western Front may have imported the disease to Europe, earning it the name 'Chungking fever.'[27] At the time, there was speculation as to whether the disease might have been related to the 1910 Manchurian plague epidemic (discussed in the previous chapter), which had been 'modified by racial and topographic differences.'[28]

Influenza is now understood to be a viral respiratory infection. While there are three main types of influenza viruses (A, B, and C), type A viruses, which infect humans and animals, are the most adaptable. Like the other two types of viruses, type A belong to a family of RNA (ribonucleic acid) viruses that have high mutation rates as they replicate (antigenic drift). Type A viruses can also combine with other viruses inside a host cell to create further subtypes (antigenic shift). In 2005, researchers succeeded in reconstructing the genetic sequence of the 1918 flu strain, using frozen lung tissue from victims of the pandemic. This confirmed the hypothesis that the 1918 virus was an avian strain and an ancestor of subsequent H1N1 influenza viruses. If studies of the viral genome have indicated that later influenza type A pandemics have been lineal descendants of the 1918 virus, historical analysis has also pointed to the distinctive epidemiological characteristics of the 1918 pandemic, including the unusually high death rates, particularly amongst healthy young adults.[29]

Viruses and the undead: Zombie pandemics

The term 'virus' derives from the Latin word meaning 'poison.' Subsequently it came to denote the venom of a snake and a man's

---

[27] Mark Osborne Humphries, 'Paths of Infection: The First World War and the Origins of the 1918 Influenza Pandemic,' *War in History*, vol.21 no.1 (January 2014): 55–81; Christopher Langford, 'Did the 1918–19 Influenza Pandemic Originate in China?' *Population and Development Review*, vol.31, no.3 (September 2005): 473–505.

[28] James Joseph King, 'The Origin of the So-Called "Spanish Influenza",' *Medical Record*, vol.94 (October 12, 1918): 632–633 (632).

[29] Jeffery K. Taubenberger and David M. Morens, '1918 Influenza: The Mother of All Pandemics,' *Emerging Infectious Diseases*, vol.12, no.1 (January 2006): 15–22 (15, 16); Jeffery K. Taubenberger and David M. Morens, 'Influenza: The Once and Future Pandemic,' *Public Health Reports*, vol.125, Supplement 3 (2010): S16–S26.

semen. Over the centuries, the term acquired other meanings. Studying the cause of an epidemic of 'tobacco mosaic disease' in the Netherlands – so named after the mottled appearance of the infected plant's leaves – Martinus Beijerinck (1851–1931) coined the term 'virus' to refer to the submicroscopic agent that could pass through a fine filter but could not be seen. It was not until the 1930s that the tobacco mosaic virus particles (virions) were isolated and electron microscopy enabled the first images of viruses. Viruses consist of genetic material (DNA or RNA) wrapped in protein. They are acellular and replicate by appropriating the machinery and metabolism of a host cell. Given this parasitic mode of replication, there is debate as to whether viruses are in fact life-forms. Viruses are part of our genetic constitution. So-called 'junk DNA' in the human genome may be evidence of past infections or possibly indicate a symbiotic relationship with viruses. The ambiguous status of viruses as non-living organisms has led to their association with zombies in popular culture – the 'undead' that reproduce by feeding off the living. In Max Brooks's bestselling novel, *World War Z* (2006), a zombifying plague threatens the world with annihilation. The story begins in the 'United Federation of China,' where a zombie bites a young boy. Here, the plot line draws on familiar globalization and emerging disease narratives, recalling avian influenza and SARS. The origin of the plague appears to be in East Asia, and the Chinese government fabricates a crisis involving Taiwan in order to conceal its draconian interventions. China becomes the epicenter of an infection that radiates globally as the zombifying pathogen spreads to other countries via refugees and a burgeoning black-market organ trade. While Asia is often imagined as the place where viral threats originate, the virus has become closely identified with the global. Today, we speak of 'going viral' to refer to information that circulates rapidly and widely.

Max Brooks, *World War Z: An Oral History of the Zombie War* (New York: Three Rivers Press, 2006).

Jeremy R. Youde, 'Biosurveillance, Human Rights, and the Zombie Plague.' In: Sara E. Davies and Jeremy R. Youde, eds., *The Politics of Surveillance and Response to Disease Outbreaks: The New Frontier for States and Non-state Actors* (Farnham and Burlington, VT: Ashgate, 2015), pp.57–69.

By 1918, experiments using Chamberland filters had suggested the existence of submicroscopic infectious agents, invisible under the microscope. In 1892, the botanist Dmitri Ivanovsky (1864–1920) had used one such filter to show that sap from an infected tobacco plant remained infectious even after it had been filtered. In 1898, the microbiologist Martinus Beijerinck confirmed the presence of a filterable 'contagious living fluid,' later coining the term 'virus' to refer to the invisible agent. Despite these advances, however, in 1918 the etiology of human influenza had not been established. Scientists attributed the infection to a bacterium, dubbed 'Pfeiffer's bacillus' (or *Bacillus influenzae*) after the German bacteriologist Richard Pfeiffer (1858–1945), who claimed to have isolated it from infected patients in 1892.

Three waves of influenza struck in quick succession over a period of roughly 12 months: from March to August 1918; from September to November 1918; and from December 1918 to March 1919.[30] The second wave was the most lethal, with most deaths caused by bacterial pneumonia. While there is now a substantive literature on the impact of the influenza in Europe and the United States, little has been written about the disease in the region where it struck the hardest, namely British India. As the cultural historian Mike Davis has observed, 'This oversight is analogous to the history of the First World War having been written with a vivid, sustained focus on the campaigns in the Balkans and Gallipoli while devoting only an occasional aside or footnote to the slaughter on the Western Front.'[31]

According to a report by Major F. Norman White, the Government of India's sanitary commissioner, influenza arrived in India via troops from Mesopotamia disembarking at Bombay in the summer of 1918. It was police sepoys who were the initial victims, followed by dock workers. Influenza then spread along the rail network into the hinterland and to port cities, such as Madras and Calcutta. An estimated 12 million perished in the subcontinent – with some historians pushing the number upwards to 20 million.

What accounts for the high mortality on the subcontinent? Colonial authorities repeatedly emphasized the insalubrious living conditions of native dwellings in Indian cities, 'which lend themselves to the rapid spread of disease' (Chapter 2). As one health officer noted in 1918, Bombay was a 'huge incubator, with suitable media, already prepared for

---

[30] R. Edgar Hope-Simpson, *The Transmission of Epidemic Influenza* (New York: Springer, 1992), pp.26–27.

[31] Mike Davis, *The Monster at Our Door: The Global Threat of Avian Flu* (New York: The New Press, 2005), p.25.

the insemination of germs of disease.'[32] Drought and famine exacerbated the situation. In June, the southwestern monsoon failed to arrive and the resulting drought led to crop failure and soaring grain prices. Famine conditions prevailed across much of the country. In September, as the famine was worsening, the second more fatal wave of influenza struck, leading to in excess of a million deaths in the Bombay Presidency alone between October and November. The highest mortality, however, was in the rural Central Provinces, where it has been estimated that over 102 per thousand of the population died. Refugees from famine-affected districts flocked to the cities from the countryside, driving the infection. Poverty, malnutrition, together with chronic illness and co-infections, such as pneumonia, were all contributory factors in the high mortality.[33] Many medical personnel had also been enlisted in the war effort, depleting the health services.

It is, perhaps, surprising, given the high mortality figures, that the pandemic in India did not precipitate widespread social unrest and panic, as was the case during the plague pandemic between 1896 and 1898 (Chapter 2). A number of reasons have been suggested to account for this discrepancy. For one, the two pandemics elicited very different responses from the colonial authorities. While the Government of India and its provincial administrations implemented drastic interventionist measures in the early years of the plague, their response to the influenza pandemic was far less draconian. Secondly, the two diseases were viewed very differently by the local population. In contrast to the plague, which was familiar, influenza 'carried very little cultural or political baggage. It had no anticipatory "aura." It was not a disease extensively discussed in Unani and Ayurvedic texts.'[34]

The 1918–1919 influenza pandemic did not only affect the Indian subcontinent. Infection traveled across the Indian Ocean from India to Southeast Asia, through Malaya, the Dutch East Indies, the Philippines, and Indochina.[35] Its demographic impact is hard to assess, but at least 1.5 million died in the Dutch East Indies, and perhaps 400,000 perished in Burma. In some areas of Vietnam, Cambodia, and Laos, morbidity was

[32] Mridula Ramanna, 'Coping with the Influenza Pandemic: The Bombay Experience.' In: David Killingray and Howard Phillips, eds., *The Spanish Influenza Pandemic of 1918–1919: New Perspectives* (Abingdon and New York: Routledge, 2003), pp.86–98 (87).

[33] I. D. Mills, 'The 1918–1919 Influenza Pandemic – The Indian Experience,' *Indian Economic and Social History Review*, vol.23, no.1 (1986): 1–40.

[34] David Arnold, 'Disease, Rumor, and Panic in India's Plague and Influenza Epidemics, 1896–1919.' In: Robert Peckham, ed., *Empires of Panic: Epidemics and Colonial Anxieties* (Hong Kong: Hong Kong University Press, 2015), pp.111–129 (120).

[35] Colin Brown, 'The Influenza Pandemic of 1918 in Indonesia.' In: Owen, ed., *Death and Disease*, pp.235–256.

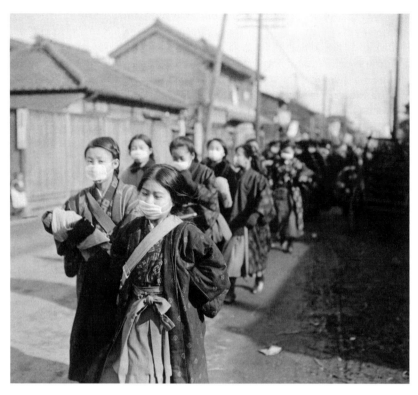

Figure 5.1. 'Japanese school girls wear protective masks to guard against the influenza outbreak (1920).' Courtesy: Bettmann/Corbis.

as high as 50 percent. Preliminary research in China has suggested that while the influenza struck the country's eastern ports and cities, 'it did not explode from there into the interior, as elsewhere in Asia.'[36] In Japan, where the disease spread by rail and steamer, the rate of infection was 6.4 per thousand, a number comparable to those of Europe and North America (Figure 5.1).[37] Influenza commonly causes death in infants and the elderly. The 1918 pandemic, however, followed a markedly different pattern. Mortality impact was highest amongst young adults. In Japan,

---

[36] Wataru Iijima, 'Spanish Influenza in China, 1918–20: A Preliminary Probe.' In: Killingray and Phillips, eds., *The Spanish Influenza Pandemic*, pp.101–109 (109).

[37] Geoffrey W. Rice, 'Japan and New Zealand in the 1918 Influenza Pandemic: Comparative Perspectives on Official Responses and Crisis Management.' In: Killingray and Phillips, eds., *The Spanish Influenza Pandemic*, pp.73–85.

excess mortality rates peaked in children aged below five and in young adults aged between 25 and 34 years.[38]

As Arnold has observed: 'No disease illustrated so dramatically the way in which the Indian Ocean region was now not only bound together by steamship and by rail, but also integrated into wider imperial networks of communication and control.'[39] The 1918 pandemic exposed the vulnerability of colonial powers and underscored the dangers posed by epidemics in a globalized world. By the first quarter of the twentieth century, the world was increasingly meshed by global flows. However, while some historians view such disruptions as inhibiting or undermining globalization, others argue that globalization manifests itself precisely through these often dislocating processes.[40] In the latter case, globalization is itself the result of a liquefaction of order and an escalation of violence. Moreover, like 'new and emerging' infections, globalization is construed in terms of its novelty. As Krause observed, globalization creates new ecologies of disease: 'Microbes thrive in these "undercurrents of opportunity" that arise through social economic change, changes in human behavior, and catastrophic events.'[41] The First World War was such a catastrophic event, presenting 'undercurrents of opportunity' for influenza to spread. Whatever the origins of the virus, its global dispersion was certainly facilitated by troop movements across continents and oceans.

The pandemic has been considered more 'equalizing' than other infections in that every social class was affected. Given this, people are likely to have reacted differently to influenza than to other diseases, such as plague, which were associated with dirt and the native poor, and led to stigmatization. Yet influenza's demographic impact varied greatly, at the same time as the pandemic gave rise to widespread panic, called forth discriminatory policies, and resulted in the abandonment of the sick.[42] As we have seen in our discussion of India above, there the influenza resulted in millions of deaths, far in excess of mortality rates in Europe and North America. In other words, local and regional circumstances determined how the global pandemic played out in specific places. The emphasis on the extent and speed of the influenza's global circulation can obscure the disparities in mortality, which were determined by a complex array

---

[38] S. A. Richard, et al., 'A Comparative Study of the 1918–1920 Influenza Pandemic in Japan, USA and UK: Mortality Impact and Implications for Pandemic Planning,' *Epidemiology and Infection*, vol.137, no.8 (August 2009): 1062–1072.

[39] Arnold, 'The Indian Ocean as a Disease Zone,' p.12.

[40] James L. Watson, 'SARS and the Consequences of Globalization.' In: Arthur Kleinman and James L. Watson, eds., *SARS in China: Prelude to Pandemic?* (Stanford, CA: Stanford University Press, 2006), pp.196–202.

[41] Krause, 'Foreword.' In: Morse, ed., *Emerging Viruses*, p.xvii.

[42] Barrett and Brown, 'Stigma in the Time of Influenza,' pp.S35–S36.

of variables, including: environmental factors, the presence of secondary infections, social and economic status, and access to healthcare. Preoccupations with influenza's global nature may also mask the distinct ways in which the disease was experienced in different countries and in different populations within specific localities. If the pandemic highlighted globalizing systems, it also drew attention to how local circumstances could shape the outcome of larger global processes.

While the 1918–1919 influenza revealed the globalized nature of the world and the inability of existing quarantine measures to halt the infection's progress, this was nonetheless still 'a world of compact powers and contending blocs' characterized by 'the arrangements and rearrangements of macro-alliances.' The 1918–1919 pandemic was propelled globally along shipping routes and railway lines, but the advent of commercial air travel in the 1950s and 1960s significantly accelerated this process. Furthermore, what came into being at the end of the twentieth century, particularly during the 1980s and following the disintegration of the Soviet Union in 1991, was a world 'of obscure divisions and strange instabilities.' As the anthropologist Clifford Geertz has expressed it, political and economic developments in the last quarter of the century 'produced a sense of dispersion, of particularity, of complexity, and of uncenteredness.'[43] This was a world of global multinationals and decentered communication networks, dominated by commodity production and characterized by fragmentation. It is the implication for infectious diseases of this 'world in pieces' that we turn to now.

Globalization and economies of HIV/AIDS in China

A profound change was inaugurated in East Asia by the policies of market liberalization adopted by Deng Xiaoping in the PRC after Mao's death in 1976. Deng repudiated the Cultural Revolution and from 1978 – the same year as the Declaration of Alma-Ata – a program of economic reform was announced with the institution of a number of 'Special Economic Zones.' The commune system was gradually dismantled and agriculture decollectivized, with farmers given the latitude to plant cash crops and sell their products in rural markets. China's economy opened to foreign trade and investment was courted. The United States finally recognized the PRC, leading to developing business ties between China and the West, and Western companies setting up production plants in China.

---

[43] Clifford Geertz, 'The World in Pieces: Culture and Politics at the End of the Century.' In: *Available Light: Anthropological Reflections on Philosophical Topics* (Princeton, NJ: Princeton University Press, 2000), pp.218–263.

As Deng put it, the aim was to combine aspects of a socialist 'planned economy' with the 'free market.' 'There are no fundamental contradictions between a socialist system and a market economy,' he informed a US journalist in 1985. 'If we combine a planned economy with a market economy,' he declared, 'we should be in a better position to release productive forces and accelerate economic growth.'[44]

In Chapter 3, we saw how agriculture was collectivized under Mao, and how state control of society was tightened through ambitious modernizing initiatives during the Great Leap Forward. In the late 1970s, these processes of socialist modernization were reversed. China's reintegration into the global markets was symbolized by the reopening of the Shanghai Stock Exchange in 1990 after its closure in 1949. Membership of the global community was reaffirmed when China joined the World Trade Organization (WTO) in December 2001. In the 1990s, as surplus US, Western European, and Japanese capital chased low-wage Chinese labor, the PRC became the second largest recipient of foreign direct investment after the United States.[45]

This market orientation led to momentous changes in the country: to mass migration from rural areas to cities, where capital investment in industry created an expanding need for labor. As state control over the economy loosened, entrepreneurial activities burgeoned in the 1980s. During the early phase of reform many rural communities enjoyed a better standard of living as they took advantage of new market incentives offered to rural households. But as the cost of industrial goods rose, the agricultural sectors stagnated, inflation skyrocketed, and student-led demonstrations erupted – culminating in the Beijing Tiananmen Square incident of June 4, 1989. However, Deng's 'South China Tour' in January and February 1992 served to re-accelerate the pace of economic reform. During visits to the key cities of Wuchang, Shenzhen, Zhuhai, and Shanghai, Deng delivered speeches that hammered home the message of economic reform as a means of unleashing China's productive potential.

While the structural changes associated with the shift to a market economy fueled astonishing growth, they also brought new challenges, including growing inequalities, a fragmentation of the healthcare system, and an attenuation of social relations, which was one result of mass urban migration and a depopulation of rural areas. As local governments took on more

[44] Henry Grunwald, 'An Interview with Deng Xiaoping: You Should Give Them the Power to Make Money,' *Time* (November 4, 1985).

[45] Nicholas R. Lardy, *Integrating China into the Global Economy* (Washington, DC: Brookings Institution Press, 2002), p.4

responsibility for their funding, they sought to meet their new obligations by imposing additional levies and fees for services. How were these changes related to the emergence and re-emergence of infectious diseases? The syphilis epidemic in the PRC suggests one answer to this question. China's shift towards a largely unregulated market-based economy in the 1980s had far-reaching repercussions, driving a booming commercial sex industry. Young women from rural China drifted to the cities, working as prostitutes to service businessmen in nightclubs, hair salons, and massage parlors. The migration of rural workers to the city also boosted a demand for commercial sex amongst a so-called 'floating population' (*liudong renkou*) with little awareness of risk or access to safe-sex measures.[46] Ironically, after it had assumed power in 1949, the Party had made it a priority to 'eradicate' prostitution through a campaign of labor re-education and imprisonment. The Rural Cooperative Medical System, launched in the 1950s, along with the 'barefoot doctors' in the 1960s, had brought infectious disease threats under control. The Party's clampdown on prostitution and its push against disease were much vaunted as evidence of its effectiveness.[47] It was under the new post-reform conditions, however, that STIs, including syphilis and gonorrhea, began to spread. The first case of HIV/AIDS was reported in China in 1985, when an Argentine tourist from the United States died in a hospital in Beijing. The first domestic cases were reported four years later in Yunnan province when 146 heroin users were diagnosed with the disease.

The spread of STIs in China was thus closely connected to the country's shift towards a market-orientated economy and the social transformations that this produced. In the first of three official phases of the HIV/AIDS epidemic from the mid 1980s, the disease was viewed primarily as an 'imported disease of affluence' since those infected were principally foreigners or Chinese who had lived overseas, or those who had become infected through the use of imported blood products. In the film *AIDS Victims* (1988), directed by Xu Tongjun and disseminated as part of a public health awareness campaign, for example, three Chinese women who are residents of a 'Special Economic Zone' contract HIV through intercourse with a foreign teacher. From 1989, however, infection began to diffuse through drug use and trafficking routes: from Vietnam, Laos, and Burma into Yunnan, Guangxi, and Xinjiang. In the course of the third 'expansion' phase, from the mid 1990s, infection diffused north

---

[46] Joseph D. Tucker, Xiang-Sheng Chen, and Rosanna W. Peeling, 'Syphilis and Social Upheaval in China,' *New England Journal of Medicine*, vol.362 (May 10, 2010): 1658–1661.

[47] Zhang Heqing, 'Female Sex Sellers and Public Policy in the People's Republic of China.' In: Elaine Jeffreys, ed., *Sex and Sexuality in China* (Abingdon and New York: Routledge, 2006), pp.139–158 (142).

along the country's main transport routes, with cases reported across provinces and autonomous regions. Infection spread via IV drug users, sex workers, and commercial blood donors.[48]

As of 2015, the number of reported cases of people living with HIV and AIDS in China is estimated by PRC authorities to be 501,000. Alarming predictions made about the likelihood of a dramatic increase in infections as HIV/AIDS spreads from high-risk groups to the general population appear not to have materialized. A report commissioned by the UN in 2002, entitled *HIV/AIDS: China's Titanic Peril*, had concluded that the country was facing an 'explosive HIV/AIDS epidemic.' As the report declared: 'A potential HIV/AIDS disaster of unimaginable proportion now lies in wait to rattle the country, and it can be feared that in the near future, China might count more HIV infections than any other country in the world.'[49] Although such forecasts about the substantial and rapid spread of HIV/AIDS in China did not eventuate, there continues to be an issue with high HIV/AIDS infection rates amongst certain communities. While IV infections remain low among the general population, sexual transmission of the infection is rising rapidly among men who have sex with men (MSM).[50]

In her study of sex workers and their clients in the town of Jinghong in southern Yunnan – the ground zero of the epidemic in China – the anthropologist Sandra Teresa Hyde has shown how changing economic relations led to a growing demand for paid sex and a drift of women into sex work with consequences for the spread of HIV/AIDS. As Hyde notes, HIV/AIDS in China during the 1980s and 1990s became 'embedded in political and economic relations.'[51] What such ethnographic research has demonstrated is the way in which a global disease is manifest in distinct ways in local settings. Jinghong is situated in the Sipsongpanna (or Xishuangbanna) Autonomous Tai Minority Prefecture bordering Burma and Laos. The emerging HIV/AIDS epidemic there was understood by PRC health officials to be a minority problem, affecting the Tai-Lüe, a non-Han Chinese ethnic population. This spatialization of disease – its location in the ethnic borderlands of the state – recuperated earlier,

[48] Johanna Hood, 'Untangling HIV in China: Social, Political, Economic, and Global-Local Factors.' In: Mark McLelland and Vera Mackie, eds., *Routledge Handbook of Sexuality Studies in East Asia* (Abingdon and New York: Routledge, 2015), pp.356–371 (357–358).

[49] *HIV/AIDS: China's Titanic Peril: 2001 Update of the AIDS Situation and Needs Assessment Report* (Geneva: UNAIDS, June 2002), p.7.

[50] Kathryn E. Muessig and Myron S. Cohen, 'China, HIV, and Syphilis Among Men Who Have Sex With Men: An Urgent Call to Action,' *Clinical Infectious Diseases*, vol.57, no.2 (July 15, 2013): 310–313.

[51] Sandra Teresa Hyde, *Eating Spring Rice: The Cultural Politics of AIDS in Southwest China* (Berkeley: University of California Press, 2007), p.2.

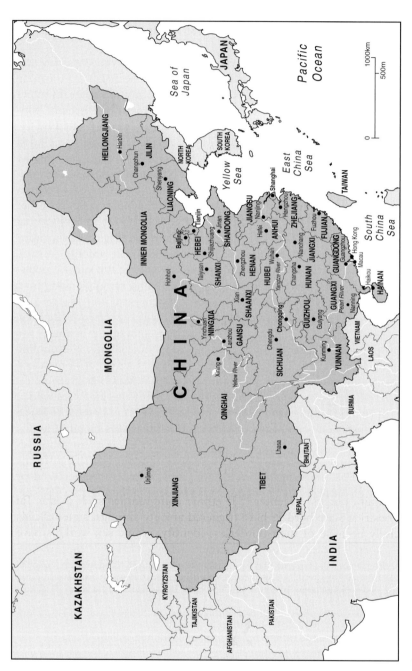

Map 5.1. Contemporary China

Healthcare and infectious disease control in the PRC

The PRC extends to some 3.6 million square miles and has a population of 1.36 billion, making it a significant contributor to the global burden of infectious disease (Map 5.1). China's population size and vast land area – it shares a border with 14 other countries – pose challenges for ensuring effective healthcare and disease surveillance. Since market liberalization began in the late 1970s, much of China's healthcare system has been privatized. As a result of major healthcare reforms over the last decade, the country has adopted a health insurance system. Wide disparities exist, however, particularly between cities and impoverished rural areas where there is often basic or no healthcare coverage. In 2013, the PRC spent an estimated 5.6 percent of its GDP on healthcare, far below that of countries such as Japan, which spent 10.3 percent on health. In addition to poor public health and hospital systems, and inadequate access to healthcare, a lack of coordination between ministries and agencies, and a mobile population also pose challenges for preventing and managing epidemics.

Longde Wang, et al., 'Emergence and Control of Infectious Diseases in China,' *Lancet*, vol.372, no.9649 (November 1, 2008): 1598–1605.

historic associations of Yunnan with plague, leprosy, and malaria. In this sense, while recognizing HIV/AIDS as a new global disease, the epidemic was recast as a highly location-specific event with historical antecedents. As Hyde puts it, 'the cultural politics of HIV/AIDS in late-twentieth-century China can be understood as a disease of geography,' with border communities at its epicenter.[52] If ethnic communities such as the Tai that bestride state borders have triggered anxiety amongst state officials precisely because of their borderless identity, ethnic sex workers have become emblematic of the 'capricious and promiscuous' character of emerging viruses that cross species barriers to infect the Han-Chinese.[53] It is precisely this border-crossing propensity of disease that produces fear, calling forth concerted efforts to maintain and reinforce boundaries

[52] Hyde, *Eating Spring Rice*, p.170.
[53] Erica Weir, 'The Ecology of Avian Influenza,' *Canadian Medical Association Journal*, vol.173, no.8 (October 11, 2005): 869–870.

between 'healthy' self and 'unhealthy' other, even though such boundary lines are never secure.[54]

IV drug users were identified in China as a group at particular risk from contracting HIV/AIDS. The anthropologist Shao-hua Liu has explored the dynamics of the epidemic among heroin addicts in rural Sichuan, a province in the southwest of China. During the market reforms in the 1980s and 1990s, young men from the Nuosu people, a minority group officially categorized as 'Yi' according to China's ethnic identification project, drifted to the nearby cities to take advantage of new economic opportunities. However, lacking the requisite skills for survival in the cities, they invariably fell into a downward spiral of petty crime and drug use. Marginalized and cut off from regular sources of income, many ended up turning to heroin and contracting HIV through contaminated needles. On the one hand, Liu's research suggests that this is a clash between tradition – the tradition of the Nuosu – and modernity. However, responses to the epidemics of HIV and IV drug use also reflect older forms of marginalization. Historically viewed by the majority Han-Chinese as hopelessly backward and prone to delinquency, the Nuosu were largely left behind during China's modernization drive from the 1950s. Opium and heroin have long been familiar among the Nuosu, with drug users suffering little stigmatization.[55] Following the medical anthropologist Merrill Singer, instead of viewing HIV/AIDS and substance addiction as '*concurrent* epidemics,' we should perhaps regard them as phenomena that 'emerge among the poor as closely intertwined threads in an often tattered fabric of their daily lives.'[56]

It was also in the context of market liberalization that the selling of blood took off. While the state's response had been principally directed at public health surveillance on the ethnic borderlands, another epidemic was unfolding in Henan and Anhui in central and eastern China, and elsewhere across the country. Blood selling had existed in China before the 1980s and 1990s. Yu Hua's novel, *Chronicle of a Blood Merchant* (1995), follows the life of a worker, Xu Sanguan, who sells his blood to support his family from the early years of the PRC in the 1950s through the Cultural Revolution in the 1960s and 1970s.[57] After market liberalization, however, blood selling assumed a new form. A character in Ma

---

[54] Robert Crawford, 'The Boundaries of the Self and the Unhealthy Other: Reflections on Health, Culture and AIDS,' *Social Science & Medicine*, vol.38, no.10 (May 1994): 1347–1365.

[55] Shao-hua Liu, *Passage to Manhood: Youth Migration, Heroin, and AIDS in Southwest China* (Stanford, CA: Stanford University Press, 2011).

[56] Singer, *Introduction to Syndemics*, p.xiv.

[57] Yu Hua, *Chronicle of a Blood Merchant*. Translated by Andrew F. Jones (New York: Pantheon, 2003).

Jian's novel *The Noodle Maker*, published in Hong Kong in 1991, for example, sells his blood to hospitals for money and sets up a blood donor agency to exploit the growing demand.[58] Perhaps most memorably, in the director Zhou Xiaowen's dark satire *Ermo* (1994), the eponymous protagonist moves from rural Hebei to the city, where she sells her blood in order to buy a new television. Blood selling and post-socialist consumerism are here intertwined and set against the pre-reform era embodied in Ermo's impotent husband, the former village head.[59]

The unimpeded growth of a semi-official 'blood market' in the 1980s and 1990s, along with deregulation, piecemeal privatization of health services – with the introduction of user charges – was to lead to an epidemic of HIV/AIDS. Particularly in the impoverished but densely populated province of Henan, many thousands were infected with HIV through blood collection programs, which were conceived as a 'novel development approach.' The profits to be had from the selling of plasma to private companies for commercial use sparked a rush to set up blood collection centers. Villagers were encouraged to sell their blood by officials eager for a way to plug the shortfall in the province's funding, as the central government devolved responsibilities to regional authorities. 'Provincial authorities found in biotechnology the illusory promise of big profits that could revitalize a devastated landscape left in the wake of the rural economic reforms,' observes Ann Anagnost. In 1992, the head of the Henan Provincial Department of Health established a company to meet the growing pharmaceutical demand for human albumin, the main protein in human blood plasma. Health workers were dispatched to rural areas to collect blood, fueling an underground network of middlemen who sought to profit from this new commercial appetite for blood.[60]

Blood selling also became an important source of household revenue for destitute farmers. Donors were not screened for disease and the extracted blood was re-infused after being pooled. As one witness noted: 'Some blood stations were composed of just a centrifuge, some plastic tubes reused many times and some needles carried on a tractor. They would go into the village to draw blood, bringing blood collection services right to the door and paying on the spot.'[61] As a result, many donors became infected with HIV/AIDS and hepatitis B and C (Figure 5.2). As

[58] Ma Jian, *The Noodle Maker*. Translated by Flora Drew (London: Chatto & Windus, 2004).

[59] Tang Xiaobing, *Visual Culture in Contemporary China* (Cambridge: Cambridge University Press, 2015), pp.126–135.

[60] Ann S. Anagnost, 'Strange Circulations: The Blood Economy in Rural China,' *Economy and Society*, vol.35, no.4 (2006): 509–529 (516).

[61] John Gittings, *The Changing Face of China: From Mao to Market* (Oxford: Oxford University Press, 2005), p.282.

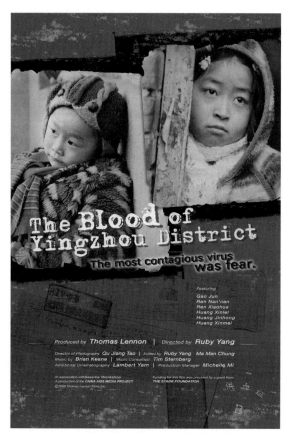

Figure 5.2. *The Blood of Yingzhou District* (2006). A documentary short directed by Ruby Yang, produced by Thomas Lennon.

HIV/AIDS on film

Set in the Yingzhou District of Fuyang, Anhui, the short documentary by Ruby Yang (Figure 5.2) explores the effect of HIV/AIDS on orphans whose parents died after contracting the disease from donating their blood to earn income. Film has become an important medium for drawing attention to the HIV/AIDS problem in the PRC and globally, and for exploring the social issues that the disease raises. The 2005 Canadian movie *3 Needles*, directed by Thom Fitzgerald, interweaves stories of persons around the world who are dealing with HIV/AIDS. One of the protagonists, played by Lucy Liu, is a blood smuggler, who persuades villagers to give their blood for $5 each. As a result, many in the village become infected. When government officials arrive to test people for HIV/AIDS at a cost of $10 per person, one character quips that it 'cost $5 when she gave me the virus.' The director Gu Changwei's *Love for Life* (2011), a romance set in a rural community in the 1990s, was the first mainstream movie in the PRC to tackle the issue of HIV/AIDS. Gu recruited HIV-positive supporting cast and crew members to make his movie, and he invited the documentary filmmaker Zhao Liang to shoot on set. Zhao's film *Together*, supported by the Ministry of Health, was also released in 2011.

stories of the blood selling began to leak out, Henan officials attempted to cover up. Gao Yaojie, a gynecologist and professor at Henan University, who had taken a lead in exposing the scandal, was debarred from traveling to the United States to receive an award from the Global Health Council, while the AIDS activist Wan Yanhai was arrested for publishing an official memo that confirmed the scale of the epidemic.

The blood selling scandal is poignantly evoked in the semi-fictional work *Dream of Ding Village* by Yan Lianke, which caused considerable controversy on its publication in 2006. A native of Henan, Yan Lianke had met HIV/AIDS patients through Gao Yaojie in the mid 1990s and began his research on the blood selling trade. In *Dream of Ding Village*, he explores the disintegration of a community in rural Henan as a result of HIV/AIDS infections contracted through blood selling:

What happened to Ding Village was unthinkable: in less than two years, this tiny village of fewer than 200 households and 800 people had lost more than 40 people to the fever. Over the last year, there had been an average of two or three deaths per month. Hardly a week went by without someone dying. The oldest were in their fifties and the youngest just a few years old. In each case, the sickness started with a fever lasting several weeks, which is how the disease got its nickname 'the fever'. It had spread until it had the village by the throat, and now there seemed no end to the stranglehold. No end to the dying, and no end to the tears.

Yan Lianke places this extractive blood economy within the context of the socio-political and economic changes that took place in the 1980s and 1990s PRC, as new market-oriented policies converged with a Party politics that continued to emphasize regional quotas. One of the characters in the book, Ding Hui, has made a fortune as a 'bloodhead,' recruiting poor villagers to give their blood in return for money. As a result of the wealth he has accrued through this trade in blood, Ding Hui has built himself a three-story house, equipped with all the modern accoutrements of a city-style Western house, including a laundry room, washing machine, refrigerator, freezer, and 'an indoor toilet made of white porcelain.'[62] The impetus for this entrepreneurial blood trade, we learn, has come from the 'higher-ups' in provincial government who are competing with other provinces to set up 'blood plasma resource centres.' As Carlos Rojas has observed, in *Dream of Ding Village* human blood is the principal commodity but one produced, however, not through labor. The selling of blood results in infection and death, not in life. Moreover, the role of the state is inverted in this labor-free commodity production. In Yan Lianke's narrative, Rojas notes, 'the epidemic is a direct result of the state's efforts to capitalize on the economic desperation of some of its citizens in order to advance an agenda that is ostensibly intended to help benefit the nation's population as a whole.'[63]

What do the cases discussed above – of Tai 'sex workers,' Nuosu IV drug users, and rural blood donors and 'bloodheads' in Henan – reveal about the HIV/AIDS epidemic in China? For one, that the identification of HIV/AIDS with non-Han Chinese minorities and the rural poor has led to the stereotyping of such communities as backward and disease-prone. This association of specific groups with disease in public health and consumer culture also points to continuities in the ways that inherited ethnic and class divisions have shaped – and continue to shape – how infectious diseases are researched, understood, and represented. A feeling of powerlessness in the face of an unknown disease may be mitigated by attributing a cause to specific individuals or 'high-risk groups.' Images of those infected with HIV/AIDS help to construct counter-images of a healthy self. The prevalence in the Chinese media of analogies that identify HIV/AIDS victims with Africa and Africans also suggests how the disease has been racialized even as it has been spatialized and imagined to infect only certain bodies in certain places.[64] Regional and local spaces are refracted through a global cartography that places Africa – the continent with the highest burden of HIV/AIDS – at its epicenter. The abject HIV/AIDS-infected person is constructed as a 'foreigner' who dwells on the other side of the border.[65]

---

[62] Yan Lianke, *Dream of Ding Village*. Translated by Cindy Carter (New York: Grove Press, 2009), pp.13, 20.

[63] Carlos Rojas, *Homesickness: Culture, Contagion, and National Transformation in Modern China* (Cambridge, MA: Harvard University Press, 2015), pp.185–189 (188).

[64] Johanna Hood, *HIV/AIDS, Health and the Media in China: Imagined Immunity Through Racialized Disease* (Abingdon and New York: Routledge, 2011).

[65] Carol S. Goldin, 'Stigmatization and AIDS: Critical Issues in Public Health,' *Social Science & Medicine*, vol.39, no.9 (November 1994): 1359–1366.

Beyond this, the cases considered in this chapter underscore a number of interrelated themes, critical to the argument about the relationship between epidemics and globalization. First, they suggest how the global and the local increasingly interconnect. This is brought out in Zhou's satirical movie *Ermo*, where a panning shot of Ermo traveling to town in a truck along a remote and snaking mountain road suggests the gulf that remains between village and city. At the same time, the characters' use of a local Hebei dialect (the film was released with subtitles) is juxtaposed to the foreign films that are screened on television. In other words, a consumer commodity brings local and global together in sometimes violent ways.

Second, the 'markets' unleashed by Deng's economic reforms in the PRC did not only involve foreign capital investments and big industry, but extended to local consumer markets and mushrooming illicit trades: the commodification of blood, sex, and drug trafficking represent the clandestine side of globalization. In the case of the blood contamination scandal, the selling of blood to service a nascent biotechnology industry hungry for human albumin became another dimension of a global market in which products manufactured in China depended on a 'floating' rural population to provide cheap labor. The marginalization of high-risk communities also reflected 'a skewed process of redistribution.'[66] As Shao Jing has observed, the HIV/AIDS blood contamination scandal 'uncovers the pathological confluence of spheres of economic circulations that have created the conditions for value to be extracted not through labor but from human plasma harvested from agricultural producers.'[67]

Third, the HIV/AIDS epidemic demonstrates the central role of the state and its institutions in mediating between the individual and the collective, the local and the global. Above all, though, it reveals the country's uneven socio-economic landscape and the increasing disparity between the wealthy and the poor. Although economic growth has improved the living standards for many, there is a widening income gap. The transition from a planned to a market economy has resulted in worsening inequality that has increased the vulnerability of certain sections of the population to disease.[68] China's Gini coefficient – a measurement of income

---

[66] Heather Xiaoquan Zhang and Richard Sanders, 'Introduction: Marginalisation and Globalisation in Transitional China.' In: Bin Wu, Heather Xiaoquan Zhang, and Richard Sanders, eds., *Marginalisation in China: Perspectives on Transition and Globalisation* (Aldershot and Burlington, VT: Ashgate, 2007), pp.1–11 (2).

[67] Shao Jing, 'Fluid Labor and Blood Money: The Economy of HIV/AIDS in Rural Central China,' *Cultural Anthropology*, vol.21, no.4 (2006): 535–569 (569).

[68] Heather Xiaoquan Zhang, 'The Gathering Storm: AIDS Policy in China,' *Journal of International Development*, vol.16, no.8 (November 2004): 1155–1168.

distribution with 0 indicating complete equality and 1 denoting complete inequality – stood at an estimated 0.55 in 2014, compared with 0.30 in 1980. HIV/AIDS is dependent, not only on biological determinants, but also on complex social determinants, which are impacted by globalization: income, social status, education, culture, and effective governance.

Ecologies of disease: Avian influenza in Asia

From the late nineteenth century, environmental changes associated with industrialization had profound implications for human health in Asia as forests were felled for commodity production and migrant labor was brought in to work in new expanding economies (Chapter 3). By the same token, in the PRC from the 1950s, Mao launched a concerted drive to remodel an agrarian society into a model socialist state by promoting rapid industrialization and collectivization – in effect, waging 'a war against nature.' This Great Leap Forward, writes Judith Shapiro, 'led China on a self-destructive rush toward ecosystem collapse and famine.'[69]

In the 1980s, an intensification of market-driven agricultural activities and resource extraction industries were to have similarly profound environmental impacts, not just in China, but in countries across Asia. The deeper integration of East and Southeast Asia into the global economy and the substantial profits to be derived from meeting global consumer demand had major ecological repercussions across the region. Focusing on Hong Kong and Vietnam, this section explores how globalization has driven environmental changes, which are implicated in the emergence of avian influenza. We began the chapter by discussing the 1918–1919 influenza pandemic. There were to be another two influenza pandemics in the second half of the twentieth century: the Asian flu pandemic of 1957–1958 and the so-called Hong Kong flu pandemic of 1968–1970. Both of these are thought to have emerged in China. The 1957 strain (H2N2), which is likely to have originated from a viral mutation in wild aquatic birds, was first reported in Guizhou province in the southwest of China in February of that year. Estimates vary widely, but perhaps over a million people died as a result of infection, with mortality highest among infants and the elderly. The Hong Kong (H3N2) flu pandemic of 1968–1970 killed an estimated 500,000 to one million people worldwide.[70] These pandemics reprised fears of the 1918–1919 catastrophe and led,

---

[69] Shapiro, *Mao's War Against Nature*, p.195.
[70] Bernd Sebastian Kamps and Gustavo Reyes-Terán, 'Influenza 2006.' In: Bernd Sebastian Kamps, Christian Hoffmann, and Wolfgang Preiser, eds., *Influenza Report 2006* (Paris: Flying Publisher, 2006), pp.17–47 (18, 22).

in turn, to a reappraisal of the 'Spanish flu.' While avian flu was linked back to the past, it was also heralded as a 'coming plague.' As noted in the Introduction, 'new and emerging' infections are typically framed in terms of both their novelty and historicity. Research has shown that people are inclined to fear a threat that is novel and fatal, regardless of the probability that it will occur – particularly a threat that comes from a force beyond human agency.[71] At the same time, however, associations of a 'new' viral disease with histories of past pandemics – the 1918–1919 influenza pandemic, for example, or the Black Death – suggest a process of entropic slippage back to a forbidding world before science. The influential report *Emerging Infections*, published by the US Institute of Medicine in 1992, used the 1918 pandemic as a reference point for planning responses to future pandemics. As virologists Richard J. Webby and Robert G. Webster declared: 'An old foe has again raised its head, reminding us that our worst nightmare may not be a new one.'[72] It is this novelty of the old that most disturbs, and Webster – celebrated in the media as the 'pope' of influenza – has spent a career warning of the 'killer strain lurking in the shadows.'

In May 1997, a novel strain of highly pathogenic avian influenza was identified in Hong Kong. As the name suggests, avian influenza or 'bird flu' is an infectious disease that primarily affects birds, although influenza A(H5N1) and A(H7N9) are recent examples of strains that have crossed species to cause lethal infections in humans. First detected in Guangdong in 1996, avian influenza spread through live poultry markets in Hong Kong the following year, infecting 18 people, with six dying as a result of viral pneumonia and multi-organ failure.

The 1997 influenza outbreak occurred during a financial crisis suggestively dubbed the 'Asian flu.' Beginning with the devaluation of the Thai baht in July 1997, emanating financial shockwaves appeared to be 'contagious,' spreading to Malaysia, Indonesia, South Korea, and Japan, with the Hong Kong stock market crashing in October. Many commentators drew links between these concurrent events – the financial crisis and the H5N1 outbreak – viewing them both as examples of the volatility produced by an increasingly interconnected world. The economist Paul Krugman summed up this convergence of contagious anxieties when he observed of the crash: 'It was as if bacteria that used to cause deadly plagues, but had long been considered conquered by modern medicine,

---

[71] George M. Gray and David P. Ropeik, 'Dealing with the Dangers of Fear: The Role of Risk Communication,' *Health Affairs*, vol.21, no.6 (November 2002): 106–116.

[72] Richard J. Webby and Robert G. Webster, 'Are We Ready for Pandemic Influenza?' *Science*, vol.302, no.5650 (November 28, 2003): 1519–1522.

had re-emerged in a form resistant to all the standard antibiotics.'[73] Co-incidentally, 1997 was also the year in which Hong Kong was 'handed back' to the PRC by the former colonial power, Britain – an event that exemplified China's growing geopolitical importance across the region.

Globalization and historical transitions

The relationship between human societies and disease has changed over time. The theory of the 'epidemiological transition' was formulated in 1971 by Abdel Omran to explain mortality decline and changing disease profiles in terms of demographic shifts. In its classic definition, three transitions or 'ages' were identified, but today four transitions are often described, specifically in relation to the history of human–infectious disease interactions. The first occurred when *Homo sapiens* transitioned from hunting and gathering to agriculture and the domestication of animals during the Neolithic period some 10,000 years ago. Higher population densities and greater exposure to zoonotic pathogens contributed to a rise in infectious diseases. The second transition took place when Eurasian civilizations came into military and commercial contact, creating a common pool of infections to which Eurasians became increasingly adapted. The third transition occurred as a result of European exploration and empire from the end of the fifteenth century, when transoceanic travel spread infectious diseases globally. During the late 1970s and early 1980s, we entered a fourth transition characterized by the quickening pace and intensity of globalization, which has enabled emerging and re-emerging infections to spread with unprecedented speed. There are problems, of course, with this schema. Dividing history into transitional stages imposes a uniformity on the heterogeneity of human experience, over-simplifying the historical complexities of human–environmental interactions. The notion of 'transition' suggests a linear trajectory and a sequential crossing over from one stage to another.

Anthony J. McMichael, 'Environmental and Social Influences on Emerging Infectious Diseases: Past, Present, and Future.' In: Angela R. McLean, et al., eds., *SARS: A Case Study in Emerging Infections* (Oxford: Oxford University Press, 2005), pp.4–15 (7–10).

---

[73] Robert Peckham, 'Contagion: Epidemiological Models and Financial Crises,' *Journal of Public Health*, vol.36, no.1 (2014): 13–17 (14).

From the 1990s, national and international preventive measures have focused on targeting poultry since contact with poultry is considered the primary animal-to-human transmission route. During the 1997 outbreak, 1.5 million birds were culled in Hong Kong in three days. In subsequent outbreaks, images of workers wearing personal protective equipment – masks, gloves, and gowns – were transmitted around the world, invariably juxtaposed with pictures of caged fowl, wild animals in crowded wet markets, and the disposal of slaughtered birds in black trash bags. Such images created a visual repertoire, helping to shape what has since become a stock motif of the pandemic thriller, which ascribes highly pathogenic avian influenza to Asian cultural habits. Southeast and East Asia have borne the brunt of infection. From the first appearance of H5N1 in 1997, the region has become a focal point for disease prevention efforts and is portrayed in the international media as 'the incubator for a global epidemic of avian influenza.'[74] Politics and public health converged as H5N1 became a locus of contention, particularly in relation to Western accusations of China's lack of international cooperation, transparency, and poor case reporting.[75]

The association of China and Southeast Asia with disease was reinforced when H5N1 resurfaced in early 2003 at the same time as SARS. In February of that year, a father and son were hospitalized in Hong Kong with severe flu-like symptoms after returning from a trip to Fujian province in mainland China. Tests confirmed that they had contracted avian influenza and the father subsequently died. The following year, outbreaks of H5N1 occurred on commercial poultry farms in Vietnam and Thailand, with simultaneous cases in numerous countries across Asia, including South Korea, Japan, and China. Twenty people died in Vietnam after contracting the disease, with 12 deaths confirmed in Thailand. Outbreaks in poultry continued across the region through 2005. Meanwhile, in April 2005, Qinghai Lake became a focus of concern when over 6,000 wild birds died of H5N1. As China's largest lake and an important stopover for many species of migratory birds, the confirmed presence of the virus there raised fears about its global diffusion. Indeed, since 2005, it is believed that migratory birds and trade in poultry account for the spread of the virus to Russia, the Indian subcontinent, the Middle East, Africa, Europe, and North America.

---

[74] Joan A. Kaufman, 'China's Health Care System and Avian Influenza Preparedness,' *Journal of Infectious Diseases*, vol.197, Supplement 1 (February 18, 2008): S7–S13 (S9).

[75] Theresa MacPhail, 'The Politics of Bird Flu: The Battle over Viral Samples and China's Role in Global Public Health,' *Journal of Language and Politics*, vol.8, no.3 (2009): 456–475.

These outbreaks of H5N1 have suggested connections between the evolution and emergence of new viral strains of influenza and the role of anthropogenic change. Evidence points to a number of interrelated factors driving viral subtype dynamics in Asia: population growth, changes in climate and land use, agricultural intensification, and global trade.[76] All of these factors are in fact linked to globalization and to the issues discussed earlier in relation to HIV/AIDS and market liberalization in the PRC. The ecological impact of the urban–industrial 'revolution' in south China has been profound. The Pearl River Delta has become a global manufacturing hub and the principal engine of China's spectacular growth. As noted in the conclusion to Chapter 2, the Delta may be regarded as an emerging megacity and according to the World Bank has become the largest urban conglomeration in the world. Economic development has entailed a transformation in the scale of production and in patterns of consumption: 'From 1990 through 2005, China's production of chicken nearly quadrupled, as did that of duck and goose. The amount of pork more than doubled.'[77] In the decade between the early 1990s and 2000s, 'Asia more than doubled its egg production,' achieving a global market share of 50 percent.[78] Poultry production has increasingly concentrated in agribusinesses outside major urban centers, particularly in Guangdong province in the south.

This intensification of farming practices is not unique to southern China. Across Asia, in Indonesia, Malaysia, Thailand, and Vietnam, the late twentieth century has witnessed similar growth in broiler chicken production and the corporatization of the livestock industry. Today, the poultry business is increasingly dominated by large multinational companies geared to a new global consumer demand for cheap meat. While the number of farms has decreased by half, production has increased six-fold – with Asia at the forefront of this development. In Indonesia, the government statistics agency has calculated that while the annual production of eggs was 59,000 tons in 1970, it had risen to 783,000 tons by 2000.[79] Thailand, in particular, has been at the forefront of this scale-up. Asia's largest agriculture conglomerate with core interests in livestock and aquaculture is the Thai-based company Charoen Pokphand (CP). 'By the mid-1990s,' notes Mike Davis, 'Thailand (which

[76] Kurt J. Vandegrift, et al., 'Ecology of Avian Influenza Viruses in a Changing World,' *Annals of the New York Academy of Sciences*, vol.1195 (May 2010): 113–128.

[77] Sipress, *The Fatal Strain*, p.144.

[78] H. Steinfeld, T. Wassenaar, and S. Jutzi, 'Livestock Production Systems in Developing Countries: Status, Drivers, Trends,' *Scientific and Technical Review*, vol.25, no.2 (August 2006): 505–516 (513).

[79] Sipress, *The Fatal Strain*, p.144.

had adopted CP's corporate slogan, 'Kitchen of the World') had the most corporatized livestock industry in Asia. CP and a handful of other vertically-integrated exporters controlled 80 percent of production, with chicken farming concentrated in a dense, polluted belt 60 to 150 kilometers outside Bangkok.'[80] In tandem with a concerted government drive to increase poultry exports, companies such as CP were crucial in persuading rice farmers to shift to chicken production, providing them with chicks and feed, as well as guaranteed prices for broilers. At the same time, Thailand's economic development and double-digit growth led to rising incomes and increasing demand for a better diet among an urban middle class.[81]

Despite the rise of a transnational poultry industry in China and Southeast Asia, the presiding images that sum up the threat of H5N1 in the Western media – aside from masked officials and 'wet markets' – are 'backyard' poultry, cock fights, and wild birds. The practice of keeping poultry is widespread across the region, sustaining families and providing food security. The accumulated imagery of backyard chickens and ducks reinforces assumptions that small farms are prime sites for biosecurity breaches and the emergence of highly pathogenic avian influenza, and that unsavory native practices may be fueling a future pandemic. These equations are further promoted by government departments and international agencies, such as the WHO and the UN Food and Agriculture Organization (FAO). Meanwhile, the policy emphasis has been on 'restructuring' small-scale poultry farms and encouraging the acceleration of larger, industrial-scale farms. A joint report published in 2005 by the FAO and the World Organisation for Animal Health (OIE), in collaboration with the WHO, noted that for the long-term success of efforts to control highly pathogenic avian influenza it was essential to reorganize poultry production:

It is also becoming increasingly apparent that many reservoirs of infection can be found in the developing world, in particular amongst the lower-income livestock farming segments; i.e. among the rural poor. This poses serious risks to the livestock sector, which is faced with a rapidly expanding demand for dietary animal protein in many developing countries, driven by growing urbanisation, increasing disposable income, and shifts from starch-based to protein-based foods. There are substantial opportunities for economic growth, particularly in rural areas, to be fuelled by this process, widely termed 'Livestock Revolution.'[82]

---

[80] Davis, *The Monster at Our Door*, pp.97–114.   [81] Sipress, *The Fatal Strain*, p.134.
[82] *A Global Strategy for the Progressive Control of Highly Pathogenic Avian Influenza (HPAI)* (Rome: UN Food and Agriculture Organization, November 2005), p.1.

In 2005, one FAO official is reported to have declared: 'The backyard chicken is the big problem . . . and the fight against bird flu must be waged in the backyard of the world's poor.'[83] Declarations such as these by epidemiologists and other 'experts,' which are invariably reaffirmed by state officials, underscore the authoritarian nature of disease prevention and often provoke distrust and resentment on the part of local communities towards what they regard as intrusive health measures.

Vietnam has been one of the countries most affected by H5N1. In the wake of the outbreaks there, the Vietnamese government implemented a draconian policy of culling and vaccinating flocks, along with an intensive disease surveillance program. In 2004, some 66 million birds were culled. Small-scale poultry operations were particularly targeted as potential reservoirs of infection.[84] Following WHO and FAO biosecurity recommendations, there was a concerted drive to discourage wet markets and promote supermarkets, where birds could be purchased that had been slaughtered in government-approved facilities. FAO reports emphasized the public health and surveillance challenges posed by small household flocks. While they acknowledged that 'scavenging poultry production' was important for local livelihoods, they anticipated that such practices would be discontinued when 'the overall benefit to society can be clearly shown to outweigh the cost and compensatory measures are established for the losers.'[85] Despite these qualifications, however, the overwhelming emphasis has been on standardizing operations and restructuring the poultry industry away from household farms towards mass production. This reorientation has involved substantial expenditure, technical developments, and interventions, including a mass vaccination program.

A major part of the Vietnamese government's policy to control avian influenza has focused on 'eliminating backyard operations and reorganizing poultry production along a Western model into large, biosecure agri-businesses.'[86] As a result of this, the market has become progressively restricted for small-scale farmers, who find it harder to trade and transport their poultry. Meanwhile, government-sanctioned commercial farms have been upheld as clean, safe, and efficient. Evidence suggests,

[83] Tran Dinh Thanh Lam, 'Health-Vietnam: Bird Flu Strategy Will Hit Poultry Farmers,' *Inter Press Service* (November 15, 2005).

[84] Stacy Lockerbie and D. Ann Herring, 'Global Panic, Local Repercussions: Economic and Nutritional Effects of Bird Flu in Vietnam.' In: Robert A. Hahn and Marcia C. Inhorn, eds., *Anthropology and Public Health: Bridging Differences in Culture and Society*. Second edition (New York: Oxford University Press, [1999] 2008), pp.566–587 (575).

[85] Nick Honhold, et al., *Biosecurity for Highly Pathogenic Avian Influenza: Issues and Options* (Rome: UN Food and Agriculture Organization, 2008), p.34.

[86] Lockerbie and Herring, 'The Coming Plague of Avian Influenza.' In: Herring and Swedlund, eds., *Plagues and Epidemics*, p.190.

however, that these very enterprises may be implicated in disease emergence: 'The influenza virus spreads slowly among small village chicken flocks and fades out under low-density conditions, but it amplifies rapidly in densely packed factory farms.'[87] Factory farms may not solve the challenge of highly pathogenic influenza, given that: 'Some of the largest outbreaks of avian influenza have been in some of the best-managed poultry operations in the world, in some of the wealthiest countries.'[88]

Humans and animals: One health?

More than half of all new emerging infections are zoonotic. Particularly since the 1990s, there has been an increasing awareness of the close connection between animal and human health, as well as the need to integrate veterinary and human medicines through interdisciplinary collaborations. A symposium convened at Rockefeller University in New York in 2004 by the Wildlife Conservation Society (WCS) popularized the phrase 'One World – One Health.' The aim of the meeting was to examine the interrelationship between humans, livestock, and wildlife – and to determine ways of combating epizootic disease. The notion that human health is interconnected with animal health was not new. Many cultures do not in fact draw a clear distinction between human and animal spheres. 'One health' is premised on a human–animal separation, which it seeks to bridge. Histories of 'one health' invariably ascribe an exclusively Western lineage to the 'one health' concept: from the ancient Greek physician Hippocrates to the veterinary epidemiologist Calvin W. Schwabe (1927–2006). Much of the non-Western world, including Asia, is left out of this canonical history.

Michael Bresalier, Angela Cassidy, and Abigail Woods, 'One Health in History.' In: Jakob Zinsstag, et al., eds., *One Health: The Theory and Practice of Integrated Health Approaches* (Wallingford: CABI, 2015), pp.1–15.

Research has thus suggested that industrial farming practices may be a significant driver of avian influenza. While the stocking densities in commercial broiler houses may enable the rapid spread of pathogenic

---

[87] Lockerbie and Herring, 'The Coming Plague of Avian Influenza.' In: Herring and Swedlund, eds., *Plagues and Epidemics*, pp.189–190.
[88] David Waltner-Toews, *The Chickens Fight Back: Pandemic Panics and Deadly Diseases that Jump from Animals to Humans* (Vancouver: Greystone Books, 2007), p.111.

viruses, the use of genetic selection and incentives for an efficient feed-to-meat ratio may reduce genetic diversity. And finally, spillover events have raised concerns about the biosecurity of these large-size poultry farms.[89] The policy in Vietnam of curtailing backyard poultry rearing in favor of larger farms runs counter to an earlier emphasis on improving rural livelihoods, reducing poverty, and ensuring food security by promoting sustainable local production. While the last two decades have seen an expansion of industrial-scale production systems, much of the public health and media focus has remained on the biosecurity risks posed by village poultry. The consequences of this for some of the poorest populations in Southeast Asia have been significant. Policy has been formulated in a context of widespread Western fear centered on an anticipated viral storm – the 'coming plague' – silently brewing in the backyards and markets of Southeast Asia. Ironically, anxieties about globalization have led to a crackdown on the local, which is viewed as dangerously unregulated – a policy that is likely to be accelerating the very global forces that are driving infection.

Globalization and the shock of history: SARS

At the same time as H5N1 was giving rise to concerns about a potential pandemic, there were reports of a new respiratory disease in China, sparking further fears that the H5N1 virus had mutated enabling human-to-human transmission. It transpired, however, that this was a hitherto unknown disease caused by a novel coronavirus – a species of virus characterized by projecting receptors on its surface, giving it a crown-like appearance (*corona* is the Latin word for 'crown' or 'halo'). SARS made its first appearance in the fall of 2002 in Guangdong before reaching Hong Kong on February 21, 2003, where it gained global media attention, spreading across the world with some 774 confirmed fatalities in 26 countries before the chain of human-to-human transmission was declared broken by the WHO in May 2004. The new 'syndrome' was referred to as 'SARS' by the WHO in a press release on March 15, 2003, while identification of the causative coronavirus was confirmed on April 16, 2003. The catchy acronym SARS invoked another four-syllable viral syndrome – AIDS – suggesting that SARS, too, might explode into a pandemic on an AIDS-like scale. SARS was also uncannily close to the abbreviation by which Hong Kong was known as a Special Administrative Region (SAR)

---

[89] Vandegrift, et al., 'Ecology of Avian Influenza Viruses in a Changing World,' pp.120–122; Horby, et al., 'Drivers of Emerging Zoonotic Infectious Diseases.' In: Yamada et al., eds., *Confronting Emerging Zoonoses*, p.19.

of China. Dubbed the 'Special Administrative Region Syndrome,' Hong Kong officials were reluctant to use the term SARS, choosing instead to call it 'atypical pneumonia,' with consequences for the implementation of quarantine measures.[90]

Hong Kong's reputation as an exceptionally disease-prone city was treated comically by the director Samson Chiu in his movie *Golden Chicken II*, released immediately after SARS in 2003. Set in 2046, the end of the 50-year 'one country, two systems' arrangement, which grants Hong Kong administrative autonomy from the PRC, the movie traces the life of the prostitute Ah Gum (the 'chicken' of the title is a derogatory term in Cantonese to describe a prostitute) in flashbacks, incorporating real news footage of the unfolding SARS crisis. We see the city in virtual lockdown, with citizens resorting to drastic measures to prevent infection: wearing gas masks during sex, shaving their body hair, with one character wrapping himself in plastic cling-film to avoid fatal body contact.

Media commentators invariably viewed SARS as exemplary of the new globalized world: the first 'plague' of the twenty-first century. It illustrated how infection could spread through transnational networks, imperiling global security.[91] The disease's rapid diffusion from East Asia to North America highlighted the challenges that emergent diseases posed for public health, exposing the vulnerabilities of state-centric health governance in controlling epidemics.[92] Cases from Vietnam to Canada and the United States could all be traced back to a doctor – regarded by the WHO as the 'superspreader' – who had traveled from Guangzhou to Hong Kong. In many ways, however, SARS might be understood not as the first plague of the twenty-first century but as a threat that recapitulated earlier fears. It highlighted an incongruity between global networks and a public health machinery reliant on historical measures to combat epidemics. In the PRC, doctors trained in TCM treated over half of all patients admitted to hospital with Chinese herbal medicine, which they combined with biomedical therapeutics.[93] Summarizing the lessons learned from 2003,

So what?

---

[90] Gwendolyn Gong and Sam Dragga, '"SARS" versus "Atypical Pneumonia": Inconsistencies in Hong Kong's Public Health Warnings and Disease-Prevention Campaign.' In: John H. Powers and Xiaosui Xiao, eds., *The Social Construction of SARS: Studies of a Health Communication Crisis* (Amsterdam: John Benjamins, 2008), pp.53–68.

[91] Deborah Davis and Helen F. Siu, eds., *SARS: Reception and Interpretation in Three Chinese Cities* (New York: Routledge, 2104); Ho-fung Hung, 'The Politics of SARS: Containing the Perils of Globalization by More Globalization,' *Asian Perspective*, vol.28, no.1 (2004): 19–44.

[92] David P. Fidler, *SARS, Governance, and the Globalization of Disease* (Basingstoke and New York: Palgrave Macmillan, 2004).

[93] Marta E. Hanson, 'Conceptual Blind Spots, Media Blindfolds: The Case of SARS and Traditional Chinese Medicine.' In: Leung and Furth, eds., *Health and Hygiene in Chinese East Asia*, pp.228–254.

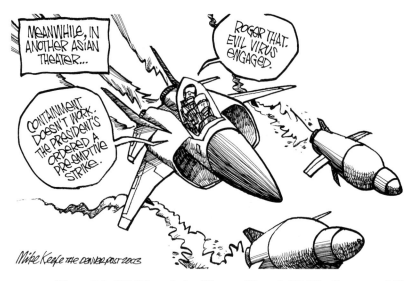

Figure 5.3. 'SARS and the War on Terror' (2003). Courtesy: Mike Keefe.

Viral terror: SARS and the invasion of Iraq

The US-led invasion of Iraq took place in March 2003 as SARS was unfolding. Both events became entangled in the media through metaphors that associated the stealthy coronavirus with a 'killer' and likened the public health response to a military operation (Figure 5.3). President George W. Bush had launched the war on Iraq following the al-Qaeda initiated attacks on New York and Washington in September 2001. The war on terror was envisaged as a military conflict, but also as a counter-insurgency struggle (Chapter 4). Analogies worked both ways as terrorists were equated with lethal viruses. As Richard N. Haass of the US State Department put it in the aftermath of 9/11:

Terrorism lives as part of the environment. Sometimes dormant, sometimes virulent, it is always present in some form. Like a virus, international terrorism respects no boundaries – moving from country to country, exploiting globalized commerce and communication to spread. It can be particularly malevolent when it can find a supportive host. We therefore need to take appropriate prophylactic measures at home and abroad to prevent terrorism from multiplying and check it from infecting our societies or damaging our lives. We need, for instance, better border control regimes and improved international counterterrorism cooperation across the board. We also need to make sure that the virus does not mutate into something even more deadly through the acquisition of nuclear, biological, or chemical weapons of mass destruction.

One justification for the invasion of Iraq had been a concern that Saddam Hussein's regime had acquired and was stockpiling small-pox, which it intended to use indiscriminately. The events of 9/11, along with the anthrax letter scare, had created a context of anxiety and suspicion. The military and counter-insurgency-like responses to SARS were manifest in the Singapore government's establishment of a special 'SARS Combat Unit' and in its institution of a joint 'nerve center' to coordinate intelligence with its US counterpart. 'SARS outbreak is like Singapore's 9/11,' declared the *Straits Times*. By coincidence, 911 was the room number in the Metropole Hotel, Hong Kong, where 64-year-old Liu Jianlin, a doctor from mainland China, stayed in February 2003 to attend a wedding, infecting 16 of the other hotel guests and disseminating the virus in Hong Kong and globally.

Wen-Yu Chiang and Ren-Feng Duann, 'Conceptual Metaphors for SARS: "War" between Whom?' *Discourse & Society*, vol.18, no.5 (2007): 579–602.

the WHO stressed the low-tech and historical nature of the containment strategies adopted:

While modern science had its role, none of the most modern technical tools had an important role in controlling SARS. Sequencing the genetic code of the virus, for example, helped identify the origin and spread of the virus but did not really help to control it ... Most important in controlling SARS were the 19th-century public health strategies of contact tracing, quarantine, and isolation ... [94]

As Alfred Crosby observed, a joke circulating among infectious disease experts at this time went: 'The nineteenth century was followed by the twentieth century, which was followed by ... the nineteenth century.'[95]

Amoy Gardens, a middle-class, high-rise housing estate built in the 1980s in Kowloon Bay, became the symbolic center of the 'fight' against SARS in Hong Kong. Between March and April 2003, 42 residents in

[94] *SARS: How a Global Epidemic Was Stopped* (Geneva: World Health Organization, 2006), p.247.
[95] Crosby, *America's Forgotten Pandemic*, p.xiii.

Amoy Gardens died of SARS, with some 329 residents infected. Apartments were pictured in the media with all the color-coded banality of real estate particulars, including the identikit bathrooms into which, it has been conjectured, the virus fatefully insinuated itself to infect its victims. In Hong Kong, the terms 'Amoy Gardens' and 'Block E,' where 41 percent of the cases of infection had been identified, were employed in common parlance as a shorthand for SARS and its victims, while the entrance to Block E served in the media as a graphic stand-in for the outbreak.[96]

During the first months of the epidemic, authorities in the PRC suppressed news of the disease. In Beijing, the National People's Congress, which had assembled to elect a new president, continued its business as usual and made no official announcement. As the number of SARS cases grew, officials including the minister of health, Zhang Wenkang, minimized the threat. At the beginning of April 2003, Li Liming, director of the Chinese CDC, went as far as to claim that the causative agent was likely not a coronavirus but a 'chlamydia-like agent.' Despite the PRC's economic takeoff, SARS underlined the challenges posed to the status quo by the mass internal migration of workers. Intensified internal mobility provided new opportunities for microbial traffic. Authorities were also conscious that burgeoning networks spawned by the mass movement of workers could serve as conduits for social unrest and panic. The danger presented by migrant labor was frequently reiterated. Rather than viewed as an individual's right, health was promoted as an individual's duty to the state.[97]

Other kinds of connectedness were revealed during SARS. While the authorities imposed a partial news blackout, citizens in the affected areas of southern China used their cell phones to text. In the early 1990s, few rural families had televisions – as we saw in the brief discussion of Zhou's 1994 movie *Ermo* – let alone phones. By the end of the decade, however, China had experienced a communications revolution with the proliferation of digital technologies. For migrants, in particular, phones were an essential purchase. 'In a universe of perpetual motion,' writes journalist Leslie Chang, 'the mobile phone was magnetic north, the thing that fixed a person in place.' The streets of booming cities such as Dongguan were crowded with mobile phone stores catering to migrant workers. As

---

[96] Arthur Kleinman and Sing Lee, 'SARS and the Problem of Social Stigma.' In: Kleinman and Watson, eds., *SARS in China*, pp.173–195 (176).

[97] Christos Lynteris, 'State of Exception, Culture of Medical Police: SARS and the Law of No Rights in the People's Republic of China.' In: Alex Mold and David Reubi, eds., *Assembling Health Rights in Global Context: Genealogies and Anthropologies* (Abingdon and New York: Routledge, 2013), pp.169–185.

Chang observes: 'People referred to themselves in the terminology of mobile phones: *I need to recharge. I am upgrading myself.*'[98] According to the *Southern Weekend*, a newspaper published in Guangzhou, an SMS text message was sent 40 million times on February 8, 2003: 'There is a fatal flu in Guangzhou.' Over the course of the next two days, a further 86 million text messages were sent.[99]

Another development was the advent of the Internet. China was linked to the Internet in 1994 but by 2003 the number of users exceeded those in Japan and soon stood just behind the United States.[100] This digital connectivity opened new channels for citizens to communicate. It also spurred the state to develop a system for monitoring and censoring Internet traffic that was deemed 'sensitive' by officials. In 1998, the Ministry of Public Security launched the Golden Shield Project (nicknamed the Great Firewall of China) with precisely this aim.

The withholding and censoring of information during SARS had several effects: while it led to the circulation of wild rumors, it also gave rise to increasingly innovative tactics for sharing intelligence. In Hong Kong, a dearth of official information prompted the creation of popular open-platform, information-sharing websites such as sosick.org, which recorded 1.8 million hits in a single week in April 2003. The circulation over the Internet of lists of buildings where SARS patients lived and worked obliged the government to release updates on SARS on a more regular basis. In the PRC, Internet users also found ways of circumventing restrictions. In Hu Fayun's novel *Ruyan@SARS.come*, published online in 2006, the central protagonist plays a cat-and-mouse game with the authorities, uploading posts that are then removed. Information spreads on the Internet in a manner analogous to a virus or 'like a self-replicating monster in a horror movie': 'Postings were deleted, even as these deletings were followed in turn by new postings. As the tide washed up, those monster's footprints on the beach were erased – but as soon as it receded, the invisible monster would leave a new set of footprints.' As Carlos Rojas notes, 'official efforts to restrict and quarantine information about the epidemic had the paradoxical effect of helping to stimulate a wide array of new discursive modes and social contacts.'[101] The multiplying meanings, which the disease–syndrome acquired in 2003 as it migrated online and across media, remind us that SARS should be

---

[98] Chang, *Factory Girls*, pp.95–97.
[99] John Pomfret, 'Outbreak Gave China's Hu an Opening,' *Washington Post* (May 13, 2003).
[100] Deborah Davis and Helen Siu, 'SARS: Reception and Interpretations in Three Chinese Cities.' In: Davis and Siu, eds., *SARS*, pp.1–18 (11).
[101] Rojas, *Homesickness*, pp.162, 164–165.

understood simultaneously as 'an epidemic of a transmissible lethal disease and an epidemic of meanings or signification.'[102]

Hu Fayun's novel *Ruyan@SARS.come* and the use of the Internet as a critical source of public information during SARS suggest the complex ways in which epidemic prevention is being reconfigured in an era of digital surveillance. Today, public health agencies, including the WHO through its Global Public Health Intelligence Network (GPHIN), are developing global alert and monitoring systems that mine 'informal' sources of online information, trawling discussion groups to gather 'epidemic intelligence.' Co-opting citizens into a real-time epidemic surveillance system in this way, however, may produce a contagious loopback effect. Online behavior is picked up by intelligence systems that issue early warnings, which may in turn feed back to influence online activity. Commenting on SARS in 2003, the American biologist David Baltimore highlighted the counter-productive effects of media coverage and the dangers of a media-induced 'epidemic of concern': 'The Internet, e-mail, and satellite-enabled media coverage have put public fear on steroids – and lent a dark twist to the old dot-com hype about the promise of "viral marketing."'[103]

'SARS has been our country's 9/11,' one Chinese journalist observed during the crisis. 'It has forced us to pay attention to the real meaning of globalization . . . China's future seemed so dazzling [that it] lulled people into thinking that our country was immune from the shocks of history.'[104] The PRC government was widely censured in the international media for its inertia and lack of transparency, and particularly for its failure to cooperate fully with the WHO investigation. Frustrated by the lack of disclosure, a retired military physician, Jiang Yanyong, fed information to the foreign press, including *Time* magazine. In a piece entitled 'Beijing's SARS Attack' published on April 8, the journalist Susan Jakes stated that based on Jiang's leaked information, 'the number of patients infected with SARS in Beijing may be significantly higher than those totals made public by China's Ministry,' and she asked: 'How many cases are unreported?' Against this mounting criticism, and as the epidemic worsened, Beijing changed its policy. A national SARS meeting was convened at which Premier Wen Jiabao called for intensified efforts to combat the epidemic. Minister Zhang and the mayor of Beijing, Meng Xuelong, were

[102] Paula A. Treichler, *How to Have Theory in an Epidemic: Cultural Chronicles of AIDS* (Durham, NC: Duke University Press, [1999] 2004), p.11.
[103] David Baltimore, 'SAM – Severe Acute Media Syndrome?' *Wall Street Journal* (April 28, 2003).
[104] Erik Eckholm, 'Spread of SARS Acts as a Rude Awakening for China,' *New York Times* (May 13, 2003).

sacked on April 20. On May 1, the Chinese government launched what President Hu called a 'people's war against SARS' – a 'war' that rapidly assumed the character of a Maoist-era health campaign (Chapter 3).

Migrancy in the PRC is regulated through a household registration system (*hukou*) introduced in 1958, which obliges rural-born citizens to register with the police upon arrival in a city. Attempts to cover up the beating to death by police of an illegal migrant, Sun Zhigang, in February 2003, served to highlight the connection between SARS and the plight of migrants, as well as the lack of transparency in the handling of both issues. The government moved to tighten its surveillance of the so-called 'floating population' (*liudong renkou*), estimated to be well over 100 million. Strict quarantine measures were imposed and special treatment centers for SARS patients were set up. In May, directives were issued that allowed for the detention in quarantine for up to 14 days of travelers returning home from SARS-affected regions. Equipment for monitoring the temperature of travelers was installed at public transport hubs. Health registration forms tracked migrant returnees and immediate isolation was imposed on those showing SARS-like symptoms. Asymptomatic returnees were kept under medical inspection in their home villages. Since the vast majority of migrants to the cities had little access to healthcare, the government reserved a special fund to cover the cost of emergency treatment and avert a panicked exodus to the countryside. Businesses were also required to pay salaries to those who were quarantined or being treated for SARS.

A system of rural neighborhood surveillance, which harked back to the pre-reform era, was instated. Residents were mobilized to prevent the disease from entering their communities. Roadblocks were set up and patrolled at the entrance to villages. Local anti-SARS teams disseminated information about the disease, checked up on the health of residents, and routinely disinfected the environs. In some instances, surveillance was even more intense. An information-collector was appointed to monitor households in order to gather 'SARS-related information among the families,' including names of the recent returnees and the health conditions of those under home quarantine. In May 2003, the *People's Daily* – an official organ of the Party – reported that following an inspection of villages in Hebei province, WHO health officials had praised the 'rigorous strategies' and 'community involvement,' which had prevented SARS from spreading further.[105]

Legal measures, as we have seen, were also imposed to stem the infection. As Wen asserted, the priority was to 'bring fully into play legal

---

[105] Ding, 'Transnational Quarantine Rhetorics,' pp.198–199.

weapons to win the war in preventing SARS.' In the absence of any provision dealing explicitly with the deliberate and criminal spreading of infectious disease, the State Council promulgated 'The Emergency Provisions in Dealing with Public Health Crises,' which was followed by 'The Explanations Concerning the Issues in the Application of Law Regarding Criminal Cases on the Prevention and Control of Outbreaks of Infectious Disease.' An array of activities were defined as criminal, including – to the consternation of the WHO – the 'deliberate spreading of infectious disease pathogens and virus [sic] and endangering public security.' Military metaphors were ubiquitous in descriptions of the 'fight' against SARS. A five-episode documentary entitled *The Battle of Guiwei*, broadcast in July 2003, concluded with a triumphalist celebration of China's collective fight against the 'enemy' and a laudation of the nation's brave healthcare warriors (Figure 5.4).[106]

Such war analogizing was not, of course, unique to the PRC. Militaristic metaphors were employed by the media across much of East and Southeast Asia, in contrast to the coverage in Britain, where they were largely absent.[107] In the report produced by the Pacific West Region of the WHO after SARS, public health operations were described as a war, replete with battlegrounds, frontlines, and allies. In a characteristic bellicose pronouncement, Tung Chee-hwa, Hong Kong's Chief Executive, asserted 'we are confident that we can win the war,' while Malaysia's health minister, Chua Jui Meng, proclaimed 'we must remember that in this region, we are more likely to be invaded by microbes than by a foreign army.' In Singapore, as in the PRC, 'wartime' dedication to service was commemorated in ceremonies that accentuated the heroism of workers on the 'frontlines' of the campaign against SARS.

Military conceptualizations in Asia co-existed with another figuration of the virus: SARS-as-insurgent. In the preface of the WHO account, the epidemic is described as if it were an omnipresent terrorist. 'It showed explosive power,' writes Shigeru Omi, director of WHO's Western Pacific Region, 'setting off multiple outbreaks around the world, often zeroing in on hospitals, attacking doctors and nurses and bringing some public-health systems to their knees.'[108] The sense of SARS as an 'unidentified' adversary, particularly in the early stages of the epidemic, created further associations with the elusive terrorist networks involved in the

---

[106] Ronald C. Keith and Zhiqiu Lin, *New Crime in China: Public Order and Human Rights* (Abingdon and New York: Routledge, 2006), pp.155, 157.

[107] Patrick Wallis and Birgitte Nerlich, 'Disease Metaphors in New Epidemics: The UK Media Framing of the 2003 SARS Epidemic,' *Social Science & Medicine*, vol.60, no.11 (June 2005): 2629–2639.

[108] *SARS: How a Global Epidemic Was Stopped*, p.vii.

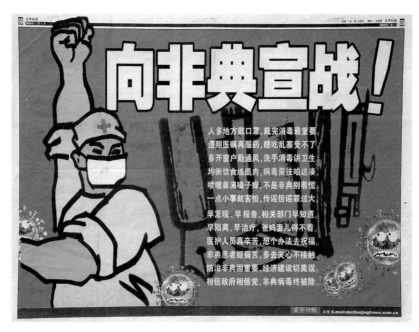

Figure 5.4. 'Declare War on SARS!' *Beijing Times* (2003). Courtesy: US
National Library of Medicine.

SARS and Maoist public health

This SARS poster (Figure 5.4), which appeared on Labor Day
2003, draws on earlier Maoist propaganda posters from the Great
Leap Forward and the Cultural Revolution in the 1950s, 1960s,
and early 1970s. In our discussion of the schistosomiasis campaign
in Chapter 3, we saw how rural populations were mobilized in the
'fight' against disease, which was also a means of promoting unity.
As Marta Hanson has observed, the phrase in the SARS poster
echoes the slogan of the Communist Revolution 'Serve the People!' The poster presents SARS as a national enemy to be subdued
through a concerted people's campaign. The final line in the poster
declares: 'Trust the Government, Trust the Party; the SARS virus
will ultimately be eliminated.'

Marta Hanson, 'Maoist Public-Health Campaigns, Chinese
Medicine, and SARS,' *Lancet*, vol. 372, no. 9648 (October 25, 2008):
1457–1458.

9/11 attacks on the United States. The Tan Tock Seng Hospital in Singapore, where Esther Mok was admitted to Ward 5 on March 1, 2003 to become the first SARS patient in the island city-state, was the center of the 'battle' against 'an unknown enemy,' which turned the hospital into 'SARS' ground zero.'[109] In Hong Kong, Amoy Gardens flashed on television screens around the world as yet another instance of global shock. The public health operation launched to contain the epidemic reinforced this linkage of epidemic and terror: the rushed rewriting of legislation; the lockdown with barricades and tape; the brown-bagged victims bussed out under escort to an isolated camp in the New Territories; the parading of armed police in surgical masks on the perimeters; the hunt for 'infected' residents who had fled the scene. As the epidemiologist Thomas Tsang of the Hong Kong Department of Health subsequently confided: 'At one moment we thought it might be a biological attack because of the vertical arrangement of cases.'[110]

The emphasis on the 'fight' against the virus in many official versions of the SARS narrative converged with an iconography reminiscent of avian influenza. Pictures of wet markets, eviscerated civet cats, surgically gowned officials, and quarantined buildings preponderated. Different versions of the 'primitive farm' narrative, as we saw in our discussion of avian influenza, also pervaded the reporting of SARS. An article in *Newsweek* on May 5, 2003, which appeared after the masked cover image the previous week ('SARS: What You Need to Know – The New Age of Epidemics'), attributed the disease to unhealthy Chinese living conditions: 'Pigs, ducks, chickens and people live cheek-by-jowl on the district's primitive farms, exchanging flu and cold germs so rapidly that a single pig can easily incubate human and avian viruses simultaneously.' Aside from the dubious biology, this passage recuperates a nineteenth-century sanitarian and Orientalist discourse, wherein Asia and the working poor of industrial cities were imagined as perilously teeming multitudes with herd-like propensities for 'overcrowded' living. 'One thing China hasn't learned from its SARS experience,' *Newsweek* noted later that year, 'is that its eating habits – particularly the taste for freshly killed meat – might have to change. Scientists found that civets, a cat-size creature and a local delicacy, can harbor the SARS virus . . . This winter the battle will be shaping up between China's tradition and the world's safety.' Such texts juxtapose Chinese 'tradition' to the 'modern' world. SARS is

---

[109] Mui Hoong Chua, *A Defining Moment: How Singapore Beat SARS* (Singapore: Ministry of Information, Communications and the Arts; Institute of Policy Studies, 2004), pp.26, 34.

[110] Thomas Abraham, *Twenty-First Century Plague: The Story of SARS* (Hong Kong: Hong Kong University Press, 2004), p.73.

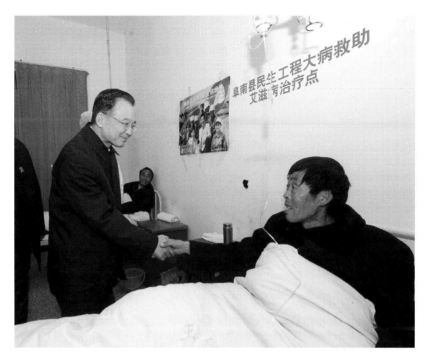

Figure 5.5. 'Wen Jiabao publicly shakes the hand of an AIDS patient on World AIDS Day' (2003). Courtesy: Rao Aimin/Xinhua Press/Corbis.

SARS and HIV/AIDS

After SARS, there was a new openness to other diseases in the PRC, including HIV/AIDS. On December 1, 2003 – World AIDS Day – Premier Wen Jiabao shook hands with AIDS patients on state television, urging citizens to treat AIDS sufferers with 'care and love.' This symbolic encounter and official pronouncement marked an important shift in policy: no senior Chinese figure had hitherto broached the issue of HIV/AIDS so publicly.

Yanzhong Huang, 'The SARS Epidemic and its Aftermath in China: A Political Perspective.' In: Stacey Knobler, et al., eds., *Learning from SARS: Preparing for the Next Disease Outbreak* (Washington, DC: National Academies Press, 2004), pp.116–136.

conceived as the product of a dangerous cultural self-centeredness that has little regard for the security of the wider community. What is glossed over is the West's complicity: an insatiable appetite for cheap Chinese produce, the push for an expansion of capital markets, and a tolerance of conspicuous inequalities.

In the reporting of SARS, the international media's focus was on masked, anonymous Asian crowds; lone passengers on empty trains; airports and other mass transit hubs devoid of people; deserted streets, guestless hotels, and vacant commercial spaces.[111] Hong Kong and Singapore were conjured as eerily frozen: bereft of tourists, with business at a stand-still. This imagery of vacancy and abandonment suggested the global city working in reverse, transformed from a center of capital and commerce into a node of global infection. The sense of loss that pervaded these visual depictions of SARS derived, not so much from the loss of life, as from the loss of business and the disorientation that this forfeiture induced in a city that exists for the sole purpose of global trade.

Conclusion: Globalization inside out

The emergence of pathogens in human societies, as we have seen, is not a new phenomenon. What is of particular concern today, however, is the frequency of this emergence and the speed with which infectious diseases are now able to spread globally. Cases of emerging and re-emerging infections since the 1980s have suggested a new dynamic of pathogenic evolution and transmission. The cross-border threats posed by recent pandemics – notably the 2009 H1N1 influenza pandemic – have also underscored the importance of instituting public health approaches that are global. 'The same forces of globalization that birthed the Asian tiger economies,' writes Sipress, 'can now speed the flu virus around the world within a day.'[112]

This chapter has explored a number of interconnections between infectious disease emergence and globalization across Asia. While globalization has been considered in relation to the extension and intensification of global interconnectedness, I have also emphasized the relationship between highly local circumstances and global flows, the impact of economic liberalization, and the social and environmental transformations that this liberalization has produced. The effects of globalization are evident in the PRC, where since the late 1970s profound realignments have

---

[111] David Serlin, 'Introduction: Toward a Visual Culture of Public Health: From Broadside to YouTube.' In: David Serlin, ed., *Imagining Illness: Public Health and Visual Culture* (Minneapolis: University of Minnesota Press, 2010), pp.xi–xxxvii (xiv–xvii).

[112] Sipress, *The Fatal Strain*, p.136.

taken place between state institutions, society, and the broader global community. The country has been transformed from a collectivized society to a society that has – often uncomfortably – sought to combine one-party socialism with market capitalism. The ramifications of this process across Asia and globally have been profound, as East and Southeast Asia become a leading force of economic change.

A central argument in the chapter has been that the timespan of these political and economic changes has coincided with an explosion of viral diseases in epidemics of HIV/AIDS, SARS, and avian influenza, which have prompted contradictory responses. On the one hand, these epidemics have been attributed to development: to rampant industrialization, for example, and to an unprecedented scale of urbanization. On the other hand, epidemics have been viewed as an increasing impediment to necessary development. According to this last view, more not less development is required: urbanization may provide a more efficient setting for healthcare delivery and disease surveillance, while the industrialization of agriculture and food production may enhance biosecurity. Efforts at epidemic prevention have been driven by economic concerns. A priority for governments in Asia (and elsewhere) has been to safeguard their economic standing. In Hong Kong after SARS, the emphasis was principally on the loss of business and on revitalizing the economy.[113] The cost of SARS to the PRC is estimated to have been US$17.9 billion. There is now much greater consciousness of the economic fallout that such events would have in the rapid-growth economies across Asia.

Connected to the issue of development and economic performance is a tension between globalization and modernity, which has been underlined by recent epidemics in East Asia. This tension is manifest in each of the case studies presented above. First, globalization may be conceived as the erosion of national and state autonomy. China's decision to work with the WHO during SARS – as well as with other national and international agencies –amounted to a recognition by the PRC leadership of the need for collaboration in the face of a 'supra-territorial' threat. If SARS demonstrated the globalization of disease, it also revealed a new governance context, which enabled the success of a global effort against SARS.[114] Second, however, modernity may be understood as a largely state-driven process of development, which is in turn powered by globalization. Confronted by an epidemic of HIV/AIDS, PRC officials responded to the

---

[113] John Nguyet Erni, 'SARS, Avian Flu, and the Urban Double Take.' In: Davis and Siu, eds., *SARS*, pp.45–73.
[114] Fidler, *SARS, Governance, and the Globalization of Disease.*

infection in developmental terms. The 'fight' against disease was waged as a national campaign, even though the disease was borderless. In this last case, globalization may be considered, in effect, as a force that extends modernity, reaffirming a developmental model, with the state as the central actor. The equation in the Chinese media of areas of impoverished rural China, where HIV prevalence is high, with sub-Saharan Africa is telling. It suggests that there is a developing world within China: a world where the only solution may be a form of neocolonial intervention.

In *Epidemics in Modern Asia*, I have examined Asia as a space of interaction, tracking epidemics from the subcontinent to the Russian Far East. Asian diasporas outside Asia have, of course, been crucial to the rise of countries such as India and China. In the twenty-first century, the Chinese involvement in Africa has marked an important shift in the balance of power. The PRC has overtaken the United States to become Africa's biggest trade partner.[115] Zambia has been at the forefront of this Chinese expansion, and since the late 1990s there has been substantial Chinese investment in Zambia's copper mines, as well as in manufacturing and agriculture.[116] China has begun to play a more active role, too, in infectious disease prevention work on the continent, and has launched a number of anti-malaria initiatives.[117] In 2015, the Chinese pharmacologist Youyou Tu was awarded the Nobel Prize for her discovery in 1971 of the antimalarial properties of artemisinin, a compound extracted from the sweet wormwood or *qinghao* (*Artemisa annua*). While artemisinin had long been used as a herbal remedy for fevers in TCM, modern artemisinin-based drugs have proven highly effective in combating malaria in Africa – although resistance has become a growing problem in areas of Southeast Asia, with fears that the drug-resistant parasite could spread to infect Africa's *Anopheles coluzzii* mosquitoes. In 2014, Chinese doctors, nurses, technicians, and engineers were dispatched to Liberia to run a new multi-million dollar Ebola clinic built by the PRC. 'Up to now in Liberia, China is the only country which provides not only the construction of an ETU (Ebola treatment unit), but also the running and operation and the staffing of an ETU,' Zhang Yue, the Chinese ambassador to Liberia announced. He added: 'They experienced SARS (severe

[115] Howard W. French, *China's Second Continent: How a Million Migrants Are Building a New Empire in Africa* (New York: Alfred A. Knopf, 2014); Juan Pablo Cardenal and Heriberto Araújo, *China's Silent Army: The Pioneers, Traders, Fixers and Workers Who are Remaking the World in Beijing's Image*. Translated by Catherine Mansfield (London: Allen Lane, 2013).

[116] French, *China's Second Continent*, p.43.

[117] Peilong Liu, et al., 'China's Distinctive Engagement in Global Health,' *Lancet*, vol.384, no.9945 (August 30, 2014): 793–804.

acute respiratory syndrome). They are very knowledgeable in this area.'[118] On a state visit to Britain in October 2015, President Xi Jin-ping, speaking before the British Parliament, noted China's intervention to save the life of Corporal Anna Cross who had contracted Ebola in Sierra Leone earlier in the year. The British Army reservist and nurse was the first person to be given the experimental Ebola drug MIL 77 after the PRC 'promptly responded' to British requests for help.

For some observers, China has come of age and is stepping up to its global humanitarian responsibilities. To others, however, China's disease prevention work is nothing more than a form of strategic health diplo-macy, closely connected to its expanding trade and resource interests across the continent. Chinese banks, businesses, and construction com-panies are expanding their markets, finding in Africa an outlet for their capital, goods, and services. Africa is also providing China with valuable raw materials to sustain its growth. The bridges, roads, and other basic infrastructure constructed by Chinese companies are part of a project-finance barter system wherein China invests in African countries in return for long-term supplies of hydrocarbons and minerals.

The rising number of Chinese laborers working in Africa has also raised the specter of disease transmission back to China. Chikungunya, a viral disease transmitted by mosquitoes, has extended its reach from Africa to Indonesia. There have been fears that malaria may be reintroduced to China, and there are increasing calls within the PRC for a more robust surveillance and response system to prevent the importation of infections back from Africa.[119] Schistosomiasis has been reintroduced from Chi-nese workers in Tanzania and Angola.[120] On a visit to China in 2014, the microbiologist Peter Piot – part of the team that first identified Ebola in 1976 – warned that the country was at risk from Ebola, given the number of Chinese workers in West Africa. Security at airports in China's boom towns of southern Guangdong province, where there are sizeable African communities, was bolstered.

Of course, China is not the only country in Asia to be affected. There are Indian and Filipino workers in West Africa. And as the Ebola epi-demic unfolded in 2014 and 2015, Asian countries with relatively few

---

[118] 'Chinese Team Arrives in Liberia to Staff Ebola Clinic,' *Reuters* (November 16, 2014).

[119] Yaobao Liu, et al., 'Malaria in Overseas Labourers Returning to China: An Analysis of Imported Malaria in Jiangsu Province, 2001–2011,' *Malaria Journal*, vol.13, no.29 (January 25, 2014): doi:10.1186/1475-2875-13-29.

[120] Poh Lian Lim, 'Schistosoma Haematobium in China, ex-Africa: New Populations at Risk?' *Journal of Travel Medicine*, vol.20, no.4 (July/August 2013): 211–213.

connections to the region, such as Malaysia, drew up preparedness plans modeled on their past experience – in this case, the NiV outbreak in 1998. Today, Asia's intensifying connections with Africa are providing a new dynamic to epidemic infections: both in terms of an Asian global presence and in terms of new, ramifying global pathways of disease.

Conclusion: Epidemics and the end of history

Until recently, and with a few notable exceptions, social and political histories of Asia had surprisingly little to say about disease. Despite the historical impact of epidemics on human societies in terms of mortality and morbidity, there has been a reluctance to invest such episodes with the significance attached to a war or a dynastic change. Epidemics take center stage only when they cannot be avoided, and even then they are most often invoked as contextual material for narratives that hinge on social, political, and economic developments. This has led to a striking asymmetry: while pages in textbooks on China are devoted to the collapse of the Ming dynasty in the 1640s, only a few sentences are included in passing on the loss of life that resulted from catastrophic epidemics. Similarly, while tomes are written about the First World War, comparatively little attention is paid to the 1918–1919 influenza pandemic in India, which may have killed up to 20 million people – far more than the sum total of those who perished in combat.

One reason for this relegation of epidemics in history has been that they have tended to be viewed as exceptional occurrences. They have been construed as exogenous events, extrinsic to the societies they affect. Like natural disasters, epidemics are understood to crash into communities from without: they belong, accordingly, to a space outside human history. Another reason is that examining the history of infectious disease is deemed to require specialized knowledge and expertise that goes beyond textual scrutiny of the historical archive. How can we write about infections if we have no formal training in, say, epidemiology or microbiology? Because epidemics are intertwined with environmental issues that are vast and complex, they are difficult to grapple with. To engage with such issues and the incommensurable scales they comprise (the very focused and the expansive), history would need to become radically transdisciplinary.[1] It would also involve uncertainty since many

---

[1] 'AHR Conversation – How Size Matters: The Question of Scale in History,' *American Historical Review*, vol.118, no.5 (2013): 1431–1472.

questions about the origin and identity of diseases in history cannot be readily answered. William McNeill has expressed this tension succinctly: 'We all want human experience to make sense, and historians cater to this universal demand by emphasizing elements in the past that are calculable, definable, and, often, controllable as well. Epidemic disease, when it did become decisive in peace or in war, ran counter to the effort to make the past intelligible. Historians consequently played such episodes down.'[2]

Over the last two decades, however, there has been a new interest in the history of epidemic disease in Asia. What has driven this? In part, it has stemmed from recognition of the role of nonhuman agency in explaining historical change. History has conventionally been concerned with humans as actors who effect change in the world. Technology and the nonhuman world, including animals, plants, and the broader biosphere, are understood to be the objects with which – and upon which – humans act. Increasingly, however, attention is being paid to the impact of nonhuman forces. Understood as environmental events, epidemics are invested with an agency to the extent that they exert a determining influence upon human societies.

Linked to this has been a further expansion of history from the social and environmental approaches of the 1960s and 1970s to 'deep' histories that draw on physics, biology, and archaeology in order to resituate the human past in an all-encompassing evolutionary and planetary context.[3] As we saw in our discussion of the Anthropocene in Chapter 3, both of these new directions have developed out of concerns about climate change and the degradation of the environment. In Southeast Asia, a region of exceptional biodiversity, as well as in the PRC, the environmental crisis triggered by interconnected anthropogenic causes is particularly pronounced and is leading to a new concentration on the history of human–environment interactivity.

Recent scholarship on colonial medicine and hygienic modernity has also demonstrated the importance of biomedicine and public health in the operations of the modern state. This work has shown how medical institutions and epidemic control measures functioned as crucial mechanisms for managing populations and extending centralized state-power: from China and Japan, to India and the Philippines. Above all, perhaps, the threat posed to the contemporary world by emerging infections is fueling a new interest in past epidemics. Asia is widely conceived as a

---

[2] McNeill, *Plagues and Peoples*, p.12.
[3] David Christian, *Maps of Time: An Introduction to Big History* (Berkeley: University of California Press, [2004] 2011).

hotspot for such diseases. Histories of epidemics reflect a recognition of the imperative to understand the nature of this challenge and what role history might play in mitigating future threats.

Epidemics in Modern Asia has been concerned with disease in history but would it be possible to write an equivalent history that centered on the non-diseased or 'healthy' condition? If so, what would such a history look like? The issue of what constitutes health remains as problematic as the issue of how disease is defined (Introduction). As oppositional categories, 'health' and 'disease' imply that there are only two human states whereas, as we have seen, diseases are socially and culturally contingent. The concept of 'health' itself has been eroded: for example, by the identification of gene mutations that determine an individual's susceptibility to specific infectious diseases.[4] Are such individuals healthy or does their pre-diseased state make them unhealthy? This book has sought to examine the evolution of biomedical ideas about infectious disease, tracking the transfer of technologies across Asia through different local, national, and transnational circuits. In other words, although the focus has been on infectious disease, the book has also been concerned with the provision of healthcare – with shifting ideas about what 'health' is and arguments about how it might be safeguarded, maintained, and promoted through practices of preventive medicine, public health, and hygiene.

Epidemics and themes in Asian history

A number of broad themes, reflected in the organization of this book, have tended to dominate modern Asian histories. The first theme is the transition from Western empire-building to the formation of sovereign nation-states. Here, the emphasis has been on tracing the continuities and discontinuities between the expansion of Western colonial powers in Asia from the sixteenth century, the rise of anti-colonial movements, and the institution of postcolonial states in the aftermath of the Second World War. Another interrelated theme is Asia's economic transformation as a result of capitalist expansion, which witnessed the rise of industry and urbanization, as well as the reorganization of agriculture. Third, is the emergence of the modern state and the bureaucratic restructuring of Asian societies that it precipitated, particularly from the late nineteenth century. A new form of governmentality was imposed through regulatory state apparatuses, along with technologies of information-gathering and the production of specialized knowledge. Fourth, is a focus on Asia's

---

[4] S. J. Chapman and A. V. Hill, 'Human Genetic Susceptibility to Infectious Disease,' *Nature Reviews Genetics*, vol.13, no.3 (February 7, 2012): 175–188.

uneven development and the striking disparities that it has given rise to. And fifth, is the importance of migration in the history of modern Asia and the fresh perspectives that migration studies offer on state-formation and the development of modern ideas about citizenship.

The aim of this book has not been to endorse a new sub-discipline – that of epidemic history. Rather, I have argued that studying epidemics may provide new ways of approaching these key themes and, in so doing, of reframing historical change. Empires in Asia produced conduits for disease, even as colonial agencies sought to regulate circulations with the imposition of border controls and quarantines. The growth of cities, the expansion of industry, and the development of large-scale and intensive agriculture transformed Asia's ecology with consequences for human health and disease. Medicine and technologies of epidemic prevention and control were integral to the process of state-formation. Mass migrations across Asia from the nineteenth century also had a profound role in accelerating microbial traffic, while flows of ideas and the transfer of knowledge shaped the ways in which diseases were understood and managed.

Studying infectious disease episodes in the past encourages us to rethink conventional historical parameters, both chronological and geographical. Epidemics highlight the contingency of state borders, while they suggest the interconnected nature of historical change, in so doing de-provincializing national narratives. As Rosenberg would have it, epidemics 'enable us to see, at one moment in time, the configuration of values and attitudes that, in less-stressful times, are so fragmented or so taken for granted that they are not easily visible.' An epidemic crisis 'illustrates the way in which its components – namely, technical understanding and available therapeutic options, epidemiological contours, policy responses, and cultural values – have intersected in ever-changing patterns.'[5] The danger of such a view, of course, is that we imagine epidemics to be portals onto the past; that is, we imagine that they offer unobstructed vistas onto otherwise obscure historical processes, cutting through accumulated cultural layers to some deep, abiding truth. In contrast, however, epidemics underscore the messiness of history and the complex entanglement of biology and culture.

Epidemics and historical scale

I began this book with a view over Victoria Harbour, Hong Kong, so it seems fitting to conclude with another local perspective: a view over the

---

[5] Rosenberg, 'Siting Epidemic Disease,' p.S6.

Hong Kong Museum of Medical Sciences in Sheung Wan. Inaugurated in 1906 as the colony's first Bacteriological Institute, the Museum is a large red-brick building sited on a buff above Taipingshan, the poor Chinese quarter that was the epicenter of the 1894 bubonic plague epidemic in Hong Kong Island's Central and Western District. The tenement buildings, regarded as insanitary by the government, were demolished under the Taipingshan Resumption Ordinance and the area was subsequently redeveloped with the construction of Blake Gardens – named after the governor of Hong Kong, Sir Henry Arthur Blake (1840–1918) – and the Bacteriological Institute.

There had been repeated calls for the establishment of such a laboratory, particularly given the recrudescence of plague at the turn of the century. By then, laboratory science increasingly underpinned medicine and public health. As Governor Blake observed in 1901, in a dispatch to the Colonial Office: 'It is felt to be of cardinal importance that there should be a laboratory for original research in the Colony, in which it is feared that plague, of which a serious epidemic is now raging, may become endemic, the effect of which would be disastrous for this Colony as a great port of call.'[6] The laboratory was envisioned as a key instrument in the fight against epidemic threats, even as it was viewed as a defensive institution that would help to preserve Hong Kong's commercial vitality and its global pre-eminence as an imperial port city.

In the history of the 1894 plague outbreak, the laboratory occupies a critical site: it was, after all, the place where the causative microorganism of the disease was first identified. A correspondent for the *Hongkong Daily Press* who visited Yersin's makeshift laboratory set up by the Alice Memorial Hospital in Kennedy Town marveled at the disease's new visibility. The germ, he reported excitedly in July 1894, had been cultured in an agar plate 'like a little plant': 'It is of a cloudy amber colour and spreads in numerous small blotchy looking branches.' Observed through the microscope, '"colonies" of bacillus [sic] are differentiated into tiny dots of uniform size and appearance.'[7]

How was it possible to reconcile this new, microscopic scale of disease with a pandemic that was sweeping the globe, inflicting millions of deaths across continents? The sizeable structure of Hong Kong's first Bacteriological Institute underscores this tension between the conspicuousness of colonial power and the indiscernible pathogenic agents the building was designed to isolate. The divergent scales on which the epidemic occurred

---

[6] Henry A. Blake to Joseph Chamberlain (June 12, 1901), Great Britain, Colonial Office, General Correspondence: Hong Kong, 1841–1951, Series 129, CO129/305, pp.350–356 (353).
[7] 'The Plague,' *Hongkong Daily Press* (July 6, 1894), p.2.

are evident, too, in Yersin's seminal paper on the plague, published in the *Annales de l'Institut Pasteur*, in which he zooms in and out from the micro-scale of the laboratory to the macro-scale of the disease's interregional diffusion. Plates of the magnified bacteria sit alongside a narrative that establishes an encompassing geographical context for the plague in Yunnan and along China's southwestern frontiers with Indochina. From this geopolitical setting, Yersin 'follows a rhythm of expanding and contracting scales: from macro to micro and back again.' While he focuses on the pathology of the disease as the trained clinician, he shifts perspective to consider the epidemiological evidence, with discussion of the native Chinese dwellings and the flawed sewerage system.[8]

The differing scales in Yersin's plague description, like the imposing red-brick colonial laboratory built in 1906 to make invisible microbes visible, remind us of the incongruent dimensions that epidemics involve. Infectious diseases occur on a micro scale: on the scale of the microscopic pathogenic organism and further, on molecular and atomic nanoscales. However, pandemics occur on a global scale; they are planetary crises, stretching across territorial extents that cannot be defined by categories such as the nation-state. In the late nineteenth century, as the microscope was expanding the parameters of the visual, new forms of steam-powered transportation and telegraphic communication were shrinking the world. In an article on 'The Shrinkage of the World,' in 1894, the *Spectator* was in awe at China's new proximity to London and wondered 'what the ultimate result' of this shrinkage might be.[9] Newspapers, journals, and scientific reports were full of it: the world was officially contracting. How should we connect these discordant scales? Is it possible to develop a new approach to multi-scalar phenomena, wherein history may be studied simultaneously on the micro-scale and along ecological and planetary timelines? As the historian Edmund Burke has noted, although environmental historians may be 'aware that ecology is a global and holistic science, [they] have tended to frame their work more narrowly and to focus on the impact of anthropogenic change on ecological regions or even particular eco-niches. Few have sought to make broader connections to world-historical forces.'[10]

---

[8] Robert Peckham, 'Matshed Laboratory: Colonies, Cultures, and Bacteriology.' In: Robert Peckham and David M. Pomfret, eds., *Imperial Contagions: Medicine, Hygiene, and Cultures of Planning in Asia* (Hong Kong: Hong Kong University Press, 2013), pp.123–147 (142).

[9] 'The Effects of the Shrinkage of the World,' *Spectator* (September 15, 1900), p.9.

[10] Edmund Burke III, 'Preface.' In: Edmund Burke III and Kenneth Pomeranz, eds., *The Environment and World History* (Berkeley: University of California Press, 2009), pp.xi–xiv (xi–xii).

Diffusing across Asia from China to India, plague accentuated this ambiguity of proportion. In the words of Louis Pasteur (1822–1895), it showed up 'the infinitely great power of the infinitely small.'[11] Plague was an invisible 'germ,' newly discovered and observable under the microscope; plague was a disease manifest in bodily symptoms and distinctive clinical conditions; plague was a local event and a global phenomenon, which decimated millions. Plague was infinitesimal and it was colossal. The question that preoccupied contemporaries, then, was not so much what *was* plague? As: *Where* was plague? What space did plague exist in? Grappling with this coincidental multi-dimensionality – not so much sliding scales as a simultaneity of the minuscule and the monumental – compels us to rethink conventional spatial units in history.[12]

Today, technologies are accelerating and extending this scalar range further. During the 2014 Ebola virus outbreak, remote sensing technology was deployed to map hitherto unmapped regions of West Africa in order to assist with public health interventions. Orbiting satellites and remote imaging are increasingly used as tools to monitor environmental conditions, such as relative levels of vegetation, temperature, rainfall, and soil moisture, which are associated with particular pathogens and disease vectors. Environmental data from satellite imagery is fed into other data sources to produce epidemic risk maps with a view to tracking and pre-empting outbreaks.[13] In Asia, satellites are co-opted to monitor environments for avian influenza and to better understand the vector transmission of malaria. In the Malaysian state of Sabah on Borneo, drones have been used to map areas affected by a malaria parasite (*Plasmodium knowlesi*), which infects macaque monkeys and is spread via mosquitoes. The use of such satellite technology in public health points to military models of surveillance, tactical intelligence, and targeting systems. These are precisely the kinds of drone technology utilized by the United States against the Taliban in the tribal areas along the Afghan–Pakistan border where, as we have seen, a counter-insurgency struggle has become fatefully entangled in a polio immunization campaign. The push to understand the sub-molecular and genetic structure of pathogens co-exists today with a global vantage epitomized by the view of the earth from orbit.

[11] René J. Dubos, *Louis Pasteur: Free Lance of Science* (Boston: Little, Brown and Co., 1950), p.45.

[12] Robert Peckham, 'Hong Kong Junk: Plague and the Economy of Chinese Things,' *Bulletin of the History of Medicine*, vol.90, no.1 (2016): 32–60; Jennifer Tucker, *Nature Exposed: Photography as Eyewitness in Victorian Culture* (Baltimore, MD: Johns Hopkins University Press, 2005), pp.156–193.

[13] Timothy E. Ford, 'Using Satellite Images of Environmental Changes to Predict Infectious Disease Outbreaks,' *Emerging Infectious Diseases*, vol.15, no.9 (2009): 1341–1346.

The oscillating scales of infectious disease are particularly evident in popular culture. In movies such as *Contagion* (2011), montage sequences of magnified coronaviruses are juxtaposed to global transit hubs, such as airports. Digital maps, telephones, and airplanes convey long, deep space and the dangers of connectivity, while roosting fruit bats and the muddle of close-up human relations spell the perils of intimate contact. Such plot lines intimate an affective structure where defeating disease involves more than biomedical know-how but depends upon the successful management of anxiety, resilience, and sacrifice. The heroines and heroes are those who can think big but are also able to read the lethal small print, since global contagion arrives with an olive in a cocktail, the throw of a dice, a handshake, and a taxi tip.

On her way back to Minneapolis from China, already manifesting flu-like symptoms, Beth Emhoff, the 'super-spreader' in *Contagion*, stops off in Chicago to have sex with a former lover, thereby spreading the infection further. Here, the movie deploys a familiar trope: that of the morally loose woman, whose sexual proclivities are putting society at risk. The Chinese casino is a fitting setting for infective transmission, recalling the cocktail lounges, bars, and nightclubs that are haunted by women of dubious virtue in Hollywood film noirs of the 1940s and 1950s. The question of the movie's authenticity raises broader issues about the processes through which scientific explanations work their way from specialized institutions to affect the everyday practices of 'ordinary' people.[14] The rhetorical techniques used in the narrative of *Contagion* recall those employed in early twentieth-century public health films, which sought to educate viewers to discern invisible contaminants by tracking global circulations of infected bodies.[15] Recasting an airborne viral infection as a sexually transmitted disease spread by wanton women is also reminiscent of Second World War disease prevention films, such as *Borne on Two Wings* (1945), where malarial mosquitoes are portrayed as predatory and promiscuous women: 'Noffie the Skita' is a sexy, blond mosquito, as is her blood-lusting daughter, 'Anophelina.'[16]

In *Contagion*, a zoonotic disease, which is the outcome of complex social, economic, and ecological processes, is reimagined as a sexually transmitted disease. Why is this? Perhaps because the issues that

---

[14] Herring and Swedlund, 'Plagues and Epidemics in Anthropological Perspective.' In: Herring and Swedlund, eds., *Plagues and Epidemics*, p.19.

[15] Kirsten Ostherr, *Cinematic Prophylaxis: Globalization and Contagion in the Discourse of World Health* (Durham, NC: Duke University Press, 2005), pp.4–11.

[16] Marianne Fedunkiw, 'Malaria Films: Motion Pictures as a Public Health Tool,' *American Journal of Public Health*, vol.93, no.7 (July 2003): 1046–1057.

the movie is contending with are just too big to see – their scale precludes plausible representation. How is it possible to fully comprehend or visualize the multiple, interconnected processes that have produced the spillover event and precipitated the pandemic, at least in a way that viewers would pay to watch? A global event, which leads to mass mortality, is shrunk to fit a human-scale drama because it is only at this individual level that death becomes emotionally comprehensible. As Mike Davis observes in his account of H5N1: 'No one mourns a multitude or keens at the graveside of an abstraction.'[17]

There is a politics to this scalar view of disease. As it developed from the late 1980s, the concept of emerging infections 'offered journalists a powerful scalar resource for characterizing individual outbreaks as incidents of global significance.' Scientists and public health experts constructed a narrative of disease emergence that brought together different scales. The US virologist Stephen S. Morse was instrumental in promoting the term 'emerging infections' and espoused 'viral traffic studies' as a field devoted to explicating the causal links between the microbial and the global. Although novel infections were viewed as the consequence of globalizing processes, the threat they posed called for intervention on the micro-scale, through laboratory research: 'Whether the object was "global health" or national security, interventions would involve "passing through" American laboratories, biotechnology firms, pharmaceutical manufacturers, and information science experts.'[18]

These scales have now expanded further to include the history of the planet. The notion of the Anthropocene, a new geological and ecological era triggered by human activities, is challenging many of the assumptions about the human that inform the discipline of history. For one, the distinction between human history and natural history has collapsed. Conventionally, history has involved studying human actions, practices, and institutions. As the British historian R. G. Collingwood articulated it, in contrast to the history of human affairs, nature does not have an 'inside': 'In the case of nature, this distinction between the outside and the inside of an event does not arise. The events of nature are mere events, not acts of agents whose thought the scientist endeavours to trace.' However, the contemporary climate-change crisis has eroded this difference. The human impact on the planet has been scaled-up through an exploding population and the use of technologies to an extent that it can now be

---

[17] Davis, *The Monster at Our Door*, p.3.
[18] Nicholas B. King, 'The Scale Politics of Emerging Diseases,' *Osiris*, vol.19 (2004): 62–76 (64–66, 69).

considered a geological force – 'a force of nature.'[19] As I noted in the previous chapter, conceptualizing the world in terms of sliding scales cannot help to elucidate complex, overlapping micro and macro processes. Studying the history of infectious disease thus poses fundamental methodological issues about how to think simultaneously across different dimensions: the biological and the ecological, the local and the global, the particular and the general. It challenges our assumptions about the scope and meaning of historical understanding. It forces us to grapple with the politics of scale. Once the distinction between human and natural histories has broken down, we may justifiably ask: Where does history begin and where does it end?

Viral imaginaries

This book has explored the past, but what of the future? Since the SARS outbreak in 2003, there have been growing concerns about what the future might bring. Along with panicked responses to new infections, such as H7N9 and MERS, the specter of the coming plague is often invoked. Within East Asia, concerns about infectious disease are habitually mixed up with other worries, about natural disasters, pollution, and food contamination. Geopolitical tensions in many parts of Asia continue to impede cooperation on pressing issues facing the region. In Southeast Asia, the Association of Southeast Asian Nations (ASEAN), established in 1967 and today comprising 10 countries, provides an opportunity for some degree of concerted response. However, faced with growing domestic issues, including population pressure and inadequate healthcare financing and resources, many countries are ill-equipped to deal with a future pandemic.

Internationally, the view of Asia as the ground zero, the place from which the next 'big one' might come, is widely promoted in documentary films, movies, news articles, novels, and non-fictional works. The bestselling book *The Viral Storm* by the virologist Nathan Wolfe, published in 2011, is a case in point. In his description of SARS, Wolfe links the disease's emergence to Hong Kong's status as a global city, as well as to Chinese social and cultural practices:

Hong Kong has a higher density of people living in it than almost any other city in the world and certainly higher than any city that existed prior to the twentieth century. Thousands of international flights going to just about any part of the world you can imagine originate in Hong Kong every day. It also sits a short

---

[19] Dipesh Chakrabarty, 'The Climate of History: Four Theses,' *Critical Inquiry*, vol.35, no.2 (2009): 197–222 (202–203, 207).

drive from the Guangdong province of China. Guangdong houses hundreds of millions of people and its culinary history includes wild animal delicacies and dishes like pig organ soup.

Hong Kong's density is unique. The city's scale as a global city is unprecedented. Or just about, since the passage above equivocates, refusing to state precisely how many other cities may be more or equally dense. This indeterminacy is carried through with the description of 'thousands' of flights to 'any part of the world you can imagine.' Hong Kong exists in an 'imagined' connection to other world cities, which the inferred cosmopolitan reader – the 'you' of the text – is free to conjure. At the same time, the use of the verb 'originate' contains within it the germ of the viral: the seed of the problem. It is a problem with which we are already familiar; one imaginatively rehearsed in Hollywood blockbusters where cities are shattered by epidemic outbreaks.

Hong Kong is proximate to the whole world and, more worryingly, it is a ride away from Guangdong, a place of 'hundreds of millions of people.' And a place where 'history' is boiled up and served as an offending 'pig organ soup.'[20] Pigs, of course, are a staple Chinese food and in Western commentaries are invariably linked to emergent viral threats. While pigs are viewed as intermediaries in the transmission of avian viruses to humans, Chinese animal husbandry practices are also understood to be a factor driving the spread of infection. When thousands of pig carcasses were discovered floating in tributaries of the Huangpu River near Shanghai in 2013, some speculated that there might be a connection to the emergence of H7N9. 'The mystery is deep, the clock is ticking, and the world wants answers,' wrote the journalist and science writer Laurie Garrett, a consultant – along with Wolfe – on the movie *Contagion*. 'If we were imagining how a terrible pandemic would unfold,' she added, 'this could certainly serve as an excellent script.'[21] The mysterious actions of an invisible quasi-species – a virus – here produce a troubling fungibility; a reassortment of identities as humans, animals, institutions, cities, and nations are drawn into the pandemic script, 'remaking biological and political relations along the way.'[22]

Having identified the distinctive features of Hong Kong and Guangdong, Wolfe's narrative backtracks to state: 'While an interesting example, Guangdong is by no means unique.' Southern China thus occupies

---

[20] Nathan Wolfe, *The Viral Storm: The Dawn of a New Age* (London: Allen Lane, 2011), p.160.

[21] Laurie Garrett, 'Is This a Pandemic Being Born?' *Foreign Policy* (April 1, 2013).

[22] Celia Lowe, 'Viral Clouds: Becoming H5N1 in Indonesia,' *Cultural Anthropology*, vol.25, no.4 (2010): 625–649 (625–626).

a doubly ambiguous position. On the one hand, it is viewed as distinctive with particular socio-environmental configurations that are driving disease. On the other hand, it is seen as exemplary: as simply one more example of a general condition. While southern China is hyper-modern, epitomizing the mass living and rapid connectivity of the world today, it is also steeped in antique ways. Above all, it is this spillover of history into the present that is seen as the nub of the problem. Hotspots such as Hong Kong and Guangdong occupy an ambivalent temporality: in their hyper-modernity they are redolent of the future, but they are also throwbacks to a pre-modern world of unhygienic practices. From an epidemiological perspective, they are places where future epidemics may be forestalled by identifying diseases as they emerge but before they spread. A temporal ambiguity reflects a fundamental epistemological uncertainty about what the virus is, where it has come from, and what it might become (Figure 6.1).[23] We are pushed towards a revelatory moment when the epidemic threat will finally be disclosed. The viral storm in this genre of pandemic writing is invariably evoked in quasi-prophetic terms, since the not-yet-emergent pathogen occupies a mysterious space between the known and the unknown. In this sense, it comes to mirror Hong Kong's own indeterminacy as a global city on the border.[24]

To be sure, *The Viral Storm* is a highly readable and informative account of the pressures that are driving disease emergence across the world. But in dramatizing the threat of the 'viral storm' in this way, the book tips into the formulaic plot line of the outbreak narrative to recycle ideas about China as a locus of infection; a place with an unsavory history, but also a place strangely devoid of distinction since after all it is 'by no means unique.'[25] And what of the pig organ soup? In the movie *Golden Chicken II*, which we discussed in Chapter 5, the prostitute Ah Gum runs a local Hong Kong eatery. During the SARS epidemic, a doctor who turns up for dinner is shunned by the staff because he is wearing a face mask. However, Ah Gum befriends him and serves him pig lung soup. Here, then, we have the reverse image of the viral storm. A traditional Chinese food is not equated with death, but is associated with life: consuming the lung will preserve the lung. This is love in the time of SARS. In the words of a Chinese proverb: 'like nourishes like.'

Of course, Asia is vulnerable to epidemics. The threat they pose is both immediate and long term. The last decade and a half has seen the emergence of a number of highly pathogenic new diseases: H5N1, SARS,

---

[23] Lowe, 'Viral Clouds,' pp.625–626.

[24] Carlo Caduff, 'Pandemic Prophecy, or How to Have Faith in Reason,' *Current Anthropology*, vol.55, no.3 (2014): 296–315.

[25] Wald, *Contagious*, pp.2–8.

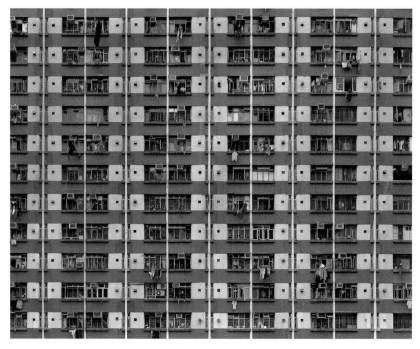

Figure 6.1. 'Architecture of Density' (Hong Kong), 2008. Photograph by Michael Wolf.

Hong Kong: Sentinel city

Hong Kong (Figure 6.1) is frequently represented in the media and in pandemic thrillers as an emerging disease hotspot. As the WHO epidemiologist Dr. Leonora Orantes (played by Marion Cotillard) puts it in the movie *Contagion*: 'Kowloon is the most densely populated area in the world and Hong Kong is a harbor. It's going to spread.' The identification of the city with infectious disease and its proximity to the 'home' of influenza in southern China has led to its inclusion as a key site in a system of global surveillance. It has become a sentinel city, where the emphasis is on gathering real-time data in order to detect imminent pandemics. Hong Kong's experience with epidemics has also acted as a spur to laboratory research and to the development of local expertise in managing acute public health events. The city has become an 'obligatory passage point' for virologists, epidemiologists, and anthropologists with interests in emerging infections. In this way, the conventional framework of the 'outbreak narrative' – wherein disease is understood to spread West from Asia, while know-how flows East from the West – is being fundamentally reconfigured.

Theresa MacPhail, *The Viral Network: A Pathography of the H1N1 Influenza Pandemic* (Ithaca, NY: Cornell University Press, 2014), pp.76–79.

Frédéric Keck, 'Hong Kong as a Sentinel Post,' *Limn*, no.3 (June 2013): 38–40.

MERS, and H7N9. Despite the often over-simplistic and problematic conceptualization of China and Southeast Asia as the 'home' of influenza, there is evidence to suggest that the region remains at particular risk from novel influenza viruses.[26] There are concerns that Zika virus disease, which is transmitted like dengue by the *Aedes* mosquito, may take hold across the region. A recent study has suggested that the Zika virus is widespread in Thailand.[27] Antimicrobial resistance poses a challenge to the treatment of a range of infectious diseases, and Southeast Asia accounts for one third of the global burden of multi-drug-resistant TB.[28] There is also increasing resistance in the malaria parasite *Plasmodium falciparum* to the use of artemisinin-based therapies in countries such as Burma, Cambodia, Thailand, and Vietnam.[29] In 2015, during a routine study on E. coli (*Escherichia coli*) by Chinese scientists, drug-resistant bacteria were identified in pigs and raw meat across southern China. A gene mutation had rendered these 'superbugs' resistant to colistin, a last-resort antibiotic used to treat serious infections. China is the world's largest pig producer and colistin is routinely fed to livestock as a means of fattening them. The discovery of the bacteria in hospital patients and recognition of the gene's potential to spread to other bacterial species has raised the

[26] Trevon L. Fuller, et al., 'Predicting Hotspots for Influenza Virus Reassortment,' *Emerging Infectious Diseases*, vol.19, no.4 (April 2013): 581–588.

[27] Rome Buathong, et al., 'Detection of Zika Virus Infection in Thailand, 2012–2014,' *American Journal of Tropical Medicine and Hygiene*, vol.93, no.2 (August 5, 2015): 380–383.

[28] Vineet Bhatia, Khurshid Alam Hyder, and Nani Nair, 'Drug Resistance in Tuberculosis in South-East Asia,' *Regional Health Forum*, vol.15, no.1 (2011): 44–51.

[29] Elizabeth A. Ashley, et al., 'Spread of Artemisinin Resistance in *Plasmodium falciparum* Malaria,' *New England Journal of Medicine*, vol.371 (July 31, 2014): 411–423.

specter of a global 'antibiotic apocalypse,' which would make common infections untreatable.[30]

As we have seen, Asia is currently experiencing a profound transition with rapid urbanization and globalization. Although the PRC has become the world's second largest economy, with an annual GDP growth rate of 10 percent over the last decade lifting many millions out of poverty, wealth disparities have also grown sharply and there is a pronounced rural-urban divide. The surge in consumption since the transition from a centrally planned to a market-based economy in the late 1970s has put further pressure on natural resources. As in other high-consumption countries, deforestation, desertification, and pollution have become critical issues. More frequent floods and prolonged droughts – the likely effects of climate change – jeopardize human health and food security. The size and complexity of China make these challenges particularly formidable.

In *Epidemics in Modern Asia*, I have sought to show how disease is interlinked with these social and environmental transformations. The purpose has been to trace the history of interwoven processes across Asia – migration, urbanization, environmental change, war, globalization – in order to demonstrate how epidemics are produced through a complex interplay of variables. Writing epidemics into history in this way opens up new perspectives on the dynamics of social, political, and economic systems; it also furnishes a means of grounding big history and rematerializing global connections. This has not been a polemical argument about history's use as a remedial tool for the present, or its indispensability for the future. Instead, I have suggested how history can challenge entrenched assumptions that inform discussions of disease emergence, and how it can help to rupture the smooth plot line of the pandemic thriller, where inherited ideas about disease coalesce, largely unopposed, and where the emphasis is increasingly on 'real time' and the 'about-to-be.' Studying past epidemics provides an invaluable critique of the now, while affording a much-needed space for reflecting on the purpose and meaning of history as a discipline and method. There is an urgency to this task since biological explanations of the world are today pushing history out of the frame. Narratives of disease emergence too often pass over the historical disparities that stoke epidemics, reimagining inequality as an insurmountable cultural difference in the present.

---

[30] Yi-Yun Liu, et al., 'Emergence of Plasmid-Mediated Colistin Resistance Mechanism MCR-1 in Animals and Human Beings in China: A Microbiological and Molecular Biological Study,' *Lancet Infectious Diseases* (November 18, 2015): doi: 10.1016/S1473-3099(15)00424-7.

Glossary

ah ku	Cantonese term for prostitute
Anthropocene	a new geological epoch brought about by the environmental impact of human activity on the planet
bacteria	single-celled microorganisms
bakufu	in Japan, the system of government under the military shoguns
biodiversity	variety of life-forms found in different ecosystems
chawls	in India, a building subdivided into working-class tenements
Chinese Protectorate	administrative agency set up in 1877 to oversee the welfare of Chinese residents in the Straits Settlements
cholera	infection caused by ingestion of the pathogenic bacterium *Vibrio cholera*
coolie	contracted laborer in the nineteenth and twentieth centuries, usually from the Indian subcontinent or southern China
Cultuurstelsel	'Cultivation System' imposed by the government of the Dutch East Indies in the 1830s, requiring farmers to pay dues to the state in specified cash crops or labor
Ebola virus disease (EVD)	infection transmitted through body fluids and caused by the *Ebola virus*, first identified in 1976 and named after the River Ebola in the Democratic Republic of the Congo (formerly Zaire)
eisei	Japanese term for health, hygiene, and sanitation
emerging disease	a disease that has appeared in a population for the first time, or that may

316

	have existed previously but is rapidly increasing in incidence or geographic range
epidemic	a disease outbreak or an unusually high occurrence of a disease or illness in a given population or area
epidemiology	the study of the distribution and determinants of health-related states or events (including disease), and the application of this study to the control of diseases and other health problems
filariasis	a disease caused by infection with a species of parasitic roundworm
gam san haak	'gold mountain seekers' in Cantonese; a term used to describe migrants to the United States and Australia during the nineteenth-century Gold Rush
hajj	Muslim pilgrimage to Mecca
haram	an act forbidden by Islamic law
HIV/AIDS	a range of conditions caused by damage to the immune system as a result of infection with the human immunodeficiency virus (HIV)
hōkō	*baojia* in Chinese, neighborhood surveillance system in colonial Taiwan
hukou	Chinese system of residential permits introduced in 1958
huoluan	'sudden turmoil' in Chinese; a term for an acute disease characterized by vomiting and diarrhea, later identified as cholera
Indios	Spanish colonial term that refers to the native peoples of the Philippines
influenza (flu)	airborne respiratory infection caused by an influenza virus, of which there are three types (A, B, and C); wild birds are the natural hosts for type A viruses
Japanese encephalitis	a mosquito-borne flavivirus, first documented in Japan in 1871
kakkebyō	Japanese for beriberi, a disease caused by a nutritional deficit in vitamin B1 (thiamine)

kakuran	a condition brought on by excessive eating and a cooling of the stomach; later applied in Japan to cholera
kala-azar	also known as *Visceral leishmaniasis*, a disease caused by protozoan parasites transmitted by the sand fly
karayuki-san	term meaning 'going to China' in Japanese; used to describe Japanese women who worked abroad as prostitutes
kawaraban	literally 'tile-block printing' in Japanese; broadsides
kokutai	Japanese term for 'national body politic'
korera	Japanese translation of cholera, also referred to as *korori*
MERS	respiratory illness caused by the highly pathogenic MERS coronavirus (MERS-CoV)
mestizo	person of mixed Chinese and Filipino ancestry
mujahideen	Muslim fighters engaged in *jihad*, or holy war; refers generally to Muslim insurgents fighting against the Soviets after their invasion of Afghanistan in 1979
Nanyang	'Southern Ocean' in Chinese, a term used to denote Southeast Asia
Nipah	neurological and respiratory disease caused by a species of henipavirus hosted by pteropid bats
Ommelanden	Dutch for 'hinterland'; the environs of Batavia
pathogen	infectious disease agent
plague	infectious disease caused by *Yersinia pestis* bacteria, identified by Alexandre Yersin and Kitasato Shibasaburō in Hong Kong in 1894
sakoku	Japanese for 'locked country,' the policy during the Tokugawa period, which restricted foreigners from entering Japan and Japanese from leaving the country
sangley	a person of Chinese ancestry in the Philippines, likely originating from the

	word for 'trader' in the Hokkien dialect of southeast China
SARS	viral respiratory disease caused by the SARS coronavirus (SARS-CoV)
schistosomiasis	infectious disease caused by a parasitic worm, also known as bilharzia
sedentism	the transition from a nomadic existence to a settled society
shantang	benevolent societies in China, literally 'charitable halls'
shogun	'military commander' in Japanese; hereditary rulers of Japan from the twelfth century to the mid nineteenth century under the nominal suzerainty of the emperor
shōki	Japanese for 'swamp gas' or 'bad air'; a miasmatic disease
syndemic	the interaction of different factors (biological and social) that produce health crises
syphilis	sexually transmitted infection caused by the bacterium *Treponema pallidum*
Taliban	from the Arabic word for 'student'; an Islamic fundamentalist political organization
treaty ports	port cities in China, Japan, Taiwan, and Korea that were opened to Western trade from the 1840s by a series of unequal treaties
tuberculosis (TB)	airborne infectious disease caused by various strains of mycobacteria
typhus	a disease caused by Rickettsia bacteria transmitted by the human louse
virus	infectious submicroscopic agent that replicates inside the cell of a host organism
weisheng	in Chinese, hygiene and health
yōjō	in Japanese, a regimen for nurturing a healthy life
zoonoses	infections transmissible from animals to humans

Select timeline

1619	Establishment of Dutch Batavia on the island of Java
1644	Collapse of the Ming dynasty in China; establishment of the Manchu Qing dynasty
1807	Abolition of Slave Trade Act passed in Britain
1815	End of the Manila–Acapulco galleon trade
1817–1824	First cholera pandemic, originating in Bengal
1819	British settlement of Singapore
1833	Abolition of slavery in the British Empire
1839–1842	First Opium War
1842	Treaty of Nanking (Nanjing); establishment of treaty ports in China and the British colony of Hong Kong
1850–1864	Taiping Rebellion
1851	First international sanitary conference held in Paris
1854	Treaty of Kanagawa (Yokohama)
1856–1873	Panthay Rebellion in Yunnan
1857	Indian Rebellion ('Mutiny')
1858	US–Japanese Treaty of Amity and Commerce; cholera epidemic in Japan; establishment of Crown rule in India
1859–1860	Second Opium War; Treaty of Peking establishes further treaty ports
1868	Meiji Restoration in Japan
1869	Opening of Suez Canal
1877	Satsuma Rebellion in Japan
1883	Robert Koch isolates the bacterium that causes cholera
1884–1885	Sino-French War
1885–1886	Burma comes under direct British rule; abdication of King Thibaw Min
1887	French Indochina established
1891	Trans-Siberian Railway construction begins
1893	Official end to Chinese ban on overseas emigration
1894	Third plague pandemic; plague bacterium identified in Hong Kong

1894–1895	First Sino-Japanese War
1895	Treaty of Shimonoseki, Japanese ceded Formosa (Taiwan); formation of the Federated Malay States
1897–1898	Ronald Ross, working in India, establishes that the malaria parasite is transmitted by mosquitoes
1898	US–Spanish War; Paul-Louis Simond discovers the role of the rat flea in the transmission of plague
1898–1902	Construction and opening of the Manchurian Railway
1899–1902	Philippine–US War
1900–1901	Boxer Rebellion
1902–1904	Cholera epidemic in the Philippines
1904–1905	Russo-Japanese War
1905	Japanese Protectorate in Korea
1910	Korea annexed by Japan
1910–1911	Manchurian plague epidemic
1911	Chinese revolution; end of the Qing dynasty
1912	Establishment of the Republic of China
1914–1918	First World War
1917	Bolshevik Revolution in Russia; indentured labor abolished across the British Empire
1918	Treaty of Bresk-Litovsk ends Russia's participation in the First World War
1918–1919	'Spanish' influenza pandemic
1918–1921	Russian Civil War
1920–1921	Second Manchurian plague epidemic
1927	Civil War begins in China between the Communist Party (CCP) and the Kuomintang (KMT)
1931	Japanese invasion of Manchuria and creation of the puppet state of Manchukuo
1934–1935	Chinese Communist Party's Long March
1937–1945	Second Sino-Japanese War
1939–1945	Second World War
1941	Bombing of Pearl Harbor by Japan; United States enters the Second World War
1947	British India partitioned into the independent states of India and Pakistan
1948	Burma gains independence from Britain; World Health Organization established
1949	Establishment of the People's Republic of China
1950–1953	Korean War
1952	Patriotic Health Campaign in China
1957	Independence of Malaya from Britain

1957–1958	Asian flu pandemic
1958–1962	Great Leap Forward and mass famine in China
1962	Military coup in Burma
1963	Establishment of Malaysia
1964–1975	Vietnam War; Gulf of Tonkin Resolution enacted by Congress in 1964 leads to the deployment of US troops in Vietnam
1966–1976	Cultural Revolution in China
1968–1970	Hong Kong flu pandemic
1969	'Race riots' in Malaysia
1971	India–Pakistan war; East Pakistan becomes the independent state of Bangladesh
1975	Khmer Rouge seize power in Cambodia
1976	Death of Mao Zedong
1978	Chinese economic reforms begin under Deng Xiaoping; Declaration of Alma-Ata
1979	Soviet invasion of Afghanistan; Vietnamese troops invade Cambodia, leading to the fall of the Khmer Rouge regime
1980	WHO declares smallpox officially eradicated
1983	Scientists discover HIV, the virus that causes AIDS
1988	Global Polio Eradication Initiative (GPEI) launched
1989	International conference on emerging viruses held in Washington, DC
1994	Polio Eradication Initiative (PEI) launched in Pakistan
1997	Asian financial crisis; avian influenza (H5N1) infects humans during a poultry outbreak in Hong Kong; handover of Hong Kong to China
1997–1998	Forest fires in Indonesia cause air pollution over Southeast Asia
1998–1999	Outbreak of Nipah virus disease in Malaysia
2001	Terrorist attacks on New York and Washington, DC; US-led invasion of Afghanistan; China joins the World Trade Organization (WTO)
2002–2003	SARS outbreak in China, which spreads globally
2003	Invasion of Iraq by US-led coalition forces
2003–2004	Re-emergence of H5N1 in China and Southeast Asia
2004	Indian Ocean earthquake and tsunami
2008	Global financial crisis; Sichuan earthquake
2009	H1N1 (swine flu) pandemic; defeat of the Liberation Tigers of Tamil Eelam by the Sri Lankan military
2011	Tohoku earthquake and tsunami

2012	MERS reported in Saudi Arabia
2013	H7N9 cases in China
2014	Ebola outbreak in West Africa
2015	MERS outbreak in South Korea; Aung San Suu Kyi's National League for Democracy (NLD) wins a landslide in the general elections in Burma
2016	The US CDC and other national health agencies issue travel alerts as a Zika virus epidemic in Brazil spreads to South and Central America and the Caribbean

Suggested reading

INTRODUCTION: CONTAGIOUS HISTORIES

A useful starting point for those interested in the history of epidemics in Asia is provided by the essays collected in Kenneth F. Kiple's *The Cambridge World History of Human Disease* (Cambridge: Cambridge University Press, 1993). See, in particular, the following entries: Shigehisa Kuriyama, 'Concepts of Disease in East Asia,' pp.52–59; Thomas L. Hall and Victor W. Sidel, 'Diseases of the Modern Period in China,' pp.362–373; David Arnold, 'Diseases of the Modern Period in South Asia,' pp.418–425; Keith W. Taylor, 'Diseases and Disease Ecology of the Modern Period in Southeast Asia,' pp.440–444; Ann Bowman Jannetta, 'Disease Ecologies of East Asia,' pp.476–482.

At the time of its publication in 1976, William H. McNeill's *Plagues and Peoples* provided a fresh perspective on world history that stressed the ecological, demographic, and political effects of disease on societies. A number of world histories of disease contain some discussion of Asia, although this tends to be limited: Michael B. A. Oldstone, *Viruses, Plagues, and History: Past, Present, and Future*. Revised edition (New York: Oxford University Press, 2010); Sheldon Watts, *Disease and Medicine in World History* (New York and London: Routledge, 2003); J. N. Hays, *Epidemics and Pandemics: Their Impacts on Human History* (Santa Barbara, CA: ABC-CLIO, 2006). For a general overview of the interrelationship between empire and disease, with sections on Asia, see: J. N. Hays, *Epidemics and History: Disease, Power, and Imperialism* (New Haven, CT: Yale University Press, 1997) and Pratik Chakrabarti, *Medicine and Empire: 1600–1960* (Basingstoke: Palgrave Macmillan, 2013). A population approach to Asian history with a section devoted to disease and mortality is contained in the volume edited by Ts'ui-jung Liu, et al., *Asian Population History* (Oxford: Oxford University Press, 2001).

There is an extensive scholarship exploring facets of colonial medicine and science on the Indian subcontinent. A pioneering volume is David Arnold's *Colonizing the Body: State Medicine and Epidemic Disease in Nineteenth-Century India* (Berkeley: University of California Press, 1993), which examines colonial responses to epidemics of smallpox, cholera, and plague. Other useful books dealing with different aspects of disease, colonial biomedicine, and public health in South Asia, include: Mark Harrison, *Public Health in British India: Anglo-Indian Preventive Medicine, 1859–1914* (Cambridge: Cambridge University Press, 1994); Pratik Chakrabarti, *Western Science in Modern India: Metropolitan Methods, Colonial Practices* (Delhi: Permanent Black, 2004); Deepak Kumar, *Science and the Raj: A Study of British India* (Oxford: Oxford University Press, 2006);

Pratik Chakrabarti, *Bacteriology in British India: Laboratory Medicine and the Tropics* (Rochester, NY: University of Rochester Press, 2012); Nandini Bhattacharya, *Contagion and Enclaves: Tropical Medicine in Colonial India* (Liverpool: Liverpool University Press, 2012). The essays collected in the volume edited by David Hardiman and Projit Bihari Mukharji, *Medical Marginality in South Asia: Situating Subaltern Therapeutics* (New York and London: Routledge, 2012), provide a novel perspective on the world of popular healing – 'subaltern therapeutics' – in South Asia.

Less has been written about the history of infectious disease in Southeast Asia. A number of chapters in Norman G. Owen's edited collection *Death and Disease in Southeast Asia* (Singapore: Oxford University Press, 1987) deal with infectious disease and the introduction to the volume provides a discussion of key issues. David Arnold treats the Indian Ocean as a zone for the exchange of infectious disease in his article 'The Indian Ocean as a Disease Zone,' *South Asia: Journal of South Asian Studies*, vol.14, no.2 (1991): 1–21. More recent studies include: Laurence Monnais and Harold J. Cook, eds., *Global Movements, Local Concerns: Medicine and Health in Southeast Asia* (Singapore: NUS Press, 2012) and Tim Harper and Sunil S. Amrith, eds., *Histories of Health in Southeast Asia: Perspectives on the Long Twentieth Century* (Bloomington and Indianapolis: Indiana University Press, 2014). Warwick Anderson's *Colonial Pathologies: American Tropical Medicine, Race, and Hygiene in the Philippines* (Durham, NC: Duke University Press, 2006) is required reading for those with an interest in colonial medicine in Southeast Asia. For an account of the plurality of medical cultures in colonial Southeast Asia, see Sokhieng Au's excellent *Mixed Medicines: Health and Culture in French Colonial Cambodia* (Chicago, IL: University of Chicago Press, 2011).

There is a burgeoning literature on the history of disease and medicine in East Asia. The collection of essays edited by Angela Ki Che Leung and Charlotte Furth, *Health and Hygiene in Chinese East Asia* (Durham, NC: Duke University Press, 2010), provides a comparative approach to evolving ideas about hygiene across East Asia – with a particular emphasis on China and infectious disease. On China, in particular, a groundbreaking work is Ruth Rogaski's *Hygienic Modernity: Meanings of Health and Disease in Treaty-Port China* (Berkeley: University of California Press, 2004). Focusing on the treaty port of Tientsin, Rogaski tracks the shifting meaning of the term *weisheng* in the nineteenth and twentieth centuries, showing how 'hygiene' was central to the construction of Chinese modernity. Other useful volumes include: Bridie Andrews, *The Making of Modern Chinese Medicine, 1850–1960* (Vancouver: UBC Press, 2014); Bridie Andrews and Mary Brown Bullock, eds., *Medical Transitions in Twentieth-Century China* (Bloomington and Indianapolis: Indiana University Press, 2014); Sean Hsiang-lin Lei, *Neither Donkey nor Horse: Medicine in the Struggle over China's Modernity* (Chicago, IL: University of Chicago Press, 2014). Marta E. Hanson's *Speaking of Epidemics in Chinese Medicine: Disease and the Geographic Imagination in Late Imperial China* (Abingdon and New York: Routledge, 2011) is a fascinating history of *wenbing*, or 'warm diseases,' in China over the last two thousand years, and suggests the extent to which older conceptions of epidemics have been integrated into 'new' understandings of disease. On Japan, Ann Bowman Jannetta's *Epidemics and Mortality in Early Modern Japan* (Princeton, NJ: Princeton University Press, 1987) still provides a useful background to the early modern period. William Johnston's *The Modern Epidemic: A History of Tuberculosis in Japan* (Cambridge, MA: Harvard University Press, 1995) is an important work that invites us to reconsider epidemics as biomedical, political, social, and cultural events. On public health in Korea, see In-Sok Yeo's essay 'A History of Public Health in Korea,' in Milton J. Lewis and Kerrie L. MacPherson, eds., *Public Health in Asia and the Pacific: Historical and Comparative Perspectives* (Abingdon and New York: Routledge, 2008), pp.73–86. On Taiwan, two useful surveys, which include discussion of epidemics, are: Mingcheng M. Lo, *Doctors within Borders: Profession, Ethnicity, and Modernity in Colonial Taiwan* (Berkeley: University of California Press, 2002) and Michael Shiyung Liu, *Prescribing Colonization: The Role of Medical Practices and Policies in Japan-Ruled Taiwan, 1895–1945* (Ann Arbor, MI: Association for Asian Studies, 2009).

CHAPTER 1: MOBILITY

There is a substantive bibliography on the links between migration and health, but surprisingly little that deals specifically with Asia. The edited volume by Santosh Jatrana, Mika Toyota, and Brenda S. A. Yeoh, *Migration and Health in Asia* (Abingdon and New York: Routledge, 2005), however, provides helpful case studies from across Asia. For a concise overview of key issues, see Sunil S. Amrith, 'Migration and Health in Southeast Asian History,' *Lancet*, vol.384, no.9954 (November 2014): 1569–1570. For a thoughtful discussion of the importance of migration in modern Asian history, see also Sunil S. Amrith, *Migration and Diaspora in Modern Asia* (Cambridge: Cambridge University Press, 2011).

On the first cholera pandemic in Southeast Asia, see the following: Robert Peckham, 'Symptoms of Empire: Cholera in Southeast Asia, 1820–1850,' in Mark Jackson, ed., *The Routledge History of Disease* (New York: Routledge, 2016); B. J. Terwiel, 'Asiatic Cholera in Siam: Its First Occurrence and the 1820 Epidemic,' in Owen, ed., *Death and Disease in Southeast Asia*, pp.142–161; Boomgaard, 'Morbidity and Mortality in Java, 1820–1880: Changing Patterns of Disease and Death,' in Owen, ed., *Death and Disease in Southeast Asia*, pp.48–69. For a discussion of epidemic disease, including cholera, in the Philippines, see Ken De Bevoise, *Agents of Apocalypse: Epidemic Disease in the Colonial Philippines* (Princeton, NJ: Princeton University Press, 1995).

There is a growing scholarship on cholera in Japan, and in my own account I have drawn on a number of insightful journal articles and book chapters. These include: Susan L. Burns, 'Constructing the National Body: Public Health and the Nation in Meiji Japan,' in Timothy Brook and André Schmid, eds., *Nation Work: Asian Elites and National Identities* (Ann Arbor: University of Michigan Press, 2000), pp.17–50; Bettina Gramlich-Oka, 'The Body Economic: Japan's Cholera Epidemic of 1858 in Popular Discourse,' *East Asian Science, Technology, and Medicine*, vol.30 (2009): 32–73; William Johnston, 'Epidemics Past and Science Present: An Approach to Cholera in Nineteenth-Century Japan,' *Harvard Asia Quarterly*, vol.14, no.4 (2012): 28–35; Akihito Suzuki and Mika Suzuki, 'Cholera, Consumer and Citizenship: Modernisations of Medicine in Japan,' in Hormoz Ebrahimnejad, ed., *The Development of Modern Medicine in Non-Western Countries: Historical Perspectives* (London: Routledge, 2009), pp.184–203.

For a global overview of the third plague pandemic, with a chapter on Canton and Hong Kong, see Myron Echenberg, *Plague Ports: The Global Urban Impact of*

Bubonic Plague, 1894–1901 (New York: New York University Press, 2010), pp.15–77. Carol Benedict's *Bubonic Plague in Nineteenth-Century China* (Stanford, CA: Stanford University Press, 1996) is an indispensable study of the plague, which I have drawn on extensively. Elizabeth Sinn has explored the conflict between the colonial government in Hong Kong and the Chinese population, as well as the tensions within the Chinese community, in *Power and Charity: A Chinese Merchant Elite in Colonial Hong Kong*. Revised edition (Hong Kong: Hong Kong University Press, 2003), pp.159–183. For a perceptive study of the plague in Hong Kong in relation to the take-up of evolving bacteriological theories, see Mary P. Sutphen, 'Not What, but Where: Bubonic Plague and the Reception of Germ Theories in Hong Kong and Calcutta,' *Journal of the History of Medicine and Allied Sciences*, vol.52, no.1 (1997): 81–113.

CHAPTER 2: CITIES

The essays contained in the edited volume by Robert Peckham and David M. Pomfret, *Imperial Contagions: Hygiene, Medicine, and Cultures of Planning in Asia* (Hong Kong: Hong Kong University Press, 2013), explore how anxieties about infectious disease shaped urban planning in colonial Asia during the late nineteenth and twentieth centuries. For a useful overview of the challenges presented by the contemporary global city in relation to emerging infections, see Harris Ali and Roger Keil, eds., *Networked Disease: Emerging Infections in the Global City* (Malden, MA and Oxford: Wiley-Blackwell, 2008).

There are a number of histories of Jakarta, which include discussion of Dutch Batavia. See, in particular, Susan Abeyasekere, *Jakarta: A History*. Revised edition (Singapore: Oxford University Press, 1989). On colonial Batavia, specifically, see Jean Gelman Taylor, *The Social World of Batavia: Europeans and Eurasians in Dutch Asia* (Madison: University of Wisconsin Press, [1983] 2009). For a comparative study of port cities, including Batavia, see Leonard Blussé, *Visible Cities: Canton, Nagasaki, and Batavia and the Coming of the Americans* (Cambridge, MA: Harvard University Press, 2008). And for an overview of Batavia in the VOC network, see Kerry Ward, *Networks of Empire: Forced Migration in the Dutch East India Company* (Cambridge: Cambridge University Press, 2012). Epidemics are mentioned in these works, but for a more focused discussion of disease and environmental factors in the decline of Batavia, see the following by Leonard Blussé, which I have drawn on: 'The Story of an Ecological Disaster: The Dutch East India Company and Batavia (1619–1799),' in *Strange Company: Chinese Settlers, Mestizo Women and the Dutch in VOC Batavia* (Dordrecht: Foris Publications, 1986), pp.15–34; 'An Insane Administration and an Unsanitary Town: The Dutch East India Company and Batavia (1619–1799),' in Robert J. Ross and Gerard J. Telkamp, eds., *Colonial Cities: Essays on Urbanism in a Colonial Context* (Dordrecht: Martinus Nijhoff, 1985), pp.65–86. On the scourge of malaria in Batavia, see P. H. van der Brug, 'Malaria in Batavia in the 18th Century,' *Tropical Medicine and International Health*, vol.2, no.9 (September 1997): 892–902.

For a study of the politics of colonial urban design in French Indochina, which deals with Saigon and Hanoi, see Gwendolyn Wright, *The Politics of Design in French Colonial Urbanism* (Chicago, IL: University of Chicago Press, 1991), pp.161–233. Eric T. Jennings's *Imperial Heights: Dalat and the Making and Undoing of French Indochina* (Berkeley: University of California Press, 2011) also explores the politics and practical exigencies that determined the siting and planning of colonial cities. William S. Logan's *Hanoi: Biography of a City* (Seattle: University of Washington Press, 2000) gives an informative historical overview of Hanoi. On the importance of epidemic disease in Hanoi's colonial history, see the essays by Michael G. Vann, which I have found particularly helpful: 'Hanoi in the Time of Cholera: Epidemic Disease and Racial Power in the Colonial City,' in Monnais and Cook, eds., *Global Movements, Local Concerns*, pp.150–170; 'Building Colonial Whiteness on the Red River: Race, Power, and Urbanism in Paul Doumer's Hanoi, 1897–1902,' *Historical Reflections/Réflexions Historiques*, vol.22, no2. (2007): 277–304'; 'Of Rats, Rice, and Race: The Great Hanoi Rat Massacre, an Episode in French Colonial History,' *French Colonial History*, vol.4 (2003): 191–203.

James Francis Warren's *Ah Ku and Karayuki-san: Prostitution in Singapore, 1870–1940* (Singapore: NUS Press, 2003) is an accessible study of prostitution in colonial Singapore, which has informed my argument. Other works dealing with prostitution, medical surveillance, and regulation include: Lenore Manderson, 'Migration, Prostitution and Medical Surveillance in Early Twentieth-Century Malaya,' in Lara Marks and Michael Worboys, eds., *Migrants, Minorities and Health: Historical and Contemporary Studies* (London and New York: Routledge, 1997), pp.49–69; Brenda S. A. Yeoh, 'Sexually Transmitted Disease in Late Nineteenth- and Twentieth-Century Singapore,' in Milton Lewis, Scott Bamber, and Michael Waugh, eds., *Sex, Disease, and Society* (Westport, CT: Greenwood Press, 1997), pp.177–202; Philippa Levine, *Prostitution, Race, and Politics: Policing Venereal Disease in the British Empire* (New York and London: Routledge, 2003). For an original interpretation of the *karayuki-san* in relation to gender hierarchies and the political economy in Meiji Japan, see Bill Mihalopoulos, *Sex in Japan's Globalization, 1870–1930: Prostitutes, Emigration and Nation-Building* (London: Pickering & Chatto, 2011).

On the planning of colonial Bombay, see Mariam Dossal, *Imperial Designs and Indian Realities: The Planning of Bombay City, 1845–1875* (Oxford: Oxford University Press, 1997). For an overview of the bubonic plague in Bombay, see Echenberg, *Plague Ports*, pp.47–77. Other work on the Bombay plague, which I have found helpful, includes: Arnold, *Colonizing the Body*, pp.200–239; Prashant Kidambi, *The Making of an Indian Metropolis: Colonial Governance and Public Culture, 1890–1920* (Aldershot and Burlington, VT: Ashgate, 2007), pp.49–70; and Mridula Ramanna, *Western Medicine and Public Health in Colonial Bombay* (Hyderabad: Orient Longman, 2002).

CHAPTER 3: ENVIRONMENT

The field of Asian environmental history has expanded rapidly over the last decade, and the bibliography is now extensive. Useful books dealing with facets of environmental history in Asia include: Peter Boomgaard, *Southeast Asia: An Environmental History* (Santa Barbara, CA: ABC-CLIO, 2006); Robert B. Marks, *China: Its Environment and History* (Lanham, MD: Rowman & Littlefield, 2011); David Biggs, *Quagmire: Nation-Building and Nature in the Mekong Delta* (Seattle: University of Washington Press, 2012); Judith Shapiro, *China's Environmental Challenges* (Cambridge: Polity, 2012); Ian J. Miller, Julia Adeney Thomas, and Brett L. Walker, eds. *Japan at Nature's Edge: The Environmental Context of a Global Power* (Honolulu: University of Hawaii Press, 2013).

For a history of the plantation complex, see the revised edition of Philip D. Curtin's *The Rise and Fall of the Plantation Complex: Essays in Atlantic History* (Cambridge: Cambridge University Press, 1998). A general history of the rubber industry in Malaya is provided by John H. Drabble, *Rubber in Malaya: 1876–1922: The Genesis of the Industry* (Kuala Lumpur: Oxford University Press, 1973). Specifically on concerns about malaria and health on the plantations, see: J. Norman Parmer, 'Estate Workers' Health in the Federated Malay States in the 1920s,' in Peter J. Rimmer and Lisa M. Allen, eds., *The Underside of Malaysian History: Pullers, Prostitutes, Plantation Workers* (Singapore: Singapore University Press, 1990), pp.179–192; Armajit Kaur, 'Indian Labour, Labour Standards, and Workers' Health in Burma and Malaya, 1900–1940,' *Modern Asian Studies*, vol.40, no.2 (2006): 425–475; Liew Kai Khiun, 'Planters, Estate Health and Malaria in British Malaya (1900–1940),' *Journal of the Malayasian Branch of the Royal Asiatic Society*, vol.83, no.298 (2010): 91–115.

A history of malaria in East Asia is provided by Ka-che Yip, ed., *Disease, Colonialism, and the State: Malaria in Modern East Asian History* (Hong Kong: Hong Kong University Press, 2009) – specifically on Taiwan, see the essay in Yip's volume by Ku Ya Wen, 'Anti-malaria Policy and Its Consequences in Colonial Japan,' pp.31–48, and Ku's chapter 'Anti-Malaria Policy in Colonial Taiwan,' in Theo Engelen, John Robert Shepherd, and Yang Wen-Sha, eds., *Death at the Opposite Ends of the Eurasian Continent: Mortality Trends in Taiwan and the Netherlands, 1850–1945* (Amsterdam: Aksant Academic Publishers/University of Amsterdam Press, 2011), pp.203–228. Other works include: Lin Yi-ping and Liu Shiyung, 'A Forgotten War: Malaria Eradication in Taiwan, 1905–65,' in Leung and Furth, eds., *Health and Hygiene in Chinese East Asia*, pp.183–203; Liu, *Prescribing Colonization*, pp.114–125; and Akihisa Setoguchi, 'Control of Insect Vectors in the Japanese Empire: Transformation of the Colonial/Metropolitan Environment, 1920–1945,' *East Asian Science, Technology and Society*, vol.1, no.2 (2007): 167–181; Ts'ui-jung Liu and Shi-yung Liu, 'Disease and Mortality in the History of Taiwan,' in Liu, et al., eds., *Asian Population History*, pp.248–269. For an interesting article on the development of the medical police in Taiwan, see Chin Hsien-Yu, 'Colonial Medical Police and Postcolonial Medical Surveillance Systems in Taiwan, 1895–1950s,' *Osiris*, vol.13 (1998): 326–338.

On the environmental consequences of Mao's Great Leap Forward, see the classic and immensely readable study by Judith Shapiro, *Mao's War Against Nature: Politics and the Environment in Revolutionary China* (Cambridge: Cambridge University Press, 2001). For a general history of schistosomiasis and tropical medicine, see John Farley, *Bilharzia: A History of Imperial Tropical Medicine* (Cambridge: Cambridge University Press, 2003). On Mao's anti-schistosomiasis campaign, specifically, see: Ka-wai Fan, 'Schistosomiasis Control and Snail Elimination in China,' *American Journal of Public Health*, vol.102, no.12 (December 2012): 2231–2232; Ruth Rogaski, 'Nature, Annihilation, and Modernity: China's Korean War Germ-Warfare Experience Reconsidered,' *Journal of Asian Studies*, vol.61, no.2 (2002): 381–415; Miriam Gross and Kawai Fan, 'Schistosomiasis,' in Andrews and Bullock, eds., *Medical Transitions in Twentieth-Century China*, pp.106–125; Liping Bu, 'The Patriotic Health Movement and China's Socialist Reconstruction: Fighting Disease and Transforming Society, 1950–80,' in Liping Bu and Ka-che Yip, eds., *Public Health and National Reconstruction in Post-War Asia: International Influences, Local Transformations* (Abingdon and New York: Routledge, 2015), pp.34–51.

On the Nipah outbreak in Malaysia, see K. B. Chua, B. H. Chua, and C. W. Wang, 'Anthropogenic Deforestation, El Niño and the Emergence of Nipah Virus in Malaysia,' *Malaysian Journal of Pathology*, vol.24, no.1 (June 2002): 15–21; L. M. Looi and K. B. Chua, 'Lessons from the Nipah Virus Outbreak in Malaysia,' *Malaysian Journal of Pathology*, vol.29, no.2 (December 2007): 63–67; Tuong Vu, 'Epidemics as Politics with Case Studies from Malaysia, Thailand, and Vietnam,' *Global Health Governance Journal*, vol.4, no.2 (April 2011): 1–11.

CHAPTER 4: WAR

A useful starting point for exploring the connections between war and infectious disease is Matthew R. Smallman-Raynor and Andrew D. Cliff, *War Epidemics: An Historical Geography of Infectious Diseases in Military Conflict and Civil Strife, 1850–2000* (Oxford: Oxford University Press, 2004). Although dealing primarily with Europe, two important volumes that examine the place of medicine in modern warfare and society are: Roger Cooter, Mark Harrison, and Steve Sturdy, eds., *Medicine and Modern Warfare* (Amsterdam: Rodopi, 1999) and Roger Cooter, Mark Harrison, and Steve Sturdy, eds., *War, Medicine and Modernity* (Stroud: Sutton, 1999).

My discussion of the US intervention in the Philippines is much indebted to Warwick Anderson's *Colonial Pathologies*, which reconsiders the role of science and medicine in the US colonization of the Philippines. Other useful works, specifically on the Philippine–US War and epidemics, include: R. C. Ileto, 'Cholera and the Origins of the American Sanitary Order in the Philippines,' in David Arnold, ed., *Imperial Medicine and Indigenous Societies* (Manchester: Manchester University Press, 1988), pp.125–148; Rodney Sullivan, 'Cholera and Colonialism in the Philippines, 1899–1905,' in Roy MacLeod and Milton Lewis, eds., *Disease, Medicine, and Empire: Perspectives on Western Medicine and the Experience of European Expansion* (London: Routledge, 1988), pp.284–300; De Bevoise, *Agents of Apocalypse*. For an account of how US colonial practices were imported back to the US, an important work is Alfred W. McCoy, *Policing America's Empire: The United States, the Philippines, and the Rise of the Surveillance State* (Madison: University of Wisconsin Press, 2009).

William C. Summers highlights the geopolitical dimensions of the Manchurian plague in *The Great Manchurian Plague of 1910–1911: The Geopolitics of an Epidemic Disease* (New Haven, CT: Yale University Press, 2012). A valuable reappraisal of the plague is provided by Mark Gamsa in 'The Epidemic of Pneumonic Plague in Manchuria 1910–1911,' *Past & Present*, vol.190 (2006): 147–183. Christo Lynteris offers a comparative analysis of the 1910–1911 and 1920–1921 plagues in 'Epidemics as Events and as Crises: Comparing Two Plague Outbreaks in Manchuria (1910–11 and 1920–21),' *Cambridge Anthropology*, vol.32, no.1 (2014): 62–76. For a classic account of the epidemics, which has served as the basis for subsequent studies, see Carl F. Nathan, *Plague Prevention and Politics in Manchuria, 1910–1931* (Cambridge, MA: East Asian Research

Center, Harvard University, 1967). Carol Benedict has written on the plague as a catalyst for the development of medical institutions in 'Policing the Sick: Plague and the Origins of State Medicine in Late Imperial China,' *Late Imperial China*, vol.14, no.2 (2011): 60–77. On the career of Wu Lien-teh, see Carsten Flohr, 'The Plague Fighter: Wu Lien-teh and the Beginning of the Chinese Public Health System,' *Annals of Science*, vol.53, no.4 (July 1996): 361–380. Wu's autobiography *Plague Fighter: The Autobiography of a Modern Chinese Physician* (Cambridge: W. Heffer & Sons, 1959) is also highly readable.

An account of the US intervention in Siberia is contained in Betty Miller Unterberger, *America's Siberian Expedition, 1918–1920: A Study of National Policy* (New York: Greenwood Press, 1969). For an overview of typhus and typhus-control strategies in Russia, see the following: K. David Patterson, 'Typhus and its Control in Russia, 1870–1940,' *Medical History*, vol.37, no.4 (1991): 361–381; Robert Argenbright, 'Lethal Mobilities: Bodies and Lice on Soviet Railroads, 1918–1922,' *Journal of Transport History*, vol.29, no.2 (2008): 259–276. And on the 'Great White Train,' see Julia F. Irwin's excellent short article 'The Great White Train: Typhus, Sanitation, and U.S. International Development during the Russian Civil War,' *Endeavour*, vol.36, no.3 (2012): 89–96.

Nancy Leys Stepan's *Eradication: Ridding the World of Diseases Forever?* (Ithaca, NY: Cornell University Press, 2011) looks at the history of eradication, with a particular focus on debates about its benefits. For a provocative account of how terror came to be the organizing principle of the United State's security policy, extending to the threat of infectious disease, see Joseph Masco, *The Theater of Operations: National Security Affect from the Cold War to the War on Terror* (Durham, NC: Duke University Press, 2014). On the opposition to polio eradication, see William A. Muraskin, *Polio Eradication and Its Discontents: An Historian's Journey Through an International Public Health (Un)Civil War* (Hyderabad: Orient Blackswan, 2012). On resistance to the smallpox eradication program in South Asia in the 1970s, see Paul Greenough, 'Intimidation, Coercion and Resistance in the Final Stages of the South Asian Smallpox Eradication Campaign, 1973–1975,' *Social Science and Medicine*, vol.41, no.5 (1995): 633–645. And for studies of the colonial smallpox vaccination campaigns in India, see: David Arnold, 'Smallpox and Colonial Medicine in Nineteenth-Century India,' in Arnold, ed., *Imperial Medicine and Indigenous Societies*, pp.45–65; Arnold, *Colonizing the Body*, pp.116–158; Sanjoy Bhattacharya, Mark Harrison, and Michael Worboys, *Fractured States: Smallpox, Public Health and Vaccination Policy in British India, 1800–1947* (Hyderabad: Orient Longman, 2005).

CHAPTER 5: GLOBALIZATION

Stefan Kaufmann provides a helpful summary of the connections between disease emergence, globalization, and poverty in *The New Plagues: Pandemics and Poverty in a Globalized World*. Translated by Michael Capone (Frankfurt: Haus Publishing, 2009). For accessible reviews of contemporary pandemic threats and the factors that are driving them, with some discussion of Asia, see David Quammen, *Spillover: Animal Infections and the Next Human Pandemic* (New York: W. W. Norton, 2012) and Nathan Wolfe, *The Viral Storm: The Dawn of a New*

Pandemic Age (London: Allen Lane, 2011). A useful overview of infectious disease in contemporary Asia – with essays on avian influenza, SARS, and HIV/AIDS – is Yichen Lu, M. Essex, and Bryan Roberts, eds., *Emerging Infections in Asia* (New York: Springer, 2008). While there is an extensive bibliography on globalization and health, there are few works dealing explicitly with Asia.

Surprisingly, there are no authoritative book-length studies of the impact of the 1918 influenza in India or, for that matter, the pandemic's repercussions across Asia. For an overview of the influenza in India, see I. D. Mills, 'The 1918–1919 Influenza Pandemic – The Indian Experience,' *Indian Economic and Social History Review*, vol.23, no.1 (1986): 1–40. David Arnold provides a comparative treatment of responses to the plague and influenza pandemics in his essay 'Disease, Rumor, and Panic in India's Plague and Influenza Epidemics, 1896–1919,' in Robert Peckham, ed., *Empires of Panic: Epidemics and Colonial Anxieties* (Hong Kong: Hong Kong University Press, 2015), pp.111–129. For a demographic analysis and estimate of the pandemic's mortality in India, see Siddharth Chandra, Goran Kuljanin, and Jennifer Wray, 'Mortality from the Influenza Pandemic of 1918–1919: The Case of India,' *Demography*, vol.49, no.3 (August 2012): 857–865. A spatial and temporal analysis of the influenza pandemic across India is undertaken by Siddharth Chandra and Eva Kassens-Noor, 'The Evolution of Pandemic Influenza: Evidence from India, 1918–19,' *BMC Infectious Diseases*, vol.14, no.510 (2014): doi:10.1186/1471-2334-14-510. For an account of influenza in Bombay, see Mridula Ramanna, 'Coping with the Influenza Pandemic: The Bombay Experience,' in David Killingray and Howard Phillips, eds., *The Spanish Influenza Pandemic of 1918–1919: New Perspectives* (Abingdon and New York: Routledge, 2003), pp.86–98. An excellent short overview of the influenza in Southeast Asia is provided by Kirsty Walker in her chapter 'The Influenza Pandemic of 1918 in Southeast Asia,' in Harper and Amrith, eds., *Histories of Health in Southeast Asia*, pp.61–71. For a summary of the pandemic in Indonesia, see Colin Brown, 'The Influenza Pandemic of 1918 in Indonesia,' in Owen, ed., *Death and Disease*, pp.235–256. And for an exploratory survey of influenza in China, see Wataru Iijima, 'Spanish Influenza in China, 1918–1920: A Preliminary Probe,' in Killingray and Phillips, eds., *The Spanish Influenza Pandemic*, pp.101–109; K. F. Cheng and P. C. Leung, 'What Happened in China during the 1918 Influenza Pandemic?' *International Journal of Infectious Diseases*, vol.11, no.4 (July 2007): 360–364.

For an introduction to the different phases of the HIV/AIDS epidemic in China, see Johanna Hood, 'Untangling HIV in China: Social, Political, Economic, and Global-Local Factors,' in Mark McLelland and Vera Mackie, eds., *Routledge Handbook of Sexuality Studies in East Asia* (Abingdon and New York: Routledge, 2015), pp.356–371. Two perceptive anthropological accounts of the epidemic in China, which I have found particularly helpful, are: Sandra Teresa Hyde, *Eating Spring Rice: The Cultural Politics of AIDS in Southwest China* (Berkeley: University of California Press, 2007) and Shao-hua Liu, *Passage to Manhood: Youth Migration, Heroin, and AIDS in Southwest China* (Stanford, CA: Stanford University Press, 2011). Johanna Hood has explored the mediatization of HIV/AIDS in China and its portrayal as a non-Han and racialized affliction in her book *HIV/AIDS, Health and the Media in China: Imagined Immunity Through Racialized Disease* (Abingdon and New York: Routledge, 2011). For excellent discussions of the blood contamination scandal, see Ann S. Anagnost, 'Strange Circulations: The Blood Economy in Rural China,' *Economy and Society*, vol.35, no.4 (2006): 509–529 and Shao Jing, 'Fluid Labor and Blood Money: The Economy of HIV/AIDS in Rural Central China,' *Cultural Anthropology*, vol.21, no.4 (2006): 535–569. Catherine Yuk-ping Lo's *AIDS in China and India: Governing Health Security* (New York and Basingstoke: Palgrave Macmillan, 2015) offers a comparative perspective on the different approaches taken to controlling HIV/AIDS in India and China.

In *The Monster at Our Door: The Global Threat of Avian Flu* (New York: The New Press, 2005), Mike Davis provides a passionate and highly readable exposé of the role of corrupt government, agribusiness, and the fast-food industry in the emergence of H5N1. For overviews of the pandemic threat from avian influenza, see Paul Tambyah and Ping-Chung Leung, *Bird Flu: A Rising Pandemic in Asia And Beyond?* (Singapore: World Scientific, 2006) and the edited volume by Ian Scoones, *Avian Influenza: Science, Policy and Politics* (London and Washington, DC: Earthscan, 2010). The latter book contains essays on Cambodia, Vietnam, Indonesia, and Thailand that explore how viral genetics, ecology, and epidemiology intersect with economic, political, and policy processes. There is also a growing anthropological literature on avian influenza – see, for example, the special issue on 'Asian Flus in Ethnographic and Political Context: A Biosocial Approach' in *Anthropology & Medicine*, vol.15, no1 (2008) edited by Arthur Kleinman, et al.

An informative general account of the SARS outbreak – written at the time – is Thomas Abraham's *Twenty-First Century Plague: The Story of SARS* (Hong Kong: Hong Kong University Press, 2004). For SARS as a case study that highlights key issues in managing emerging infections, see the edited volume by Angela R. McLean, et al., *SARS: A Case Study in Emerging Infections* (Oxford: Oxford University Press, 2005). Two useful edited volumes, which develop comparative and cross-disciplinary approaches to the epidemic, and investigate the biomedical, social, and political dimensions of SARS, are: Deborah Davis and Helen F. Siu, eds., *SARS: Reception and Interpretation in Three Chinese Cities* (London: Routledge, 2007) and Arthur Kleinman and James Watson, eds., *SARS in China: Prelude to Pandemic?* (Stanford, CA: Stanford University Press, 2005). In *SARS, Governance and the Globalization of Disease* (Basingstoke and New York: Palgrave Macmillan, 2004), David P. Fidler considers SARS as a global challenge. Marta E. Hanson demonstrates the role of TCM in the medical response to SARS in China in her essay 'Conceptual Blind Spots, Media Blindfolds: The Case of SARS and Traditional Chinese Medicine,' in Leung and Furth, eds., *Health and Hygiene in Chinese East Asia*, pp.228–254.

CONCLUSION: EPIDEMICS AND THE END OF HISTORY

For debates about scale in history, see the AHR Conversation 'How Size Matters: The Question of Scale in History,' *American Historical Review*, vol.118, no.5 (2013): 1431–1472. For an astute paper on the politics of scale in the discourse of emerging infectious disease, see Nicholas B. King, 'The Scale Politics of Emerging Diseases,' *Osiris*, vol.19 (2004): 62–76. On notions of uncertainty, preparedness, and the 'sentinel' in research on infectious disease, see: Frédéric

Keck, 'Sentinel Devices: Managing Uncertainty in Species Barrier Zones,' in Limor Samimian-Darash and Paul Rabinow, eds., *Modes of Uncertainty: Anthropological Cases* (Chicago, IL: University of Chicago Press, 2015), pp.165–181; Andrew Lakoff, 'The Generic Biothreat, or, How We Became Unprepared,' *Cultural Anthropology*, vol.23, no.3 (2008): 399–428. On the future of epidemic disease in Asia, a decade after SARS, see Peter W. Horby, Dirk Pfeiffer, and Hitoshi Oshitani, 'Prospects for Emerging Infections in East and Southeast Asia 10 Years after Severe Acute Respiratory Syndrome,' *Emerging Infectious Diseases*, vol.19, no.6 (June 2013): 853–860. For a discussion of the 'outbreak narrative' and representations of Asia as a locus of infection, see Priscilla Wald, *Contagious: Cultures, Carriers, and the Outbreak Narrative* (Durham, NC: Duke University Press, 2008). (Ari) Larissa N. Heinrich analyzes the historical associations of China with sickness in *The Afterlife of Images: Translating the Pathological Body between China and the West* (Durham, NC: Duke University Press, 2008), a theme also developed in a recent book by Carlos Rojas, which tracks the trope of contagion in contemporary Chinese literature and cinema: see *Homesickness: Culture, Contagion, and National Transformation in Modern China* (Cambridge, MA: Harvard University Press, 2015).

Index